Cavernous Malformations of the Nervous System

Cavernous Malformations of the Nervous System

Edited by

Daniele Rigamonti

Johns Hopkins University

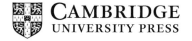

CAMBRIDGE
UNIVERSITY PRESS

CAMBRIDGE UNIVERSITY PRESS
Cambridge, New York, Melbourne, Madrid, Cape Town,
Singapore, São Paulo, Delhi, Tokyo, Mexico City

Cambridge University Press
The Edinburgh Building, Cambridge CB2 8RU, UK

Published in the United States of America by Cambridge
University Press, New York

www.cambridge.org
Information on this title: www.cambridge.org/
9780521764278

First published 2011

Printed in the United Kingdom at the University Press,
Cambridge

*A catalogue record for this publication is available from the
British Library*

Library of Congress Cataloging in Publication data
Cavernous malformations of the nervous system / edited by
Daniele Rigamonti.
   p.   cm.
ISBN 978-0-521-76427-8 (hardback)
1. Cerebral arteriovenous malformations.   2. Brain –
Hemorrhage.   I. Rigamonti, Daniele, 1951–
II. Title.
RD594.2.C385   2011
616.8′1–dc22
2011008052

ISBN 978-0-521-76427-8 Hardback

I dedicate this book to my wife and children, to the memory of my father, who exemplified for me how a physician should practice, and to Bunny and Charles Salisbury who supported my research over all these years.

Contents

Contents

Section 4.   Special aspects

Color plate section is to be found between pp. 100 and 101.

Preface

The diagnosis and the management of cavernous malformations (CMs) have been challenging and intriguing neurologists and neurosurgeons for several decades. Prior to the advent of MRI, the diagnosis of CM was often limited to patients presenting with either hemorrhage or seizures. The advent of MRI has completely transformed the field and asymptomatic as well as symptomatic CMs are now increasingly being diagnosed.

Along with an improved diagnosis, there has been an ever-improving understanding of their biology and the course of their natural history. Neurologists and neurosurgeons nowadays still face the challenge of determining the most appropriate treatment for lesions that, even when clinically quiescent, may be characterized by evidence of hemorrhage on advanced imaging. Currently, there is a general consensus on the conservative management of clinically benign CM, and on the appropriateness of surgical resection of symptomatic superficial lesions. Controversy persists regarding the most appropriate approach to treating deep or infratentorial lesions. Surgical resection performed by very experienced surgeons is a very valid option for symptomatic deep or infratentorial lesions; however, the risks associated with surgery in these locations are not negligible. The increased availability of radiosurgery as a tool for non-invasively reaching deep lesions has been therefore met with enthusiasm by some physicians and patients dealing with symptomatic CMs in deep or infratentorial lesions.

This book is an attempt to provide a foundation for an improved diagnosis and discussion of the treatment options available for CMs by critically summarizing the knowledge gained over past decades and the opinion of leading experts in the management of CMs. The book has been divided into four sections, each emphasizing specific aspects of the CMs.

Section I on basic aspects aims to provide the foundation for clinical decision-making regarding medical and surgical management: it discusses the epidemiology and natural history of cavernomas. In addition, this section contains chapters that bring to light current understanding of CM biology, molecular genetics, and the role of ionizing radiation in de novo formation of CMs and the safety of radiation sources frequently used for diagnostic and therapeutic purposes.

Section II details imaging of CMs, the inconsistencies in the criteria for defining hemorrhage in CMs, and clinical features, including specifically seizures.

Section III discusses therapy: the options available to the patient are outlined and their pros and cons discussed. The surgical chapters contain up-to-date information regarding the technique and outcomes related to a specific location and problem. A radiosurgical chapter outlines the role of radiosurgery in the management of cavernomas.

Section IV, the last section of the book, deals with special aspects encountered in the management of these patients.

This book is the result of tremendous efforts put in by authors who have provided insightful guidance critical in the discussion of the most appropriate management of these lesions at this point in time. Special thanks go to the team at Cambridge University Press whose painstaking efforts made this book possible.

Contributors

Wael Abdalla
Department of Radiology
Johns Hopkins Hospital
Baltimore, MD
USA

Nicola Acciarri
Department of Neurosurgery
Bellaria Hospital
Bologna
Italy

Issam Awad
University of Chicago
Pritzker School of Medicine
Chicago, IL
USA

Xavier Ayrignac
Hôpital Lariboisière
Université Paris
Paris
France

Sachin Batra
Department of Neurosurgery
Johns Hopkins Hospital
Baltimore, MD
USA

Michel J. Berg
Strong Epilepsy Center
University of Rochester Medical Center
Rochester, NY
USA

Gregory K. Bergey
Department of Neurology
Johns Hopkins Hospital
Baltimore, MD
USA

Helmut Bertalanffy
Professor of Neurosurgery
Center for Vascular Neurosurgery
International Neuroscience Institute
Hannover
Germany

Oliver Bozinov
Department of Neurosurgery
University Hospital
Zurich
Switzerland

Jan-Karl Burkhardt
Department of Neurosurgery
University Hospital
Zurich
Switzerland

Joaquin Camara-Quintana
Departments of Neurosurgery
Stanford University
Stanford, CA
USA

Barbara Crain
Diagnostic Neuropathology
Department of Pathology
Johns Hopkins Hospital
Baltimore, MD
USA

Mahua Dey
University of Chicago
Pritzker School of Medicine
Chicago, IL
USA

Rachel Engelmann
Department of Neurosurgery
Johns Hopkins Hospital
Baltimore, MD
USA

John C. Flickinger
Department of Radiation Oncology
University of Pittsburgh Medical Center
Pittsburgh, PA
USA

Colin B. Josephson
Clinical Neurosciences, Bramwell
University of Edinburgh
Western General Hospital
Edinburgh
UK

M. Yashar S. Kalani
Division of Neurological Surgery
Barrow Neurological Institute
St Joseph's Hospital and Medical
Phoenix, AZ
USA

Hideyuki Kano
Department of Neurological Surgery
University of Pittsburgh Medical Center
Pittsburgh, PA
USA

Ahmet Hilmi Kaya
Department of Neurosurgery
Faculty of Medicine
Ondokuz Mayis University
Kurupelit, Samsun
Turkey

Ralf Alfons Kockro
Department of Neurosurgery
University Hospital
Zurich
Switzerland

Douglas Kondziolka
Department of Neurological Surgery
University of Pittsburgh Medical Center
Pittsburgh, PA
USA

Richard Leigh
Department of Neurology
Johns Hopkins Hospital
Baltimore, MD
USA

Angela Li
Department of Neurosurgery
Johns Hopkins Hospital
Baltimore, MD
USA

Doris D. M. Lin
Department of Radiology
Johns Hopkins Hospital
Baltimore, MD
USA

Sheng-Fu Larry Lo
Department of Neurosurgery
Johns Hopkins Hospital
Baltimore, MD
USA

L. Dade Lunsford
Department of Neurological Surgery
University of Pittsburgh Medical Center
Pittsburgh, PA
USA

Leslie Morrison
Department of Neurology
UNM School of Medicine
Albuquerque, NM
USA

Eugenio Pozzati
Neurosurgery Department
Bellaria-Maggiore Hospital
Bologna
Italy

Pablo F. Recinos
Department of Neurosurgery
Johns Hopkins Hospital
Baltimore, MD
USA

Daniele Rigamonti
Department of Neurosurgery
Johns Hopkins Hospital

Baltimore, MD
USA

Rustam Al-Shahi Salman
Clinical Neurosciences, Bramwell
University of Edinburgh
Western General Hospital
Edinburgh
UK

Johannes Sarnthein
Department of Neurosurgery
University Hospital
Zurich
Switzerland

R. Michael Scott
Department of Neurosurgery
The Children's Hospital
Boston, MA
USA

Edward R. Smith
Department of Neurosurgery
The Children's Hospital
Boston, MA
USA

Robert F. Spetzler
Barrow Neurological Institute
Phoenix, AZ
USA

Elisabeth Tournier-Lasserve
Hôpital Lariboisière
Université Paris
Paris
France

Uğur Türe
Department of Neurosurgery
Yeditepe University School of Medicine
Istanbul, Ankara
Turkey

Tegan Vay
University of Rochester
School of Medicine and Dentistry
Rochester, NY
USA

Robert J. Wityk
Department of Neurology
Johns Hopkins Hospital
Baltimore, MD
USA

Jun Zhang
Department of Anesthesiology
Texas Tech University
Health Science Center
El Paso, TX
USA

Pathology of cavernous malformations

Sachin Batra, Barbara Crain, Rachel Engelmann, Joaquin Camara-Quintana and Daniele Rigamonti

Cerebrovascular malformations are classified as cavernous malformations (CMs), arteriovenous malformations (AVMs), developmental venous anomalies (DVAs) and capillary telangiectasias (CTs). CMs are the second most common form of cerebrovascular malformation and constitute up to 10–15% of the total [1,2]. In the past, CMs were not visualized on radiological examinations such as CT scanning or angiography and were therefore referred to as angiographically occult or cryptic vascular malformations. Recent studies have resurrected the old suspicion that CMs are vascular tumors [3], hence the alternative terms cavernous hemangiomas, cavernomas, or cavernous angiomas. Clinical features of CMs include epilepsy (22–50%), focal deficits (20–45%), headaches (6–34%), or hemorrhages (up to 56%); CMs may also remain clinically silent (up to 40%) [4–8].

Macroscopic and microscopic features

CMs resemble well circumscribed, multilobulated, mulberry-like structures ranging in size from a few millimeters to several centimeters in diameter [2,9,10]. Intracranial CMs are more frequently located supratentorially (64–84%) while spinal lesions are frequently located in the lower thoracolumbar region (97%) [2,11,12]. They have been observed in all cortical locations as well as in deep locations like the basal ganglia, thalamus, cerebellum and the brainstem [2,13,14]. Lesions of the cerebellopontine angle, pituitary, and periventricular region have all been reported to have intraventricular CMs [15–17].

The histological features of CMs are best understood in the context of normal vascular anatomy. Normal cerebral blood vessels are lined by endothelial cells joined by tight junctions. The endothelial layer is surrounded by a basal lamina. While capillaries have just the endothelial cell layer, all other vessels have one or more layers of smooth muscle cells as well as some pericytes immediately adjacent to the endothelial cells. Surrounding the entire vessel are astrocytic endfeet which comprise the glia limitans. Together, the endothelial cells, their tight junctions, and the astrocytic endfeet form the morphologic basis of the blood–brain barrier.

Like capillaries, the blood vessels of CMs lack smooth muscle cells and have a homogeneous, hyalinized appearance in sections stained with hematoxylin and eosin (Fig. 1A). The overall arrangement of vessels is compact, with the classic appearance being one of back-to-back vessels without intervening parenchyma. However, most lesions also contain some areas with more loosely packed vessels [18]. Thrombosis is common in these low-flow malformations as well as acute, organized, and recanalized thrombi, or even completely occluded vessels (Fig. 1B). Calcification is common both within vessel walls and within the adjacent parenchyma. In our unpublished series of 24 patients who underwent surgery for CMs, 58% had thrombosis, 41% had calcification, and 4% (one case) showed intervening parenchyma; the true incidence of these processes was likely higher, as the volume of material sampled was small.

CMs are generally surrounded by a rim of fibrosis with associated hemosiderin deposition (Fig. 1C). The appearance of this tissue is distinctive enough to be strongly suggestive of cavernous angioma in the proper setting [19]. Hemosiderin may also be present in the adjacent neuropil, where it may be responsible for occurrence of seizures [20]. In our series, 92% of CMs showed hemosiderin, with reactive astrocytosis in 29%.

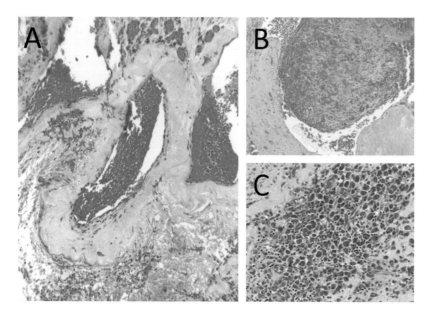

Figure 1.1. (A) The back-to-back blood vessels of cavernous malformations have thick, amorphous walls. (B) The blood vessel shown here contains a recent thrombus. (C) Densely packed hemosiderin-laden macrophages are often found within or around the rim of a cavernous angioma. See color plate section.

Immunohistochemistry of cavernous malformations

The vessels of CMs have also been studied using immunohistochemistry. Endothelial cells, astrocytes, and extracellular matrix proteins have all been studied. Expression of angiogenic growth factors, proliferation markers, and molecules associated with angiogenesis has also been examined.

Many of the common endothelial cell markers are proteins that are potentially important in endothelial cell interactions with platelets or with the coagulation system. One of the endothelial cell markers that are most commonly used for identification of endothelial cells is CD31 (platelet endothelial cell adhesion molecule PECAM 1). CD 31 is involved in endothelial migration and angiogenesis and is expressed normally in CMs by both immunohistochemical and *in situ* hybridization techniques [21]. Expression of another common marker, von Willebrand factor (a platelet-vessel wall mediator in the coagulation system), is normal [21,22], as is the expression of thrombomodulin [22]. Thus, there is no evidence from these immunohistochemical studies that endothelial cell abnormalities are responsible for the frequent thrombosis seen in CMs.

As the vessel walls within CMs contain virtually no smooth muscle cells, immunostains for smooth muscle actin-alpha show no reactivity within vessel walls. However, normal endothelial cells often contain small amounts of actin and that is also the case for the endothelial cells within CMs [23]. The subendothelial layer may also contain actin immunoreactivity, likely in the basal lamina. Kilic *et al.* have suggested that the expression of smooth muscle actin-alpha could represent an immature molecular construction in CMs compared to AVMS [23]. Collagen IV, fibronectin, and laminin were similarly present in the endothelium and subendothelium, but not in the amorphous portion of the vessel wall. There was relatively more fibronectin staining than laminin staining, a pattern that is also seen in early stages of angiogenesis. Faint staining for collagen III was present in the subendothelium only [23].

There have been a number of studies examining markers of angiogenesis in CMs. The best studied is vascular endothelial growth factor (VEGF), which is found in the endothelium and subendothelium, though more so in adults than in children [24–26]. The VEGF receptor Flk-1 is found in endothelial cell nuclei. Basic fibroblast growth factor (bFGF) and transforming growth factor-alpha (TGF-alpha) are also found in the endothelial cells of adults and children, with no difference between the two age groups [24–26].

Hypoxia inducible factor-1alpha (HIF-1alpha), which is involved in oxygen homeostasis, is present in cavernous angiomas, in all layers in a pediatric study

[26] and in endothelium in an adult study [24]. Endoglin, a normal endothelial antigen, a part of the TGF-beta1 and beta3 receptor complex and the gene mutated in hereditary hemorrhagic telangiectasia Type 1, is also present in pediatric and adult samples [24,26]. Of note, it has been suggested that endoglin may be important in vascular development and in vascular remodeling in response to increased blood flow or shear stress [26,27].

Endothelial cell proliferation has been documented by positive labeling using antibodies to proliferating cell nuclear antigen (PCNA) and the Ki-67 epitope (MIB-1) [24,26].

Etiology

Cavernous malformations are generally believed to be congenital lesions presenting at any age from the neonatal period through adulthood. They may occur sporadically or with familial clustering. The familial forms of lesions have been attributed to mutations of the CCM1, CCM2 and CCM3 genes and are expressed as autosomal dominant phenotypes with penetrances of 60–88%, 100% and 63% respectively [28]. Although the role played by the products of CCM genes is yet to be established, animal models suggest that these are critical to angiogenesis and that the loss of their function leads to dilatation of major vessels, defective endothelial association and barrier function, and dysfunctional sprouting [29]. The detailed role of these genes is discussed in the chapters "Clinical and molecular genetics of cerebral cavernous malformations" and "Molecular biology of cerebral cavernous malformation".

De novo appearance of CMs has been reported following brain irradiation [30], brain biopsy [31], and viral infection [32]. Exposure to such stimuli may initiate a reactive angiogenesis or cause mutations leading to local loss of expression of CCM genes leading to *de novo* appearance of CMs [33–35]. Some authors have associated hormonal influences with *de novo* occurrence of CM such as a case with follicle stimulating hormone producing pituitary adenoma described by Pozzati *et al.*, wherein new lesions appeared [30]. Lüdemann *et al.* also reported *de novo* appearance of CM in a pregnant patient but failed to demonstrate estrogen or progesterone receptors on immunohistochemical staining, suggesting that new lesions appear independently of hormone levels, contrary to what was widely considered [36].

CMs and other vascular malformations

Like CMs, other types of vascular malformations have characteristic macroscopic and microscopic features. Capillary telangiectasias (CTs) are composed of aggregates of thin-walled vessels indistinguishable from normal capillaries and separated by normal intervening brain parenchyma. While CMs are well circumscribed radiologically, CTs may sometimes appear as a nebulous blush [37]. Developmental venous anomalies (DVAs, sometimes termed venous malformations) are collections of abnormally dilated veins forming a caput medusa draining into a large central vein. As described below, these frequently occur with CMs in their vicinity. DVAs do not tend to bleed, and the intervening brain tissue appears normal. Arteriovenous malformations (AVMs) contain tortuous, anastomosing blood vessels. Some of the vessels resemble true arteries or veins, but most are abnormal vessels of varying diameters whose walls are formed primarily by collagen rather than by smooth muscle. Intervening parenchyma is found across the lesion but is almost absent at the densely packed nidus of the lesion. The intervening and surrounding parenchyma is often hemosiderin-stained and gliotic. Calcification is common.

Although various intracranial vascular malformations were initially described as distinct entities based on the factors described above, both MRI examinations and the histological features observed at surgery or autopsy suggest that different types of malformations may exist within the same patient. Moreover, individual lesions may have features of more than one type of malformation, suggesting intermediate forms. In the case of CMs, coexistent DVAs or CTs have been frequently reported [38–43]. Rigamonti *et al.* described the coexistence of features of typical CT as well as CM in two (10%) of 20 patients who underwent resection of CM [39]. One patient had multiple lesions including both CT and CM. Staining for smooth muscle actin revealed smooth muscle in the walls of 20% of the lesions, indicating the presence of arterial or venous differentiation. Brain parenchyma was interspersed between vessels in 35% of the patients, a feature generally attributed to CTs rather than CMs. Rigamonti *et al.* [39] and others have concluded that CM and CT constitute part of a larger spectrum of intracranial vascular malformations. For example, Awad *et al.* described two (14.2%) patients with coexisting CT and CM in a series of 14 mixed vascular malformations. Histopathological examination revealed zones of CTs in the surrounding brain parenchyma that eventually coalesced into the CMs [44].

Rigamonti *et al.* reported the first evidence of a high association between CM and DVA and suggested a possible pathogenetic relationship [38]. Abdulrauf *et al.* confirmed that 13 of 55 patients (24%) with CM had associated DVA [43]. Similarly, Wurm *et al.* reported 25.8% of CMs were associated with DVAs in a series of 58 patients [45]. In contrast, Porter *et al.* reported DVA associated with CMs in all of his surgically treated patients whereas preoperative MRI revealed such lesions in only 32% of 73 patients [46]. The latter result suggests that the association may be underestimated as MRI may not always detect DVAs [45,47]. Recognition of such combined pathology may be important as CMs associated with DVAs may have a greater predilection to bleed and be symptomatic than lesions which are purely CM [43]. The increased bleeding tendency of CMs associated with DVAs has been hypothesized to result from venous hypertension

[43,48]. Dillon cited stenosis at the junction of the DVA and central vein as a possible cause of elevated venous pressures in DVAs [41]. It has been suggested that hemorrhagic recurrences and organization of the resulting thrombus initiate the process of angiogenesis, which may cause growth of CMs through an ongoing process of hemorrhage and ischemia [48]. In support of this idea, others have demonstrated that DVAs are composed of mature blood vessels and are formed earlier in embryogenesis [49], while CMs are immature vascular lesions with active angiogenesis. More recently Abe *et al.* classified venous anomalies into two distinct types: venous malformations which are not DVAs that are angiographically occult and contain compact venous channels devoid of smooth muscle layers; and angiographically detectable dilated venous channels draining normal white matter and communicating with cortical veins [47]. Abe *et al.* suggested that angiographically occult venous malformations can be safely resected without significant sequelae, indicating anatomical

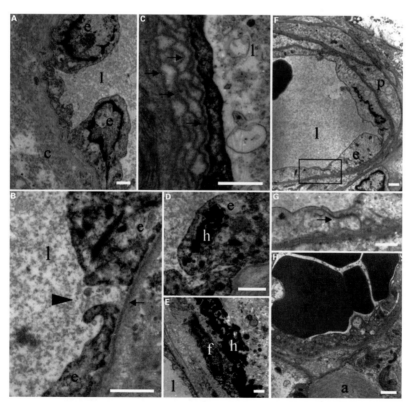

Figure 1.2. Electron micrographs of cavernous malformations (A-E) and microvessels in adjacent normal brain (F-H). (A) Ultrastructurally, these lesions consist of endothelial cells (e) lining vascular sinusoid lumens (l) and surrounded by a dense collagenous matrix (c). No perivascular cells were seen and the endothelial basal lamina was in direct contact with the collagenous matrix. (B) Gaps (arrowhead) between adjacent endothelial cells were seen in cavernous malformations where the lumen (l) was exposed directly to the basal lamina (arrow). (C) In focal areas, the basal lamina (arrows) demonstrated multiple abnormal layers. (D,E) Haemosiderin (h) could be seen within endothelial cells (D) and within microns of the lumens of the vascular sinusoids (E). A rare fibroblast profile (f) is seen in (E) in the connective tissue matrix. (F) A cerebral microvessel from brain tissue adjacent to a lesion demonstrates typical encircling pericytes (p) separating the endothelial cell basal lamina from the neuropil. A red blood cell (r) is noted in the lumen. (G) Magnification of the boxed area in F demonstrates a tight junction (arrow) between adjacent endothelial processes. (H) Another microvessel from the surrounding brain is being contacted by an astrocyte foot process (a) containing abundant intermediate filaments. Scale bar shown in all images represents 1 μm. Reproduced from [49] with permission from BMJ Publishing Group.

and pathophysiological differences from DVAs [47]. It is possible that such venous malformations may remain undetected on MRI until they are revealed on pathological examination.

Ultrastructure and pathophysiology of CMs

The ultrastructure of blood vessels within cavernous angiomas differs markedly from that of normal cerebral vessels, with abnormalities in endothelial cells that would predict an impaired blood–brain barrier, increased extravasation of red blood cells, and structural weakness.

Such changes may help explain the pathophysiology of the growth, hemorrhage, and epilepsy caused by CMs.

Like their normal counterparts, the vessels of cavernous angiomas are lined by endothelial cells, the somata of which are relatively unremarkable. However, there are associated features, which would be expected to interfere with the normal blood–brain barrier. For example, the endothelial cells have been described as having few if any tight junctions [49], with those junctions that are present being described as intermediate or poorly formed [50]. There may be gaps between endothelial cells [49–51] (Fig. 1.2). The basal lamina that underlies the endothelial cells has been reported both as present [49,50] and as thin or absent [51], perhaps depending on whether the malformation has bled [51]. Previous hemorrhage has also been associated with changes in the endothelial cells themselves, including more filopodia and increased numbers of Weibel-Palade bodies, micropinocytotic vesicles, filaments, and other organelles [51].

In the vessel walls, pericytes and subendothelial smooth muscle cells are lacking or are very poorly formed. The walls also lack organized collagen and elastic fibers, which would make them more likely to bleed [50,51]. Astrocytic endfeet are also lacking [49,51].

Summary

CMs are vascular malformations composed of endothelial lined dilated vessels (caverns) packed together without intervening neural parenchyma. CMs are both hereditary and sporadic. They can be seen with a history of previous irradiation and viral infection. The low flow rate and luminal pressures inside CMs make them angiographically occult and less likely to bleed than other vascular malformations. However, microscopic extravasations, hemorrhages, thrombosis with areas of reorganization, calcification, and inflammation are common features. Ultrastructural studies have demonstrated a dysfunctional blood–brain barrier with poorly formed tight junctions, and the presence of Weibel bodies in lesions with recurrent bleeds. CMs and other vascular malformations are known to coexist and such lesions are more likely to bleed and recur after resection. Further research in the etiopathogenesis and genetics of CMs will help elucidate the pathobiology of CMs.

References

1. Moriarity, J., Clatterbuck, R. & Rigamonti, D. The natural history of cavernous malformations. *Neurosurg Clin N Am* 1999;**10**:411–417.

2. Maraire, J. & Awad, I. Intracranial cavernous malformations: lesion behavior and management strategies. *Neurosurgery* 1995;**37**:591–605.

3. Notelet, L., Houtteville, J., Khoury, S., Lechevalier, B. & Chapon, F. Proliferating cell nuclear antigen (PCNA) in cerebral cavernomas: an immunocytochemical study of 42 cases. *Surg Neurol* 1997;**47**:364–370.

4. Porter, P., Willinsky, R., Harper, W. & Wallace, M. Cerebral cavernous malformations: natural history and prognosis after clinical deterioration with or without hemorrhage. *J Neurosurg* 1997;**87**:190–197.

5. Robinson, J., Awad, I. & Little, J. Natural history of the cavernous angioma. *J Neurosurg* 1991;**75**:709–714.

6. Zabramski, J., *et al.* The natural history of familial cavernous malformations: results of an ongoing study. *J Neurosurg* 1994;**80**:422–432.

7. Aiba, T., *et al.* Natural history of intracranial cavernous malformations. *J Neurosurg* 1995;**83**:56–59.

8. Del Curling, O. J., Kelly, D. J., Elster, A. & Craven, T. An analysis of the natural history of cavernous angiomas. *J Neurosurg* 1991;**75**:702–708.

9. McCormick, W. & Nofzinger, J. "Cryptic" vascular malformations of the central nervous system. *J Neurosurg* 1966;**24**:865–875.

10. McCormick, W., Hardman, J. & Boulter, T. Vascular malformations ("angiomas") of the brain, with special reference to those occurring in the posterior fossa. *J Neurosurg* 1968;**28**:241–251.

11. Nozaki, K., Inomoto, T., Takagi, Y. & Hashimoto, N. Spinal intradural extramedullary cavernous angioma. Case report. *J Neurosurg* 2003;**99**:316–319.

12. Er, U., Yigitkanli, K., Simsek, S., Adabag, A. & Bavbek, M. Spinal intradural extramedullary cavernous angioma: case report and review of the literature. *Spinal Cord* 2007;**45**:632–636.

13. Conway, J. E. & Rigamonti, D. Cavernous malformations: a review and current controversies. *Neurosurg Quart* 2006;**16**:15–23.

14. Baumann, C. R., *et al.* Seizure outcome after resection of supratentorial cavernous malformations: a study of 168 patients. *Epilepsia* 2007;**48**:559–563.

15. Simard, J., Garcia-Bengochea, F., Ballinger, W. J., Mickle, J. & Quisling, R. Cavernous angioma: a review of 126 collected and 12 new clinical cases. *Neurosurgery* 1986;**18**:162–172.

16. Bertalanffy, H., *et al.* Cerebral cavernomas in the adult. Review of the literature and analysis of 72 surgically treated patients. *Neurosurg Rev* 2002;**25**:1–53; discussion 54–55.

17. Wang, C., Liu, A., Zhang, J., Sun, B. & Zhao, Y. Surgical management of brain-stem cavernous malformations: report of 137 cases. *Surg Neurol* 2003;**59**:444–454; discussion 454.

18. Tomlinson, F. H., *et al.* Angiographically occult vascular malformations: a correlative study of features on magnetic resonance imaging and histological examination. *Neurosurgery* 1994;**34**:792–799; discussion 799–800.

19. Burger, P., Scheithauer, B. W. & Vogel, F. S. *Surgical Pathology of the Nervous System and Its Coverings* (New York: Churchill Livingstone, 2002).

20. Awad, I. & Jabbour, P. Cerebral cavernous malformations and epilepsy. *Neurosurg Focus* 2006;**21**:e7.

21. Uranishi, R., Awadallah, N. A., Ogunshola, O. O. & Awad, I. A. Further study of CD31 protein and messenger ribonucleic acid expression in human cerebral vascular malformations. *Neurosurgery* 2002;**50**:110–115; discussion 115–116.

22. Storer, K. P., Tu, J., Karunanayaka, A., Morgan, M. K. & Stoodley, M. A. Thrombotic molecule expression in cerebral vascular malformations. *J Clin Neurosci* 2007;**14**:975–980.

23. Kilic, T., *et al.* Expression of structural proteins and angiogenic factors in cerebrovascular anomalies. *Neurosurgery* 2000;**46**:1179–1191; discussion 1191–1172.

24. Sure, U., *et al.* Biological activity of adult cavernous malformations: a study of 56 patients. *J Neurosurg* 2005;**102**:342–347.

25. Sure, U., *et al.* Endothelial proliferation, neoangiogenesis, and potential de novo generation of cerebrovascular malformations. *J Neurosurg* 2001;**94**:972–977.

26. Tirakotai, W., *et al.* Biological activity of paediatric cerebral cavernomas: an immunohistochemical study of 28 patients. *Childs Nerv Syst* 2006;**22**:685–691.

27. Matsubara, S., Bourdeau, A., terBrugge, K. G., Wallace, C. & Letarte, M. Analysis of endoglin expression in normal brain tissue and in cerebral arteriovenous malformations. *Stroke* 2000;**31**:2653–2660.

28. Labauge, P., Denier, C., Bergametti, F. & Tournier-Lasserve, E. Genetics of cavernous angiomas. *Lancet Neurol* 2007;**6**:237–244.

29. Batra, S., Lin, D., Recinos, P., Zhang, J. & Rigamonti, D. Cavernous malformations: natural history, diagnosis and treatment. *Nat Rev Neurol* 2009;**5**:659–670.

30. Pozzati, E., Acciarri, N., Tognetti, F., Marliani, F. & Giangaspero, F. Growth, subsequent bleeding, and de novo appearance of cerebral cavernous angiomas. *Neurosurgery* 1996;**38**:662–669; discussion 669–670.

31. Ogilvy, C., Moayeri, N. & Golden, J. Appearance of a cavernous hemangioma in the cerebral cortex after a biopsy of a deeper lesion. *Neurosurgery* 1993;**33**:307–309; discussion 309.

32. Flocks, J., Weis, T., Kleinman, D. & Kirsten, W. Dose-response studies to polyoma virus in rats. *J Natl Cancer Inst* 1965;**35**:259–284.

33. Pagenstecher, A., Stahl, S., Sure, U. & Felbor, U. A two-hit mechanism causes cerebral cavernous malformations: complete inactivation of CCM1, CCM2 or CCM3 in affected endothelial cells. *Hum Mol Genet* 2009;**18**:911–918.

34. Baumgartner, J., *et al.* Pathologically proven cavernous angiomas of the brain following radiation therapy for pediatric brain tumors. *Pediatr Neurosurg* 2003;**39**:201–207.

35. Massa-Micon, B., Luparello, V., Bergui, M. & Pagni, C. De novo cavernoma case report and review of literature. *Surg Neurol* 2000;**53**:484–487.

36. Lüdemann, W., Ellerkamp, V., Stan, A. & Hussein, S. De novo development of a cavernous malformation of the brain: significance of factors with paracrine and endocrine activity: case report. *Neurosurgery* 2002;**50**:646–649; discussion 649–650.

37. Barr, R., Dillon, W. & Wilson, C. Slow-flow vascular malformations of the pons: capillary telangiectasias? *AJNR Am J Neuroradiol* 1996;**17**:71–78.

38. Rigamonti, D. & Spetzler, R. The association of venous and cavernous malformations. Report of four cases and discussion of the pathophysiological, diagnostic, and therapeutic implications. *Acta Neurochir (Wien)* 1988;**92**:100–105.

39. Rigamonti, D., Johnson, P., Spetzler, R., Hadley, M. & Drayer, B. Cavernous malformations and capillary

telangiectasia: a spectrum within a single pathological entity. *Neurosurgery* 1991;**28**:60–64.

40. Ciricillo, S., Dillon, W., Fink, M. & Edwards, M. Progression of multiple cryptic vascular malformations associated with anomalous venous drainage. Case report. *J Neurosurg* 1994;**81**:477–481.

41. Dillon, W. Cryptic vascular malformations: controversies in terminology, diagnosis, pathophysiology, and treatment. *AJNR Am J Neuroradiol* 1997;**18**:1839–1846.

42. Awada, A., Russell, N., Al Rajeh, S. & Omojola, M. Non-traumatic cerebral hemorrage in Saudi Arabs: a hospital-based study of 243 cases. *Journal of the Neurological Sciences* 1996;**144**:198–203.

43. Abdulrauf, S., Kaynar, M. & Awad, I. A comparison of the clinical profile of cavernous malformations with and without associated venous malformations. *Neurosurgery* 1999;**44**:41–46; discussion 46–47.

44. Awad, I., Robinson, J. J., Mohanty, S. & Estes, M. Mixed vascular malformations of the brain: clinical and pathogenetic considerations. *Neurosurgery* 1993;**33**:179–188; discussion 188.

45. Wurm, G., Schnizer, M. & Fellner, F. Cerebral cavernous malformations associated with venous anomalies: surgical considerations. *Neurosurgery* 2005;**57**:42–58; discussion 42–58.

46. Porter, R., *et al.* Cavernous malformations of the brainstem: experience with 100 patients. *J Neurosurg* 1999;**90**:50–58.

47. Abe, M., Hagihara, N., Tabuchi, K., Uchino, A. & Miyasaka, Y. Histologically classified venous angiomas of the brain: a controversy. *Neurol Med Chir (Tokyo)* 2003;**43**:1–10; discussion 11.

48. Wilson, C. Cryptic vascular malformations. *Clin Neurosurg* 1992;**38**:49–84.

49. Clatterbuck, R., Eberhart, C., Crain, B. & Rigamonti, D. Ultrastructural and immunocytochemical evidence that an incompetent blood-brain barrier is related to the pathophysiology of cavernous malformations. *J Neurol Neurosurg Psychiatry* 2001;**71**:188–192.

50. Wong, J., Awad, I. & Kim, J. Ultrastructural pathological features of cerebrovascular malformations: a preliminary report. *Neurosurgery* 2000;**46**:1454–1459.

51. Tu, J., Stoodley, M., Morgan, M. & Storer, K. Ultrastructural characteristics of hemorrhagic, nonhemorrhagic, and recurrent cavernous malformations. *J Neurosurg* 2005;**103**:903–909.

Epidemiology and natural history of cavernous malformations

Rachel Engelmann, Sachin Batra, Angela Li, Joaquin
Camara-Quintana and Daniele Rigamonti

Cavernous malformations (CM) are multilobulated lesions composed of sinusoids derived from endothelium embedded in collagen matrix without histological elements found in mature vasculature [1]. CMs may be found at any location in the central nervous system and therefore can present with diverse clinical presentations like seizures (23–50%), headaches (6–52%), and focal deficits (20–45%) arising from mass effect or lesion hemorrhage; however, up to 40% of patients may be asymptomatic [2]. Most CMs are found supratentorially. They are usually characterized clinically by seizures and less commonly by inconspicuous growth or intermittent bleeding. Seizures caused by perilesional deposits of epileptogenic hemosiderin may become intractable [3]. Hemorrhages associated with CMs are of low pressure and frequently clinically asymptomatic [4]. When a lesion is present in eloquent locations like the brainstem, however, even a small bleed can cause clinically significant neurological deficits [5]. The natural history of CMs is affected by several factors like gender, lesion location, and genotype. This chapter discusses the natural history of CMs and its clinical relevance.

Etiology

Cavernous malformations may be of sporadic or familial type. Familial CMs are caused by mutations of CCM1 or CCM2 or CCM3 genes [6–9]. Most reports have described familial lesions in patients of French or Hispanic descent, but familial occurrence may be more widespread than these reports suggest [9–12]. Most CMs including sporadic lesions were historically considered congenital lesions; however, several cases of their *de novo* appearance following

brain irradiation or viral infection have been reported [13,14]. It is believed that *de novo* appearance of CMs occurs in genetically predisposed individuals [15].

Prevalence

CMs constitute 10–15% of all vascular malformations and are the second most commonly found vascular malformation after developmental venous anomalies (DVAs), which are found in about 4% of the population and represent up to 63% of all cerebrovascular malformations [16–18]. The estimated prevalence of CM by MRI-based studies has been reported to be 0.4–0.53% of the general population, while on autopsy series the prevalence of CM is about 0.4% [19–21]. Up to 20% of CMs are asymptomatic, making it more difficult to accurately study their epidemiology and natural history. CMs were frequently not detected (occult) by radiological investigations like angiography or CT scans. This has changed since the advent of MRI; now these lesions are increasingly diagnosed in the asymptomatic population [16,22]. Thus accurate understanding of their natural history has become critical to appropriate management of these patients.

Asymptomatic CMs are frequently diagnosed amongst the relatives of patients harboring familial CMs [10,12,23,24]. Rigamonti *et al.* diagnosed three (27.3%) asymptomatic individuals out of 11 relatives diagnosed with familial lesions while Zabramski *et al.* found 39% (12 individuals) prevalence of asymptomatic lesions in a population of 31 relatives of patients harboring familial lesions [12,23]. Conversely, others have suggested a prevalence of symptomatic lesions (approximately 60%) amongst patients with the familial form of cavernous malformations [25,26]. At least 6–10% of all patients harboring CMs may have a pattern of inheritance consistent with familial lesions [27,28].

Furthermore, it is estimated that while 10–15% of Caucasian patients have familial lesions, 40% of Hispanic patients have familial CM [29]. Most existing studies describe the epidemiology of familial CMs based on screening of relatives of symptomatic patients with multiple CMs; however, the population prevalence of the sporadic type is yet to be studied.

Lesion characteristics

The typical measurements of cavernous malformations range from 0.01 to 1.7 cm [16,30,31]. Multiple CMs have been reported by several series, but are more frequently found in patients with a history suggestive of inherited CMs than in sporadic cases [2,16]. Multiple lesions are present in 50–84% of familial cases but in only 10–33% of sporadic cases [32,33,34]. *De novo* occurrence of lesions is more common in familial forms [35,36] and there exists an apparent association between the number of lesions and the age of the patient, with older patients having a greater number of lesions, suggesting *de novo* occurrence during the life of the patient [35,36].

CMs are more often supratentorial (64–84%) than infratentorial (19–35%) [16,37,39], with a distribution proportionate to the volume of neural tissue. The most common supratentorial locations are the frontal and temporal lobes while the most common infratentorial locations are the pons and the cerebellum [16,20]. CMs may rarely be found at locations like the cerebello-pontine angle, optic chiasm, pineal and pituitary gland, and third or fourth ventricles [33,40,41]. CMs may be found in association with other vascular malformations like developmental venous anomaly (DVAs) or capillary telangiectasia [16,42]. When associated with DVAs, CMs are more likely to bleed, with an incidence of 62% as compared to a 38% incidence of hemorrhage amongst CMs without a draining DVA [17]. These lesions also had a greater incidence of recurrent bleeding (23%) than when CMs were present with DVA (9.6%) [17]. This has been attributed to a higher intraluminal pressure within the lesion associated with DVA [43,44].

Natural history of cavernous malformations

Although the natural history of cavernous malformations has been investigated for more than 50 years, it is still difficult to clearly describe it due to a lack of comparability between studies. Most studies differ in

patient characteristics (pure familial cases versus combination of familial and sporadic cases; population-based versus hospital-based series), study design (retrospective versus prospective studies) and the criteria defining hemorrhage (extra-lesional versus intra-lesional, occult versus clinically significant bleeds) [5,12,23,38,39,45–49]. Consequently, wide variation can be observed in reported rates of hemorrhage, ranging between 0.25% per person years to 4.2% per person years [20,37,45,50]. Thus, it is impossible to make a statement regarding the natural history that is consistent with all the reports in the literature. It follows that clinical decisions based on the interpretation of these studies remain challenging.

Despite disagreements on the natural history of CM and its predictors, most studies have shown a relatively benign course of superficial lesions compared to deep lesions or those located infratentorially with respect to bleeding [16,31,45]. In an MRI-based study Del Curling *et al.* reported an overall bleeding rate of 0.25% per person years of exposure [39]. Multiple lesions were present in six (18.75%) of the patients in this series; after accounting for the multiple lesions the risk of bleeding was reduced to 0.1% per lesion per person year of exposure. Similar to these findings, Robinson *et al.* described a hemorrhage rate of 0.7% per lesion per person year of exposure in a series of 66 patients with six patients (9%) presenting with a bleed at the start of the study and only one patient suffering a bleed on follow-up of 143 lesion years of observation [20]. In contrast to this, Kondziolka *et al.* reported a higher overall bleeding rate of 2.63% per person year [47]. However, due to referral bias, deep or infratentorial lesions constituted over 50% of this study population. Thirty-five percent of patients harbored brainstem lesions, of which 62.8% had a previous hemorrhage. Another 17% had thalamic or basal ganglia lesions. Overall about 50% of the study population suffered at least one previous hemorrhage from the lesion as compared to the series by DeCurling *et al.*, which included no patients with a prior history of bleeding, and patients presented with 72% of their lesions in a supratentorial location [39]. Similarly Porter *et al.* in a series of 173 patients followed for 437 person-years reported a higher bleeding or deficit rate in deep locations as compared to superficial locations (10.6%/year versus 0%/year: $p = 0.001$) [45]. MRI-documented bleeding rates were 1.6% per year for deep versus 0% per year for superficial lesions. Furthermore, the multivariate analysis in this study revealed deep location to be a significant predictor of subsequent events but not a history of past bleeding.

A study of the natural history of CM by Kupersmith et al. described predictors of hemorrhage in brainstem lesions. Hemorrhage was more frequent in lesions associated with developmental venous anomalies, lesions symptomatic at an early age (<35 years), and those greater than 1 cm in diameter. Mathiesen et al. described outcomes of conservatively managed deep lesions and found a lower event rate (bleeding or focal deficits) in patients with asymptomatic lesions (2% per year) as compared to those with symptomatic lesions (7% per year) [49]. This observation suggests that symptomatic lesions tend to follow an aggressive course whereas incidentally found lesions with no history of related symptoms follow a more benign course even in deep locations. These data confirm the bias in interpreting the natural history based on either surgical series or series containing conservatively managed lesions. Zimmerman et al., however, reported a lower rate of hemorrhage in patients even with symptomatic brainstem lesions at presentation [48]. All of the eight conservatively managed patients who presented with symptoms due to lesions in midbrain tectum (four patients), midbrain tegmentum (one patient), and pons (three patients) recovered. However, one patient had a fatal hemorrhage 1 year after initial evaluation. Similarly, Kharkar et al. followed 14 patients harboring symptomatic spinal lesions but who were managed conservatively. Of the 10 patients (71%) who continued to be conservatively managed, nine (90%) were stable or better over a mean follow-up of 80 months since presentation [51].

Familial lesions

The bleeding rates in familial studies have varied from 1.1% per lesion per year to 4.3% per lesion per year [10,23]. The wide difference in the bleeding rates between these two studies may be related to relative differences in the prevalence of CCM genotypes. Denier et al. reported 50% of patients with mutations in CCM3 exhibiting clinical signs and symptoms before reaching 15 years of age [52], whereas only 17% and 19% of patients with mutations in CCM1 or CCM2 respectively were symptomatic by this age. Lesions expressed by CCM3 mutations had bleeding at initial presentation in 53% of cases, as compared to those due to CCM1 or CCM2 mutations, which caused

bleeding in 26% and 39% of patients respectively [52]. Furthermore, the multiplicity of lesions increased with age in individuals possessing the CCM1 genotype but not in CCM2 or CCM3 genotypes [52].

Risk of subsequent bleeding

A greater risk of subsequent hemorrhage is anticipated in patients with a prior history of bleeding or focal deficits. Most studies have reported a rebleeding rate ranging from 2.63 to 60% per person year, with most lesions rebleeding either deep or infratentorial in location [37,53–55]. Kondziolka et al. reported a hemorrhage rate of 4.5% per person year in patients with a history of prior bleeding as compared to an overall hemorrhage rate of 2.63% per person year ($p = 0.028$). Similarly, Porter et al. reported seven episodes of bleeding over the study follow-up of 427 person years, six (7.40%) of which occurred in the subgroup of 81 patients who presented with hemorrhage or focal deficit attributable to lesions located in the brainstem [45]. Aiba et al. in a series including both conservative and surgically managed patients reported a higher prospective hemorrhage rate of 22.9% per year per lesion in the subgroup of patients who presented with symptomatic hemorrhage, most of whom underwent resection of lesion. High rebleeding rates ranging from 17 to 60% have been reported in most surgical series [53–55] and may represent an aggressive subclass of lesions [49]. While risk of rebleeding is considered higher than risk of bleeding in incidental lesions, Barker et al. reported temporal clustering of hemorrhages in the lesions, suggesting that lesions may return to baseline risk within 2–3 years following the initial bleed [56].

Effect of age and sex

Cavernous malformations have been reported in patients from both extremes of life, although the average age of symptom onset is approximately 35 years [57,39]. In general, the prognosis for younger patients is worse than that for older patients as younger patients are more likely to experience hemorrhage or recurrent hemorrhage, and are more likely to be afflicted with a neurological deficit [33,58–60]. In contrast to the high rate of hemorrhage in younger patients, elderly patients rarely experience symptoms in association with cavernous malformations [33]. However, this age-associated disparity in hemorrhage rate was not confirmed by Robinson et al., who found no significant difference in hemorrhage rates between patients under age 40 and those who were over the age of 40.

Some studies have reported differences in bleeding between males and females [31,33,61]. Males harboring CMs are more likely to become symptomatic at a younger age and to experience seizures, while females are more likely to have later symptom onset and to experience neurological deficits [62]. This has been attributed to hormonal differences. Several studies have also suggested a greater likelihood of hemorrhage in females irrespective of location of lesion [33,31,61]. In a study conducted by Robinson et al. 86% of the subjects who hemorrhaged were female despite a comparable number of male and female subjects [31]. Based on more recent evidence, it is now generally accepted that CMs behave similarly in both genders [25,45,47].

Several authors have cited an increased risk of hemorrhage concurrent with pregnancy and possibly related to the effect of estrogen on angiogenesis and structural integrity of the CM [63]. Evidence suggests an increase in the size of cavernous malformations during pregnancy which could contribute to increased risk of hemorrhage [64]. Additional research is necessary to confirm this finding and to determine the best method of management for pregnant women with cavernous malformations.

Summary

CMs are vascular malformations found throughout the brain and spinal cord. They present primarily with seizures or focal deficits, often caused by perilesional hemosiderin deposition or mass effect from lesion growth or bleeding. Natural history studies have several shortcomings; however, the majority seem to suggest that most lesions have a relatively benign course. This is particularly true when the lesions are located superficially in the supratentorial compartment. Lesions at deep locations are more prone to become symptomatic, although they too may remain clinically quiescent. Several aspects of lesion behaviour, such as the influence of prophylactic anticoagulation, pregnancy, and familiality of the clinical course, remain to be clarified. Knowledge of all these aspects is critical to determining appropriate management strategies and therefore they require further investigation.

References

1. Clatterbuck, R., Eberhart, C., Crain, B. & Rigamonti, D. Ultrastructural and immunocytochemical evidence that an incompetent blood-brain barrier is related to the pathophysiology of cavernous malformations. *J Neurol Neurosurg Psychiatry* 2001;**71**:188–192.

2. Batra, S., Lin, D., Recinos, P., Zhang, J. & Rigamonti, D. Cavernous malformations: natural history, diagnosis and treatment. *Nat Rev Neurol* 2009;**5**:659–670.

3. Awad, I. & Jabbour, P. Cerebral cavernous malformations and epilepsy. *Neurosurg Focus* **21**, e7 (2006).

4. Cordonnier, C., et al. Differences between intracranial vascular malformation types in the characteristics of their presenting haemorrhages: prospective, population-based study. *J Neurol Neurosurg Psychiatry* 2008;**79**:47–51.

5. Kupersmith, M., et al. Natural history of brainstem cavernous malformations. *Neurosurgery* 2001; **48**: 47–53; discussion 53–44.

6. Bergametti, F., et al. Mutations within the programmed cell death 10 gene cause cerebral cavernous malformations. *Am J Hum Genet* 2005;**76**:42–51.

7. Laberge-le Couteulx, S., et al. Truncating mutations in CCM1, encoding KRIT1, cause hereditary cavernous angiomas. *Nat Genet* 1999;**23**:189–193.

8. Liquori, C., et al. Deletions in CCM2 are a common cause of cerebral cavernous malformations. *Am J Hum Genet* 2007;**80**:69–75.

9. Gunel, M., et al. A founder mutation as a cause of cerebral cavernous malformation in Hispanic Americans. *New Engl J Med* 1996;**334**:946–951.

10. Labauge, P., Brunereau, L., Laberge, S. & Houtteville, J. Prospective follow-up of 33 asymptomatic patients with familial cerebral cavernous malformations. *Neurology* 2001;**57**:1825–1828.

11. Brunereau, L., et al. Familial form of intracranial cavernous angioma: MR imaging findings in 51 families. French Society of Neurosurgery. *Radiology* 2000;**214**:209–216.

12. Rigamonti, D., et al. Cerebral cavernous malformations. Incidence and familial occurrence. *New Engl J Med* 1988;**319**:343–347.

13. Pozzati, E., Acciarri, N., Tognetti, F., Marliani, F. & Giangaspero, F. Growth, subsequent bleeding, and de novo appearance of cerebral cavernous angiomas. *Neurosurgery* 1996;**38**:662–669; discussion 669–670.

14. Ogilvy, C. S., Moayeri, N. & Golden, J. A. Appearance of a cavernous hemangioma in the cerebral cortex after a biopsy of a deeper lesion. *Neurosurgery* 1993;**33**:307–309; discussion 309.

15. Pagenstecher, A., Stahl, S., Sure, U. & Felbor, U. A two-hit mechanism causes cerebral cavernous malformations: complete inactivation of CCM1, CCM2 or CCM3 in affected endothelial cells. *Hum Mol Genet* 2009;**18**:911–918.

16. Maraire, J. & Awad, I. Intracranial cavernous malformations: lesion behavior and management strategies. *Neurosurgery* 1995;**37**:591–605.

17. Abdulrauf, S., Kaynar, M. & Awad, I. A comparison of the clinical profile of cavernous malformations with and without associated venous malformations. *Neurosurgery* 1999;**44**:41–46; discussion 46–47.

18. Brown Jr, R. D. Wiebers, D. O., Torner, J. C. & O'Fallon, W. M. Frequency of intracranial hemorrhage as a presenting symptom and subtype analysis: A population-based study of intracranial vascular malformations in Olmsted County, Minnesota. *J Neurosurg* 1996;**85**:29–32.

19. Otten, P., Pizzolato, G., Rilliet, B. & Berney, J. [131 cases of cavernous angioma (cavernomas) of the CNS, discovered by retrospective analysis of 24,535 autopsies]. *Neurochirurgie* 1989;**35**:82–83, 128–131.

20. Robinson, J., Awad, I. & Little, J. Natural history of the cavernous angioma. *J Neurosurg* 1991;**75**:709–714.

21. Sarwar, M. & McCormick, W. Intracerebral venous angioma. Case report and review. *Arch Neurol* 1978;**35**:323–325.

22. Morris, Z., *et al.* Incidental findings on brain magnetic resonance imaging: systematic review and meta-analysis. *BMJ* 2009;**339**:b3016.

23. Zabramski, J., *et al.* The natural history of familial cavernous malformations: results of an ongoing study. *J Neurosurg* 1994;**80**:422–432.

24. Brunereau, L., *et al.* Familial form of cerebral cavernous malformations: evaluation of gradient-spin-echo (GRASE) imaging in lesion detection and characterization at 1.5 T. *Neuroradiology* 2001;**43**:973–979.

25. D'Angelo, V. A., *et al.* Supratentorial cerebral cavernous malformations: clinical, surgical, and genetic involvement. *Neurosurg Focus* 2006;**21**:e9.

26. Labauge, P., Denier, C., Bergametti, F. & Tournier-Lasserve, E. Genetics of cavernous angiomas. *Lancet Neurol* 2007;**6**:237–244.

27. Hsu, F. P., Rigamonti, D. & Huhn,SL. *Epidemiology of Cavernous Malformation* (American Association of Neurological Surgeons, 1993).

28. Bertalanffy, H., *et al.* Cerebral cavernomas in the adult. Review of the literature and analysis of 72 surgically treated patients. *Neurosurg Rev* 2002;**25**:1–53.

29. Dashti, S. R., Hoffer, A., Hu, Y. C. & Selman, W. R. Molecular genetics of familial cerebral cavernous malformations. *Neurosurg Focus* 2006;**21**:e2.

30. Casazza, M., *et al.* Supratentorial cavernous angiomas and epileptic seizures: preoperative course and postoperative outcome. *Neurosurgery* 1996;**39**:26–32; discussion 32–24.

31. Robinson, J. R., Awad, I. A. & Little, J. R. Natural history of the cavernous angioma. *J Neurosurg* 1991;**75**:709–714.

32. Kim, D. S., Park, Y. G., Choi, J. U., Chung, S. S. & Lee, K. C. An analysis of the natural history of cavernous malformations. *Surg Neurol* 1997;**48**:9–17; discussion 17–18.

33. Maraire, J. N. & Awad, I. A. Intracranial cavernous malformations: lesion behavior and management strategies. *Neurosurgery* 1995;**37**:591–605.

34. Vinas, F. C., Gordon, V., Guthikonda, M. & Diaz, F. G. Surgical management of cavernous malformations of the brainstem. *Neurol Res* 2002;**24**:61–72.

35. Brunereau, L., Levy, C., Laberge, S., Houtteville, J. & Labauge, P. De novo lesions in familial form of cerebral cavernous malformations: clinical and MR features in 29 non-Hispanic families. *Surg Neurol* 2000;**53**:475–482; discussion 482–473.

36. Pozzati, E., Acciarri, N., Tognetti, F., Marliani, F. & Giangaspero, F. Growth, subsequent bleeding, and de novo appearance of cerebral cavernous angiomas. *Neurosurgery* 1996;**38**:662–669; discussion 669–670.

37. Kondziolka, D., Lunsford, L. & Kestle, J. The natural history of cerebral cavernous malformations. *J Neurosurg* 1995;**83**:820–824.

38. Moriarity, J., Clatterbuck, R. & Rigamonti, D. The natural history of cavernous malformations. *Neurosurg Clin N Am* 1999;**10**:411–417.

39. Del Curling, O., Jr., Kelly, D. L., Jr., Elster, A. D. & Craven, T. E. An analysis of the natural history of cavernous angiomas. *J Neurosurg* 1991;**75**:702–708.

40. Baumann, C. R., *et al.* Seizure outcome after resection of supratentorial cavernous malformations: A study of 168 patients. *Epilepsia* 2007;**48**:559–563.

41. Simard, J., Garcia-Bengochea, F., Ballinger, W. J., Mickle, J. & Quisling, R. Cavernous angioma: a review of 126 collected and 12 new clinical cases. *Neurosurgery* 1986;**18**:162–172.

42. Rigamonti, D., Johnson, P., Spetzler, R., Hadley, M. & Drayer, B. Cavernous malformations and capillary telangiectasia: a spectrum within a single pathological entity. *Neurosurgery* 1991;**28**:60–64.

43. Ciricillo, S., Dillon, W., Fink, M. & Edwards, M. Progression of multiple cryptic vascular malformations associated with anomalous venous drainage. Case report. *J Neurosurg* 1994;**81**:477–481.

44. Dillon, W. Cryptic vascular malformations: controversies in terminology, diagnosis, pathophysiology, and treatment. *AJNR Am J Neuroradiol* 1997;**18**:1839–1846.

45. Porter, P., Willinsky, R., Harper, W. & Wallace, M. Cerebral cavernous malformations: natural history and

prognosis after clinical deterioration with or without hemorrhage. *J Neurosurg* 1997;**87**:190–197.

46. Al-Shahi Salman, R., Berg, M., Morrison, L. & Awad, I. Hemorrhage from cavernous malformations of the brain: definition and reporting standards. Angioma Alliance Scientific Advisory Board. *Stroke* 2008;**39**:3222–3230.

47. Kondziolka, D., Lunsford, L. D. & Kestle, J. R. The natural history of cerebral cavernous malformations. *J Neurosurg* 1995;**83**:820–824.

48. Zimmerman, R., Spetzler, R., Lee, K., Zabramski, J. & Hargraves, R. Cavernous malformations of the brain stem. *J Neurosurg* 1991;**75**:32–39.

49. Mathiesen, T., Edner, G. & Kihlström, L. Deep and brainstem cavernomas: a consecutive 8-year series. *J Neurosurg* 2003;**99**:31–37.

50. Del Curling, O. J., Kelly, D. J., Elster, A. & Craven, T. An analysis of the natural history of cavernous angiomas. *J Neurosurg* 1991;**75**:702–708.

51. Kharkar, S., Shuck, J., Conway, J. & Rigamonti, D. The natural history of conservatively managed symptomatic intramedullary spinal cord cavernomas. *Neurosurgery* 2007;**60**:865–872; discussion 865–872.

52. Denier, C., *et al.* Genotype-phenotype correlations in cerebral cavernous malformations patients. *Ann Neurol* 2006;**60**:550–556.

53. Fritschi, J., Reulen, H., Spetzler, R. & Zabramski, J. Cavernous malformations of the brain stem. A review of 139 cases. *Acta Neurochir (Wien)* 1994;**130**:35–46.

54. Bruneau, M., *et al.* Early surgery for brainstem cavernomas. *Acta Neurochir (Wien)* 2006;**148**:405–414.

55. Ferroli, P., *et al.* Brainstem cavernomas: long-term results of microsurgical resection in 52 patients. *Neurosurgery* 2005;**56**:1203–1212; discussion 1212–1204.

56. Barker, F. N., *et al.* Temporal clustering of hemorrhages from untreated cavernous malformations of the central nervous system. *Neurosurgery* **49**, 15–24; discussion 24–15 (2001).

57. Conway, J. E. & Rigamonti, D. Cavernous malformations: a review and current controversies. *Neurosurg Quart* 2006;**16**:15–23.

58. Aiba, T., *et al.* Natural history of intracranial cavernous malformations. *J Neurosurg* 1995;**83**:56–59.

59. Kupersmith, M. J., *et al.* Natural history of brainstem cavernous malformations. *Neurosurgery* 2001;**48**:47–53; discussion 53–44.

60. Zabramski, J. M., *et al.* The natural history of familial cavernous malformations: results of an ongoing study. *J Neurosurg* 1994;**80**:422–432.

61. Wang, C. C., Liu, A., Zhang, J. T., Sun, B. & Zhao, Y. L. Surgical management of brain-stem cavernous malformations: report of 137 cases. *Surg Neurol* 2003;**59**:444–454; discussion 454.

62. Casazza, M., *et al.* Supratentorial cavernous angiomas and epileptic seizures: preoperative course and postoperative outcome. *Neurosurgery* 1996;**39**:26–32; discussion 32–24.

63. Aiba, T., *et al.* Natural history of intracranial cavernous malformations. *J Neurosurg* 1995;**83**:56–59.

64. Safavi-Abbasi, S., *et al.* Hemorrhage of cavernous malformations during pregnancy and in the peripartum period: causal or coincidence? Case report and review of the literature. *Neurosurg Focus* 2006;**21**:e12.

Chapter 3

Familial cavernous malformations: a historical survey

Leslie Morrison

In 1928, Kufs reported the first familial cavernous hemangiomas [1]. As brain imaging technology has advanced, the detection of single or multiple CCMs has facilitated our ability to identify patients with the familial form in which lesions are multiple. Obtaining detailed pedigree information remains important, but it is less informative than imaging due to incomplete penetrance of the gene mutation and variability of gene expression. Familial CCM has a disease phenotype that spans from asymptomatic to completely neurologically disabled. The high incidence of seizures, headaches and strokes within the general population and even in family members who are unaffected by the gene mutation further complicates the ability to rely exclusively on family neurological history. In this chapter, the history of familial CCM is traced through radiographic eras, followed by gene discovery, other systemic manifestations, disease variability and natural history.

Pre-CT scans

The contribution of brain imaging to identify familial cases began with plain skull radiographs showing single calcified cavernous malformations. Interestingly, there are no reports of multiple calcified cavernous malformations discovered by skull film reported in the literature. Review of the record of a New Mexico patient with epilepsy revealed the clinical use of plain skull radiographs that showed multiple calcified CCMs in a young girl with epilepsy, who was initially suspected of having multiple calcified brain tumors. Another of her relatives exhibited the same findings (personal observation Morrison 2010). Brain imaging of multiple lesions was not reported in the literature until computerized tomography (CT) became available in the 1960s.

Prior to the availability of head CT scanning, the diagnosis of CCM depended on the pathological analysis of surgical lesions or autopsy material corroborated by pedigree analysis and plain skull films. In 1936 a Swedish family was reported with multiple lesions and the familial nature was also simultaneously identified (Michael, Levin, 1936.) An Icelandic family of two generations was reported by Kidd and Cummings (Kidd, Cummings, 1947). The third report by Clark in 1970 described the first pathological study of multiple family members [2] with neuropsychiatric features in the father and episodic headaches in the daughter. CCMs were considered very rare prior to the CT era [3].

CT era

Commercial CT scans were invented by Sir Godfrey Hounsfield in Hayes, United Kingdom, at EMI Central Research Laboratories using X-rays. Hounsfield conceived his idea in 1967, and it was publicly announced in 1972 (BMJ (London, UK: BMJ Group) 2004;329:687). As use of CT expanded, multiple CCMs became easier to identify. Multiple CCMs were found in a white male with increased intracranial pressure, pathologically confirmed in both the hemorrhagic lesion, non-hemorrhagic lesion and a pulmonary hemorrhagic lesion [4]. The author notes that without CT, the multiplicity of lesions would have been missed.

An additional large kindred of Hispanic-American families from New Mexico was reported by Bicknell in 1978, introducing the utility of cranial computerized tomography and discussing the first three kindred reports [5]. Another large Hispanic family was studied by Hayman et al. through the use of CCT in 1982 [6].

Mason et al. studied a large Hispanic family and identified CCMs in 10 of 22 family members using

MRI rather than CT [7]. Rigamonti confirmed the existence in Hispanic families, reporting six new families, five of the six of Hispanic origin [8]. As brain imaging technology progressed from CT to MRI, it became much easier to identify patients with multiple lesions.

MRI era

Multiple lesions are best identified based on magnetic resonance imaging (MRI) [56,57].

Gradient-echo and susceptibility-weighted imaging techniques identify more lesions than standard MRI sequences in familial CM [9–13]. Although gradient images exaggerate the size of lesions that have a surrounding hemosiderin rim, this technique is more sensitive for the identification of smaller lesions, picking up approximately threefold the number seen on T1, T2, and intermediate sequences [14]. Up to 400 lesions have been identified in a patient by gradient sequence [15]. Whereas, SWI identifies numerous additional tiny lesions, up to threefold the number seen on gradient-echo imaging [13]. In comparing SWI and GRE, lesions may appear smaller on SWI than on GRE. Increased numbers of lesions are identified by MRI with increased age [16,17].

Contrast enhancement with current standard techniques adds minimal information to brain imaging. Early reports identified some lesions that showed "blush" with contrasted CT, even though most lesions did not enhance with contrast on standard angiogram or on contrasted CT. On MRI with gadolinium, some lesions also show mild enhancement but the significance of this finding remains undetermined.

Gene discovery

The first genetic localization was identified on chromosome 7 and included a large Italian-American family from Boston, and a large Hispanic family from New Mexico [18,19]. Further narrowing of the disease locus included a number of New Mexico Hispanic families [20] and the New Mexico cohort was attributed to a genetic founder effect [21]. In 1997, linkage of the locus for CCM to 7q was published about a family with Mexican-American descent but ancestry from Sonora, Mexico [22].

The first gene was identified as KRIT1 by Labauge in 1999 [23]. Almost simultaneously, the specific mutation that created the large Hispanic American cohort was found in the KRIT1 gene and was deemed "the common Hispanic mutation (CHM)" by Sahoo et al. in

1999. This remains the only large cohort of familial CCM worldwide, numbering in the thousands [15]. CHM along with other mutations in CCM1 accounts for a total of approximately 40% of detected mutations. Another 20% are accounted for by mutation in CCM2 [24]. The third known gene is CCM3 and there is evidence of linkage to a fourth disease-causing gene [25]. At least 10–40% of non-Hispanic cases are familial, and in Mexican-American families in the USA the familial incidence is estimated at 50% [26].

Genetic testing

Genetic testing is now available for CCM1, 2, and 3 on a commercial basis, with several labs still working on identification of a suspected fourth familial gene. Genetic testing is further discussed in Chapter 18 on genetic counseling.

CCM in New Mexico

Familial forms

In 1978, Bicknell et al. reported the first case of a New Mexican family of Hispanic descent, with four affected patients (one by historic report) ranging in age from 19 to 38. Presenting diagnoses included epilepsy, paraplegia, and hemorrhagic stroke [5]. The original genetic founder of the large southwestern US Hispanic population has not yet been identified but is suspected to be one of the original Hispanic settlers in New Mexico, possibly as early as 1598 with the Oñate expedition. In one large pedigree, the ancestors were born in New Mexico in the early 1700s (Gonzales and Gonzales, 2009). Outside the Southwestern United States and northern Mexico, the specific gene mutation CHM has not been identified in patients with origins further south in Mexico City, nor in Spain [27,28]. In Spain, a variety of other mutations have been identified in CCM1, 2, and 3.

The natural history of familial CCM was reported retrospectively [29]. A later study provided genotype–phenotype correlations. While this later study did not include patients with CCM1-CHM, these authors found that other mutations in CCM1 may have a milder clinical presentation than mutations in CCM2 or CCM3. However, the proportion of symptomatic patients under 15 years was higher in CCM3 kindreds [30]. Overall, clinical symptomatology and the number of lesions on MRI were very similar among the genetic forms of disease. Fifteen German families were reported in 2005, finding 75% symptomatic, 40–50% with epilepsy, 10–20% with chronic headache, and 30–40% with hemorrhage, and 15% with focal neurological deficits [31]. In the only study of predictive factors for intracerebral hemorrhage in CCM, familial cases had a decreased relative risk with a family history of epilepsy and lobar location of lesions [32]. Imaging features do not differ in the three known and suspected fourth genetic forms. In a large study comparing sporadic and familial forms of CCM, the incidence of associated developmental venous anomalies (DVA) was extremely low in the familial form (mostly CCM1) with nearly 50% of sporadic patients showing associated DVAs [15].

Multisystemic involvement

Association with other vascular brain malformations is rare. In 1984, Pasyk *et al.* reported 25 members of one affected family, also detailing other associated types of vascular malformations including arteriovenous malformations and capillary hemangiomas co-existing in some families [33]. However, familial forms are recognized to include lesions within other tissues. Approximately 5–10% of cases have cutaneous or subcutaneous lesions [34], retinal lesions or both cutaneous and retinal involvement.

Cutaneous

The first case report of a 32-year-old man with a retinal cavernous hemangioma, cutaneous angiomas, and CT and MRI confirmation of cerebrovascular lesions was made in 1984 [35]. Since then, several families have been reported showing this triad of involvement, but the cutaneous findings were inconsistent within families [36–39]. A case report of a 51-year-old man with familial CCM had thousands of cherry angiomas with over 150 lesions surgically removed [40]. The cutaneous findings appear in patients with mutations in all three known genes, but there seem to be no specific mutations that predispose to skin lesions [41]. A rare occurrence of associated cavernous malformation has been reported in Klippel Trenauney Weber syndrome [42]. Cutaneous and subcutaneous angiomas have also been reported with CCM1-CHM [43].

Ocular

Retinal cavernous angiomas were reported in a family with CNS and hepatic CMs in an Italian family [44]. Retinal lesions were also reported in a large four-generation family [45]. Choroidal hemangiomas were reported in a California family, with localization of the gene to 7q [46] likely CCM1, and possibly CHM. The authors did not make note of the ethnicity of the family. In one family with autosomal dominant CCM, several family members were found to have twin vessels of the retina [47]. Sixty patients with familial CCM were screened with retinal examinations, finding 5% estimated frequency in any of the three known genes [26].

Other tissues

Lesions in liver and bone are reported in occasional kindreds [41,48].

Disease variability

In most families, disease severity is remarkably variable. Family members may carry the mutation and remain unaffected lifelong in up to 25% (Siegal *et al.* 1998), some remaining asymptomatic despite single or multiple CCMs noted on imaging. Still others are left with permanent neurological disability in the form of debilitating headaches, seizures or residual neurological impairment secondary to CNS hemorrhages or their surgical management. A recent attempt to identify gene polymorphisms in the angiotensin-converting enzyme gene was suggestive of an effect on lesion number [49]. In a prospective study of 33 asymptomatic patients from 29 unrelated French families with asymptomatic lesions, subjects were evaluated with serial clinical exams and spin-echo and gradient-echo MRI over a mean of 2.1 years. Only two out of 33 patients became symptomatic but 46% of patients showed changes in MRI that included bleeding, new lesion formation in 30.3%, change in signal intensity, and changes in size [17,50]. Five Italian families were studied with clinical MRI and genetic studies. This study included 45 at-risk, symptom-free relatives. In this study, three new mutations in CCM1 were identified, and of 33 KRIT1 mutation carriers, 57.6% were asymptomatic. MRI revealed CCM lesions in only 82.3% of these asymptomatic carriers, but MRI was performed on a 1.5 tesla magnet and with gradient-echo but not SWI (1988 [51]). In another Italian study, another novel gene mutation was found in CCM1 and also in CCM2. A large Italian family with a CCM1 mutation has been reported [52] in which genetic variations were searched for in all three known genes to help explain clinical variability. The spectrum of genotype and clinical manifestation in CCM found large clinical variability in CCM1 in 22 Hispanic-American cases with the CHM. Interestingly, CCM1 may have a decreased risk of hemorrhage compared with CCM2 and CCM3 [53]. A large prospective study of CCM1 common Hispanic mutation patients will include a genome-wide association study to identify modifier genes with either beneficial or deleterious effects.

Natural history and prognosis of familial CCMs

A study of 264 consecutive patients in Helsinki, Finland, reported only 33 patients with multiple CCMs. Genotyping was not performed in this study. Only 9% had a family history of the disease. A total of 416 cavernomas were found, 70% supratentorial and 30% infratentorial. Eighteen of the 33 patients had surgery, typically to remove the largest cavernoma. Of these 18 patients, one developed temporary hemiparesis and another had permanent motor dysphasia. Of patients operated on for epileptogenic lesions, 70% had Engel class 1 outcome. From the 13 patients with follow-up MR imaging, 52 new cavernomas were found, with a mean follow-up of 7 years. An interesting finding was that no patients who underwent surgery had acute hemorrhages, and no patients had hemorrhage for more than one lesion simultaneously [54]. In a study of Hispanic CCM patients in New Mexico (presumed CCM1-CHM) by Kattapong et al., lesions increased at an average of one per decade and mean diameter decreased slightly [17]. The estimated rate of de novo lesion formation is 0.2–0.4 new lesions per patient/year.

For familial CCM, recommendations regarding routine imaging are sparse at present, especially with regard to surveillance imaging for spinal cord lesions [55]. As treatments become available, we will undoubtedly require routine imaging to assess treatment effects. Studies of lesion permeability will be essential in this outcome assessment as well.

References

1. Kufs, H. Über die heredofamiläre Angiomatose des Gehirns und der Retina, ihre Beziehung en zueinander und zur Angiomatose der Haut. *Z Neurol Psychiatrie* 1928;**113**:651–686.

2. Clark, J. V. Familial occurrence of cavernous angiomata of the brain. *J Neurol Neurosurg Psychiatry* 1970;**33**:871–876.

3. Villani, R. M., Arienta, C., *et al.* Cavernous angiomas of the central nervous system. *J Neurosurg Sci* 1989;**33**:229–252.

4. Tindall, R. S., Kirkpatrick, J. B., *et al.* Multiple small cavernous angiomas of the brain with increased intracranial pressure. *Ann Neurol* 1978;**4**:376–378.

5. Bicknell, J. M., Carlow, T. J., *et al.* Familial cavernous angiomas. *Arch Neurol* 1978;**35**:746–749.

6. Hayman, L. A., Evans, R. A., *et al.* Familial cavernous angiomas: natural history and genetic study over a 5-year period. *Am J Med Genet* 1982;**11**:147–160.

7. Mason, I., Aase, J. M., *et al.* Familial cavernous angiomas of the brain in an Hispanic family. *Neurology* 1988;**38**:324–326.

8. Rigamonti, D., Hadley, M. N., *et al.* Cerebral cavernous malformations. Incidence and familial occurrence. *New Engl J Med* 1988;**319**:343–347.

9. Rutka, J. T., Brant-Zawadzki, M., *et al.* Familial cavernous malformations. Diagnostic potential of magnetic resonance imaging. *Surg Neurol* 1988;**29**:467–474.

10. Labauge, P., Laberge, S., *et al.* Hereditary cerebral cavernous angiomas: clinical and genetic features in 57 French families. Societe Francaise de Neurochirurgie. *Lancet* 1998;**352**:1892–1897.

11. Brunereau, L., Leveque, C., *et al.* Familial form of cerebral cavernous malformations: evaluation of gradient-spin-echo (GRASE) imaging in lesion detection and characterization at 1.5 T. *Neuroradiology* 2001;**43**:973–979.

12. Cooper, A. D., Campeau, N. G., *et al.* Susceptibility-weighted imaging in familial cerebral cavernous malformations. *Neurology* 2008;**71**:382.

13. de Souza, J. M., Domingues, R. C., *et al.* Susceptibility-weighted imaging for the evaluation of patients with familial cerebral cavernous malformations: a comparison with t2-weighted fast spin-echo and gradient-echo sequences. *AJNR Am J Neuroradiol* 2008;**29**:154–158.

14. Lehnhardt, F. G., von Smekal, U., *et al.* Value of gradient-echo magnetic resonance imaging in the diagnosis of familial cerebral cavernous malformation. *Arch Neurol* 2005;**62**:653–658.

15. Petersen, T. A., Morrison, L. A., *et al.* Familial versus sporadic cavernous malformations: differences in developmental venous anomaly association and lesion phenotype. *AJNR Am J Neuroradiol* 2010;**31**:377–382.

16. Horowitz, M. & Kondziolka, D. Multiple familial cavernous malformations evaluated over three

generations with MR. *AJNR Am J Neuroradiol* 1995;**16**:1353–1355.

17. Kattapong, V. J., Hart, B. L., *et al.* Familial cerebral cavernous angiomas: clinical and radiologic studies. *Neurology* 1995;**45**:492–497.

18. Gunel, M., Awad, I. A., *et al.* Mapping a gene causing cerebral cavernous malformation to 7q11.2-q21. *Proc Natl Acad Sci USA* 1995;**92**:6620–6624.

19. Marchuk, D. A., Gallione, C. J., *et al.* A locus for cerebral cavernous malformations maps to chromosome 7q in two families. *Genomics* 1995;**28**:311–314.

20. Johnson, E. W., Iyer, L. M., *et al.* Refined localization of the cerebral cavernous malformation gene (CCM1) to a 4-cM interval of chromosome 7q contained in a well-defined YAC contig. *Genome Res* 1995;**5**:368–380.

21. Gunel, M., Awad, I. A., *et al.* A founder mutation as a cause of cerebral cavernous malformation in Hispanic Americans. *New Engl J Med* 1996;**334**:946–951.

22. Polymeropoulos, M. H., Hurko, O., *et al.* Linkage of the locus for cerebral cavernous hemangiomas to human chromosome 7q in four families of Mexican-American descent. *Neurology* 1997;**48**:752–757.

23. Laberge-le Couteulx, S., Jung, H. H., *et al.* Truncating mutations in CCM1, encoding KRIT1, cause hereditary cavernous angiomas. *Nat Genet* 1999;**23**:189–193.

24. Liquori, C. L., M. J. Berg, *et al.* Deletions in CCM2 are a common cause of cerebral cavernous malformations. *Am J Hum Genet* 2007;**80**:69–75.

25. Liquori, C. L., Berg, M. J., *et al.* Low frequency of PDCD10 mutations in a panel of CCM3 probands: potential for a fourth CCM locus. *Hum Mutat* 2006;**27**:118.

26. Labauge, P., Krivosic, V., *et al.* Frequency of retinal cavernomas in 60 patients with familial cerebral cavernomas: a clinical and genetic study. *Arch Ophthalmol* 2006;**124**:885–886.

27. Lucas, M., Solano, F., *et al.* Spanish families with cerebral cavernous angioma do not bear 742C->T Hispanic American mutation of the KRIT1 gene. *Ann Neurol* 2000;**47**:836.

28. Lucas, M., A. F. Costa, *et al.* Germline mutations in the CCM1 gene, encoding Krit1, cause cerebral cavernous malformations. *Ann Neurol* 2001;**49**:529–532.

29. Labauge, P., Brunereau, L., *et al.* The natural history of familial cerebral cavernomas: a retrospective MRI study of 40 patients. *Neuroradiology* 2000;**42**:327–332.

30. Denier, C., Labauge, P., *et al.* Genotype-phenotype correlations in cerebral cavernous malformations patients. *Ann Neurol* 2006;**60**:550–556.

31. Siegel, A. M., Bertalanffy, H., *et al.* [Familial cavernous malformations of the central nervous system. A clinical and genetic study of 15 German families]. *Nervenarzt* 2005;**76**:175–180.

32. Cantu, C., Murillo-Bonilla, L., *et al.* Predictive factors for intracerebral hemorrhage in patients with cavernous angiomas. *Neurol Res* 2005;**27**:314–318.

33. Pasyk, K. A., Argenta, L. C., *et al.* Familial vascular malformations. Report of 25 members of one family. *Clin Genet* 1984;**26**:221–227.

34. Kunkeler, A. C., Uitdehaag, B. M., *et al.* Familial cavernous haemangiomas. *Br J Dermatol* 1998;**139**:166–167.

35. Schwartz, A. C., Weaver, R. G. Jr., *et al.* Cavernous hemangioma of the retina, cutaneous angiomas, and intracranial vascular lesion by computed tomography and nuclear magnetic resonance imaging. *Am J Ophthalmol* 1984;**98**:483–487.

36. Dobyns, W. B., Michels, V. V., *et al.* Familial cavernous malformations of the central nervous system and retina. *Ann Neurol* 1987;**21**:578–583.

37. Ohkuma, A., Kuroda, T., *et al.* [Familial cavernous angioma of the central nervous system – report of a family and review of literature]. *No To Shinkei* 1992;**44**:155–161.

38. Leblanc, R., Melanson, D., *et al.* Hereditary neurocutaneous angiomatosis. Report of four cases. *J Neurosurg* 1996;**85**:1135–1142.

39. Garcia-Moreno, J. M., Gamero, M. A., *et al.* [Familial cerebral cavernomatosis associated with cutaneous angiomas]. *Rev Neurol* 1998;**27**:484–490.

40. Clatterbuck, R. E. & Rigamonti, D. Cherry angiomas associated with familial cerebral cavernous malformations. Case illustration. *J Neurosurg* 2002;**96**:964.

41. Gianfrancesco, F., Cannella, M., *et al.* Highly variable penetrance in subjects affected with cavernous cerebral angiomas (CCM) carrying novel CCM1 and CCM2 mutations. *Am J Med Genet B Neuropsychiatr Genet* 2007;**144**:691–695.

42. Pichierri, A., Piccirilli, M., *et al.* Klippel-Trenaunay-Weber syndrome and intramedullary cervical cavernoma: a very rare association. Case report. *Surg Neurol* 2006;**66**:203–206; discussion 206.

43. Zlotoff, B. J., Bang, R. H., *et al.* Cutaneous angiokeratoma and venous malformations in a Hispanic-American patient with cerebral cavernous malformations. *Br J Dermatol* 2007;**157**:210–212.

44. Drigo, P., Mammi, I., *et al.* Familial cerebral, hepatic, and retinal cavernous angiomas: a new syndrome. *Childs Nerv Syst* 1994;**10**:205–209.

45. Goldberg, R. E., Pheasant, T. R., *et al.* Cavernous hemangioma of the retina. A four-generation pedigree with neurocutaneous manifestations and an example of bilateral retinal involvement. *Arch Ophthalmol* 1979;**97**:2321–2324.

46. Sarraf, D., Payne, A. M., *et al.* Familial cavernous hemangioma: An expanding ocular spectrum. *Arch Ophthalmol* 2000;**118**:969–973.

47. Bottoni, F., Canevini, M. P., *et al.* Twin vessels in familial retinal cavernous hemangioma. *Am J Ophthalmol* 1990;**109**:285–289.

48. Toldo, I., Drigo, P., *et al.* Vertebral and spinal cavernous angiomas associated with familial cerebral cavernous malformation. *Surg Neurol* 2009;**71**:167–171.

49. Altas, M., Bayrak, O. F., *et al.* Angiotensin-converting enzyme insertion/deletion gene polymorphism in patients with familial multiple cerebral cavernous malformations. *J Clin Neurosci* 2010;**17**:1034–1037.

50. Labauge, P., Brunereau, L., *et al.* Prospective follow-up of 33 asymptomatic patients with familial cerebral cavernous malformations. *Neurology* 2001;**57**:1825–1828.

51. Battistini, S., Rocchi, R., *et al.* Clinical, magnetic resonance imaging, and genetic study of 5 Italian families with cerebral cavernous malformation. *Arch Neurol* 2007;**64**:843–848.

52. Pileggi, S., Buscone, S., *et al.* (2010). Genetic variations within KRIT1/CCM1, MGC4607/CCM2 and PDCD10/CCM3 in a large Italian family harbouring a Krit1/CCM1 mutation. *J Mol Neurosci* 2010;**42**:235–242.

53. Gault, J., Sain, S., *et al.* Spectrum of genotype and clinical manifestations in cerebral cavernous malformations. *Neurosurgery* 2006;**59**:1278–1284; discussion 1284–1275.

54. Kivelev, J., Niemela, M., *et al.* Long-term outcome of patients with multiple cerebral cavernous malformations. *Neurosurgery* 2009;**65**:450–455; discussion 455.

55. Cohen-Gadol, A. A., Jacob, J. T., *et al.* Coexistence of intracranial and spinal cavernous malformations: a study of prevalence and natural history. *J Neurosurg* 2006;**104**:376–381.

56. Rigamonti, D., Drayer, B. P., Johnson, P. C., Hadley, M. N., Zabramski, J., Spetzler, R. F. The MRI appearance of cavernous malformations (angiomas). *J Neurosurg* 1987;**67**:518–524.

57. Zabramski, J., *et al.* The natural history of familial cavernous malformations: results of an ongoing study. *J Neurosurg* 1994;**80**:422–432.

Clinical and molecular genetics of cerebral cavernous malformations

Xavier Ayrignac and Elisabeth Tournier-Lasserve

Introduction

Cerebral cavernous malformations (CCM/OMIM 116860) are vascular lesions histologically characterized by abnormally enlarged capillary cavities without intervening brain parenchyma. From large series based on necropsy and/or magnetic resonance imaging (MRI) studies, their prevalence in the general population has been estimated to be close to 0.1–0.5%. Most of them are located within the central nervous system but they sometimes affect either the retina or the skin [1].

CCMs occur both as a sporadic or familial condition. Sporadic cases showing a single lesion on cerebral MRI are not inherited and do not carry a germline mutation in CCM genes. The influence of genetics was first suspected by Kufs et al. in 1928 in a German family including a CCM patient whose 17-year-old daughter was strongly suspected to also have CCM when she presented with hemiparesis [2]. Several additional families including more than one affected member were thereafter published. However, very limited neuroradiological data were available until 1988 when Rigamonti et al. characterized the clinical and MRI features of familial CCM in a series of six large Hispanic-American families [3]. They emphasized the higher sensitivity and specificity of magnetic resonance imaging (MRI), as compared to CT scans, for the detection of CCM lesions, whose multiplicity is a hallmark of familial CCM. They also established the incomplete penetrance of this condition. In 1998, a clinical and MRI analysis of 57 consecutive, white, non-Hispanic-American probands with multiple lesions and their relatives showed that most, but not all, sporadic cases with multiple lesions have inherited their disease from one of their two asymptomatic parents and that genetic CCM is an evolutive condition as assessed by the strong correlation between patients' age and number of lesions (Ref. 4 and Fig. 4.1).

Three CCM genes have been mapped and identified in the last 10 years [5–12] (Fig. 4.2). These molecular genetics data dramatically increased our knowledge of this disease and have provided useful information for clinical care and genetic counseling. They were also an important step towards the understanding of the mechanisms of this disorder. This chapter will summarize the advances in CCM clinical and molecular genetics and the remaining gaps in this field.

Clinical genetics

Pattern of inheritance

The proportion of familial cases has been estimated as high as 50% in Hispanic-American CCM patients and close to 10–40% in Caucasian patients. However, no epidemiology-based study has been conducted so far and these numbers should be considered as estimations based on hospital-based recruitment of patients.

The CCM pattern of inheritance is autosomal dominant with an incomplete clinical and neuroradiological penetrance. The recent identification of CCM loci and genes allowed the identification of mutation carriers and helped to estimate the penetrance of this disorder. In a genetic linkage analysis conducted on 20 families Craig et al. estimated the clinical penetrance at 88% in CCM1 families, 100% in CCM2 and 63% in CCM3 families [6]. However, a recent analysis conducted in a series of 64 consecutive families showed a penetrance which was closer to 60% in CCM1 families [13]. Additional studies conducted on large series of CCM2 and CCM3 families are now needed to estimate precisely the penetrance in those families.

Many CCM patients who carry a mutation in one of the three CCM genes nevertheless present as sporadic cases, due to incomplete clinical penetrance.

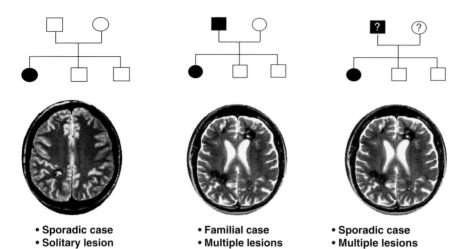

• Sporadic case
• Solitary lesion
• Non genetic

• Familial case
• Multiple lesions
• Genetic

• Sporadic case
• Multiple lesions
• Genetic in most likely all cases

Figure 4.1. Multiplicity of CCM lesions is a hallmark of the familial form of the disease. Left panel: a sporadic, non-genetic case with a unique lesion on cerebral MRI. Middle panel: a familial case with multiple lesions. Right panel: a sporadic case with multiple lesions which is most likely a genetic case due to either an incomplete clinical penetrance or a *de novo* mutation. See color plate section.

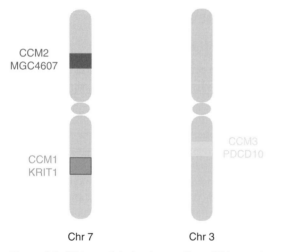

Figure 4.2. CCM genetic loci and genes. Three CCM genes have been mapped on chromosomes 7 (CCM1 and CCM2) and 3 (CCM3). The vast majority of CCM gene mutations are loss of function mutations. See color plate section.

Indeed, a clinical and neuroradiological analysis conducted prior to CCM gene identification in a series of 22 consecutive sporadic cases with multiple lesions showed that 75% of them were indeed affected with a hereditary form of the disease since one of their two asymptomatic parents showed lesions on MRI [4]. These patients are true familial genetic cases and their offspring have a 50% risk of inheriting the mutated gene.

What about the 25% remaining patients whose biological parents do not show CCM on brain MRI?

A proportion of these patients are most likely affected by a hereditary form of the disease since they were shown to carry a de novo mutation in one of the three CCM genes [14]. These patients are therefore also true genetic cases and their offspring also have a 50% risk of inheriting the mutated gene.

In some other sporadic cases with multiple lesions, screening of all three CCM genes does not detect any mutation (see below). However, the multiplicity of their lesions strongly suggests that a genetic form of the disease affects these patients and that their offspring are at risk of developing CCM lesions. Several hypotheses may be raised to explain the absence of any detected mutation, including a somatic mosaicism of a de novo mutation which occurred during gestation and is not detectable in DNA extracted from peripheral blood cells. This will be important to solve in the future since it is of interest for genetic counseling. Indeed, depending of the mosaicism ratio within the gonads of this patient, the risk for their offspring may be lower than 50%.

Altogether, these data strongly suggest that (i) the vast majority, if not all, sporadic cases with multiple lesions are true genetic cases; (ii) their offspring have a 50% risk of developing lesions; and (iii) they should be managed in the same way as familial cases.

Genetic counseling

Molecular screening of the three CCM genes is technically feasible in any routine genetics diagnostic laboratory. Sensitivity of genetic screening is above 98%

in probands having an affected relative and above 60% in sporadic cases with multiple lesions, providing that an extensive screening of all three CCM genes is conducted, looking for both point mutations and genomic rearrangements (Ref. 14 and unpublished data). Once the mutation has been identified in a proband, sensitivity is 100% when screening his/her relatives.

The main question for the clinician relates to the utility of this molecular screening in affected and/or at-risk individuals in clinical practice. Another question is that of the respective indications of MRI and genetic screening in asymptomatic individuals.

Genetic screening should carry a balanced benefit/risk ratio. This ratio varies depending on several factors including the clinical status of an individual and his/her age. Based on clinical, MRI and molecular genetic data, the following algorithm may be proposed to facilitate molecular screening decisions [15].

Sporadic case with a unique lesion on MRI

The risk of having a mutation is null or extremely low, providing that both T2-weighted and gradient-echo (GRE) MRI sequences have been performed. Genetic screening is not useful.

Symptomatic case with multiple CCM lesions and one or more affected relatives

The genetic nature of the disease is already known. Unless genetic counseling is envisioned, molecular genetic screening is not useful.

Symptomatic sporadic case with multiple CCM lesions

The genetic nature of the disease is most likely, but not proven. Genetic screening in those cases will identify a mutation in 60% of the cases. This information will not change the patient's clinical care but may be useful for genetic counseling. However, the patient has to be aware that a negative test does not exclude a genetic cause (see supra).

Asymptomatic individual with affected relatives

The first step will be to draw the genealogical tree of the family to check whether this individual is or is not at risk, depending on his/her link with the proband. In most cases, neurosurgeons recommend presymptomatic screening and, in positive asymptomatic adult individuals, MRI follow-up [16]. However, presymptomatic screening should always be envisioned with great caution since it is difficult at present to estimate the real benefit of presymptomatic screening. Parental

requests for screening an asymptomatic child should be managed even more cautiously since psychological issues are even more important than in adult asymptomatic individuals. Presymptomatic screening can be performed with cerebral MRI. Magnetic resonance imaging should include a gradient-echo (GRE) sequence to ensure a good sensitivity. Indeed, 18% of mutation carriers have only one lesion on T2-weighted MRI as compared to 6% when using GRE sequences [14]. However, a normal MRI (including normal GRE sequences) can be observed in around 3% of asymptomatic mutation carriers, as shown in a cross-sectional study. It will be interesting to know in future large series whether susceptibility weighting MR phase imaging (SWI) may decrease this false-negative proportion. Alternatively, molecular screening can be used as a first step for presymptomatic screening, providing that the mutation has been identified previously in a symptomatic member of the family; sensitivity would then be 100% with no false negative. If molecular screening is positive, MRI is recommended for follow-up.

The choice to use MRI or molecular screening depends on the availability of information on the mutation present in the family as well as practical local availability of genetic testing. With regard to ethical considerations, presymptomatic MRI screening should be considered as the equivalent of presymptomatic molecular screening.

Prenatal screening

Prenatal diagnosis requests are quite rare in CCM but may be encountered in families in which several patients have suffered severe symptoms. Prenatal diagnosis may be of benefit in such families. In all cases, all available information on the disease should be given to the parents before they make any final decision.

Genotype–phenotype correlations

The severity of CCM is highly variable from one patient to another. The outcome is not associated with the number of lesions, but rather with the location of lesions. The most severe lesions are those located within the brainstem or basal ganglia.

The identification of the three CCM genes provides a unique opportunity to analyze and compare clinical and MRI features of genetically homogeneous groups of CCM mutation carriers. A cross-sectional analysis of 163 consecutive families showed that the proportion of patients with a young age of onset (<15 years old) is

CCM1/Krit1

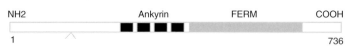

CCM2/Malcavernin

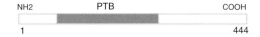

CCM3/pdcd10

Figure 4.3. The three CCM genes encode for three unrelated proteins, krit1 (CCM1) which contains several ankyrin domains and a FERM domain, CCM2, also called malcavernin, which contains a PTB (phosphotyrosine binding) domain, and CCM3/PCDCD10, a protein involved in apoptosis. See color plate section.

significantly higher in the CCM3 group (Ref. 14 and Fig. 4.2). CCM3 patients are also more prone than CCM1 and CCM2 patients to develop cerebral hemorrhages at a young age. The collection and analysis of larger series of CCM3 patients is needed to fully establish all clinical features of this group of CCM patients.

In addition to central nervous system lesions, some CCM patients show retinal and/or skin lesions. Retinal CCM has been observed in approximately 5% of CCM patients, and with all CCM genes [17]. With regard to cutaneous vascular malformations, 9% of CCM patients show either capillary malformations, hyperkeratotic cutaneous capillary venous malformations (HCCVM), and/or venous malformations [18]. CCM1 mutated patients may be affected by all the types of cutaneous vascular malformations; however, HCCVM has been shown to be associated only with CCM1/KRIT1 mutations [18–20]. Nodular venous malformations are encountered in both CCM1 and CCM3 mutants [18].

CCM molecular genetics

CCM gene germline mutations

Three CCM loci have been mapped to chromosome 7q (CCM1), 7p (CCM2), and 3q (CCM3) [5,6]. A strong founder effect has been observed in Hispanic-American CCM patients with most families linked to the CCM1 locus [7]. In Caucasian families, the proportions of families linked to each CCM locus were estimated to be 40% (CCM1), 20% (CCM2), and 40% (CCM3) [6]. The three genes located at these loci have now been identified [8–12].

The CCM1/KRIT1 gene contains 16 coding exons, which encode for Krit1, a 736 amino-acid protein containing three ankyrin and one FERM (F for 4.1 protein, E for Ezrin, R for radixin, and M for Moesin) domains (Fig. 4.3). CCM2, a 10 exon gene, encodes for the MGC4607 protein, also called malcavernin, which contains a phosphotyrosine binding (PTB) domain. CCM3 includes seven exons that encode for PDCD10 (Programmed Cell Death 10), a protein without any known conserved functional domain. Considerable progress has been made in the past 3 years in understanding the biochemical pathways in which those proteins might be involved (see Chapter 5).

Sequencing of all coding exons and exon–intron boundaries of the three CCM genes and searching for genomic rearrangements using either cDNA analysis and/or quantitative multiplex PCR such as MLPA (multiplex ligation-dependent probe amplification) or QMPSF (quantitative multiplex PCR of short fluorescent fragments) in Caucasian non-Hispanic-American CCM multiplex families led to the identification of the causative mutation in over 98% of familial CCM (Refs. 14, 21 and unpublished data). Approximately 72% of multiplex families harbored a mutation in CCM1, 18% in CCM2, and 10% in CCM3. The CCM3 proportion was much lower than expected based on previous linkage data that suggested 40% of CCM families were linked to the CCM3 locus.

The mutation detection rate is, however, much lower in sporadic cases with multiple lesions, ranging from 45% to 67% [14,21,22]. Several hypotheses may be raised to explain the absence of any detectable mutation in those patients, including a somatic mosaicism of a *de novo* mutation which occured during gestation and is not detectable in DNA extracted from peripheral blood cells, the existence of undetected regulatory mutations located far away from coding exons, epigenetic silencing events and/or additional yet unknown CCM genes. This will be important to solve in the future since it is of interest for genetic counseling of sporadic cases with multiple lesions.

With regard to sporadic CCM cases with a unique lesion on cerebral MRI, no mutation was detected in reported series [23,24]. The combination of these data with those obtained in familial CCM strongly suggests that clinically sporadic cases with a unique lesion on MRI of the brain that harbor a germline mutation are most likely very rare. Therefore, molecular screening is not indicated in these cases.

More than 150 distinct CCM1/CCM2/CCM3 germline mutations have been reported so far [8–12,21–31]. Those mutations were highly stereotyped. Almost all of them lead to a premature termination codon through different mechanisms including nonsense, splice-site, large deletions, and frameshift mutational events. These data strongly suggest that a loss of function through mRNA decay of the mutated allele is the most likely pathophysiological mechanism involved in CCM patients.

Fewer than 10 missense mutations have been reported so far in CCM genes. All of them except one actually activated cryptic splice sites and led to an aberrant splicing of CCM mRNA and a frameshift with a premature stop codon. The mutation L198R is the only known CCM missense mutation which does not affect splicing; it is located within the C-terminal part of the PTB domain of CCM2. It has been shown to abolish the interaction of CCM2 and CCM1, strongly suggesting its causality [13,33]. A total of four intragenic in-frame deletions have been reported of which two affect exons 17 and 18 of CCM1, one deleting exon 2 of CCM2, and the last one deleting exon 5 of CCM3. The last two deletions have been used to map potential relevant interaction domains of CCM2 and CCM3 [21, 34]. However, it is not known so far whether these putative truncated proteins were indeed produced and stable in vivo.

A founder effect was reported in the Hispano-American CCM population, based on microsatellite haplotyping data at the CCM1 locus; this was confirmed by the detection of a founder Q455X stop codon mutation in CCM1 in most families with this ethnic background [9]. Recurrent mutations have also been identified in a few additional populations [30,32,35]. However, in most cases despite their highly stereotyped consequences, germline CCM mutations are "private" mutations present in only one or very few families.

Biallelic somatic and germline mutations in CCM lesions

The autosomal dominant pattern of inheritance of CCM and the presence of multiple lesions in familial CCM, contrasting with the detection of a single lesion in non-hereditary cavernous angiomas, strongly suggested a "two-hit" hypothesis might be involved in CCM, as reported previously in other conditions such as retinoblastoma or other vascular malformations [36,37]. According to this hypothesis, the complete loss within an affected cell of the two alleles of a given CCM gene would lead to a CCM lesion. Loss of the first allele (first hit) would be the result of a germ line mutation and loss of the second allele (second hit) will occur somatically.

The highly heterogeneous nature of CCM lesions and the very limited number of endothelial cells lining the capillary cavities have rendered this hypothesis difficult to test. Direct sequencing of the DNA extracted from a heterogeneous lesion was initially used to screen CCM lesions from both sporadic and a few familial patients. This did not detect any somatic mutation except in one sporadic case [39]. In this latter case, two CCM1 missense mutations, F97S and K569E, were detected in the CCM lesion and were shown to be absent in the blood of the patient. However these data were difficult to interpret due to the nature of the mutations; they were not truncating mutations (a possible aberrant splicing effect of these two mutations was not investigated) and the biallelism of these mutations was not explored.

The first biallelic germ line and somatic mutations within a CCM lesion was reported by Gault *et al.* in 2005 in a CCM1 mutated patient. This work strongly supported the "two-hit" mechanism in the formation of lesions at least in CCM1 patients; this group demonstrated recently that the second hit occurred within the endothelial cells [40,41].

Biallelic somatic and germline mutations in each of the three CCM genes was recently reported by Akers *et al.* [42]. They were able to convincingly establish the presence of a biallelic somatic and germline deleterious mutation in two CCM1, one CCM2, and one CCM3 lesions from four unrelated patients. None of these mutations was detected through direct sequencing of lesions' DNA, emphasizing the lack of sensitivity of direct sequencing. These data established the existence of biallelic somatic and germline mutations, independent of the nature of the CCM gene involved. Using microdissection laser capture, they showed that the somatic mutation occurred in endothelial cells and not in the intervening neural tissue. The proportion of endothelial cells that harbor the somatic mutation was estimated in one lesion and shown to be close to 30%. This suggests the presence of mosaicism in the somatic mutation. These data are in agreement with a recent immunohistochemistry-based approach [43]. This question would need, however, additional investigation. It would also be important to analyze several lesions from a given patient to test for the presence of the same mutation in multiple lesions. A unique somatic mutation has indeed been detected in multifocal lesions in another hereditary vascular condition, suggesting a common origin for abnormal endothelial cells lying in distant sites [38].

Altogether these data strongly suggest that CCM shows predominant inheritance like several other hereditary vascular conditions. It remains to be determined when and in which endothelial cell compartments second-hit somatic events occur.

Are there additional CCM genes?

Previous linkage data suggested that the three CCM loci on 7p, 7q, and 3q would most likely account for all CCM families [6]. However, despite extensive screening of exonic sequences for point mutations and deletions, no mutation is detected in 2–5% of familial CCM cases and in around 20% of sporadic cases with multiple lesions. In addition, the proportion of families showing a mutation within CCM3/PDCD10 (10%) at the CCM3 locus on chromosome 3q25 is much lower than expected based on linkage data (40%).

The mosaicism of *de novo* mutations might likely be involved in sporadic cases with multiple lesions. Epigenetic silencing of these three genes might also be involved. Cis-regulatory mutations located far away from CCM coding sequences may explain both the very small proportion of non-mutated familial cases or sporadic cases with multiple lesions. However, the existence of additional non-identified CCM genes, one of which being possibly located close to PDCD10, cannot be excluded at this point.

Recently an additional gene, ZPLD1 (zona pellucida-like domain containing 1), has been reported to be disrupted in a CCM patient harbouring a balanced translocation between chromosome X and chromosome 3q, centromeric to CCM3/PDCD10 [44]. The expression of ZPLD1 mRNA in lymphoblastoid cell lines of the patient was shown to be significantly decreased, suggesting that the interruption of this gene may be causal. However, none of the 20 additional CCM patients (without any mutation in CCM1/CCM2/CCM3) screened by the same group showed either a point mutation or a deletion within this gene. These data suggest that either this gene is involved in a very small proportion of CCM patients or its interruption does not cause CCM but that the translocation present in this patient deregulated the expression of a gene that is still unidentified.

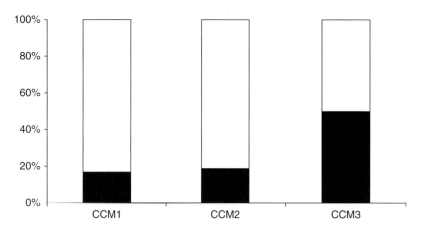

Figure 4.4. CCM3 patients are at higher risk of having a cerebral hemorrhage at a young age. In more than 50% of CCM3 patients the initial clinical manifestation is a cerebral hemorrhage [14].

The tremendous progress in sequencing technologies should help to resolve this question in the very near future [45].

Conclusions and future

Since the identification of the first family with several affected members, tremendous progress has been made in the characterization of this condition, mainly thanks to the use of the MRI tool and the identification of CCM genes, which with the use of molecular tools allows for the identification of mutation carriers. The combined use of both tools helped us to clarify several features of this condition, including its incomplete clinical and MRI penetrance as well as the molecular basis of sporadic cases with multiple lesions. Genetic counseling is now possible.

Several additional questions, however, have to be addressed. What is the molecular basis in familial CCM cases in which no mutation of the three known CCM genes has been detected? Are sporadic CCM patients with multiple lesions examples of mosaicism for a germline mutation? Are there modifying genes that may explain the intra-familial clinical variability? The ongoing progress of genotyping and sequencing will most likely help us solve these questions in the immediate future.

In addition to these questions, one main challenge is to understand the pathophysiological mechanisms of this condition. The recent identification of several of the biochemical pathways involving CCM proteins as well as the analysis of several fish and mouse CCM animal models have already provided a number of clues to this goal. These data as well as the availability of animal models mimicking this disease will be of major help for the development of new approaches to cure the most severe forms of this disease in the next 10 years.

References

1. Russell, D. S. & Rubinstein, L. J. *Pathology of the Tumors of the Central Nervous System*, 5th edn (Baltimore: Williams and Wilkins, 1989), pp. 730–736.

2. Kufs H. Uber heredofamiliare Angiomatose des Gehirns und der Retina, ihre Beziehungen zueinander und zur Angiomatose der Haut. *Z Gesamte Neurol Psychiatr* 1928;**113**:651–686.

3. Rigamonti, D., Drayer, B. P., Johnson, P. C., *et al.* Cerebral cavernous malformations. Incidence and familial occurence. *New Engl J Med* 1988;**319**:343–347.

4. Labauge, P., Laberge, S., Brunereau, L., Lévy, C. & Tournier-Lasserve, E. Hereditary cerebral cavernous angiomas: clinical and genetic features in 57 French families. *Lancet* 1998;**352**:1892–1897.

5. Dubovsky, J., Zabramski, J. M., Kurth, J., *et al.* A gene responsible for cavernous malformations of the brain maps to chromosome 7q. *Hum Mol Genet* 1995;**4**:453–458.

6. Craig, H. D., Günel, M., Cepeda, O., Johnson, E. W., *et al.* Multilocus linkage identifies two new loci for a Mendelian form of stroke, cerebral cavernous malformation, at 7p15–13 and 3q25.2–27. *Hum Mol Genet* 1998;**7**:1851–1855.

7. Günel, M., Awad, I. A., Finberg, K., *et al.* A founder mutation as a cause of cerebral cavernous malformation in Hispanic Americans. *New Engl J Med* 1996;**334**:946–951.

8. Laberge-le Couteulx, S., Jung, H. H., Labauge, P., *et al.* Mutations in CCM1, encoding KRIT1, cause hereditary cavernous angiomas. *Nat Genet* 1999;**23**:189–193.

9. Sahoo, T., Johnson, E. W., Thomas, J. W., *et al.* Mutations in the gene encoding KRIT1, a Krev-1/rap1a binding protein, cause cerebral cavernous malformations (CCM1). *Hum Mol Genet* 1999;**8**:2325–2333.

10. Liquori, C. L., Berg, M. J., Siegel, A. M., *et al.* Mutations in a gene encoding a novel protein containing a phosphotyrosine-binding domain cause type 2 cerebral cavernous malformations. *Am J Hum Genet* 2003;**73**:1459–1464.

11. Denier, C., Goutagny, S., Labauge, P., *et al.* Mutations within the MGC4607 gene cause cerebral cavernous malformations. *Am J Hum Genet* 2004;**74**:326–337.

12. Bergametti, F., Denier, C., Labauge, P., *et al.* Mutations within the programmed cell death 10 gene cause cerebral cavernous malformations. *Am J Hum Genet* 2005;**76**:42–51.

13. Denier, C., Labauge, P., Brunereau, L., *et al.* Clinical features of cerebral cavernous malformations patients with KRIT1 mutations. *Ann Neurol* 2004;**55**:213–220.

14. Denier, C., Labauge, P., Bergametti, F., *et al.* Genotype-phenotype correlations in cerebral cavernous malformations patients. *Ann Neurol* 2006;**60**:550–556.

15. Labauge, P., Denier, C., Bergametti, F. & Tournier-Lasserve, E. Genetics of cavernous angiomas. *Lancet Neurol* 2007;**6**:237–244.

16. Raychaudhuri, R., Batjer, B. A. & Awad, I. Intracranial cavernous angioma: a practical review of clinical and biological aspects. *Surg Neurol* 2005;**63**:319–328.

17. Labauge, P., Krivosic, V., Denier, C., Tournier-Lasserve, E. & Gaudric, A. Frequency of retinal cavernomas in 60 patients with familial cerebral cavernomas: a clinical and genetic study. *Arch Ophthalmol* 2006;**124**:885–886.

18. Sirvente, J., Enjolras, O., Wassef, M., Tournier-Lasserve, E. & Labaug, P. Frequency and phenotypes of cutaneous vascular malformations in a consecutive series of 417 patients with familial cerebral cavernous malformations. *J Eur Acad Dermatol Venereol* 2009;**23**:1066–1072.

19. Labauge, P., Enjolras, O., Bonerandi, J. J., *et al.* An association between autosomal dominant cerebral cavernomas and a distinctive hyperkeratotic cutaneous vascular malformation in 4 families. *Ann Neurol* 1999;**45**:250–254.

20. Eerola, I., Plate, K. H., Spiegel, R., *et al.* KRIT1 is mutated in hyperkeratotic cutaneous capillary-venous malformation associated with cerebral capillary malformation. *Hum Mol Genet* 2000;**9**:1351–1355.

21. Stahl, S., Gaetzner, S., Voss, K., *et al.* Novel CCM1, CCM2, and CCM3 mutations in patients with cerebral cavernous malformations: in-frame deletion in CCM2 prevents formation of a CCM1/CCM2/CCM3 protein complex. *Hum Mutat* 2008;**29**:709–717.

22. Liquori, C. L., Penco, S., Gault, J., *et al.* Different spectra of genomic deletions within the CCM genes between Italian and American CCM patient cohorts. *Neurogenetics* 2008;**9**:25–31.

23. Verlaan, D. J., Laurent, S. B., Sure, U., *et al.* CCM1 mutation screen of sporadic cases with cerebral cavernous malformations. *Neurology* 2004;**62**:1213–1215.

24. Verlaan, D. J., Laurent, S. B., Rouleau, G. A. & Siegel, A. M. No CCM2 mutations in a cohort of 31 sporadic cases. *Neurology* 2004;**63**:1979.

25. Cavé-Riant, F., Denier, C., Labauge, P., *et al.* Spectrum and expression analysis of KRIT1 mutations in 121 consecutive and unrelated patients with cerebral cavernous malformations. *Eur J Hum Genet* 2002;**10**:733–740.

26. Laurans, M. S., DiLuna, M. L., Shin, D., *et al.* Mutational analysis of 206 families with cavernous malformations. *J Neurosurg* 2003;**99**:38–43.

27. Liquori, C. L., Berg, M. J., Squitieri, F., *et al.* Low frequency of PDCD10 mutations in a panel of CCM3 probands: potential for a fourth CCM locus. *Hum Mutat* 2006;**27**:118.

28. Verlaan, D. J., Roussel, J., Laurent, S. B., *et al.* CCM3 mutations are uncommon in cerebral cavernous malformations. *Neurology* 2005;**65**:1982–1983.

29. Guclu, B., Ozturk, A. K., Pricola, K. L., *et al.* Mutations in apoptosis-related gene, PDCD10, cause cerebral cavernous malformation 3. *Neurosurgery* 2005;**57**:1008–1013.

30. Liquori, C. L., Berg, M. J., Squitieri, F., *et al.* Deletions in CCM2 are a common cause of cerebral cavernous malformations. *Am J Hum Genet* 2007;**80**:69–75.

31. Verlaan, D. J., Siegel, A. M., Rouleau, G. A. Krit1 missense mutations lead to splicing errors in cerebral cavernous malformations. *Am J Hum Genet* 2002;**70**:1564–1567.

32. Ortiz, L., Costa, A. F., Bellido, M. L., *et al.* Study of cerebral cavernous malformation in Spain and Portugal: high prevalence of a 14 bp deletion in exon 5 of MGC4607 (CCM2 gene). *J Neurol* 2007;**254**:322–326.

33. Zawistowski, J. S., Stalheim, L., Uhlik, M. T., *et al.* CCM1 and CCM2 protein interactions in cell signaling: implications for cerebral cavernous malformations pathogenesis. *Hum Mol Genet* 2005;**14**:2521–2531.

34. Voss, K., Stahl, S., Hogan, B. M., *et al.* Functional analyses of human and zebrafish 18-amino acid in-frame deletion pave the way for domain mapping of the cerebral cavernous malformation 3 protein. *Hum Mutat* 2009;**30**:1003–1011.

35. Cau, M., Loi, M., Melis, M., *et al.* C329X in KRIT1 is a founder mutation among CCM patients in Sardinia. *Eur J Med Genet* 2009;**52**:344–348.

36. Knudson, A. G. Mutation and cancer: statistical analysis of retinoblastoma. *Proc Natl Acad Sci USA* 1971;**68**:820–823.

37. Limaye, N., Boon, L. M. & Vikkula, M. From germline towards somatic mutations in the pathophysiology of vascular anomalies. *Hum Mol Genet* 2009;**18**(R1):R65–74.

38. Limaye, N., Wouters, V., Uebelhoer, M., *et al.* Somatic mutations in angiopoietin receptor gene TEK cause solitary and multiple sporadic venous malformations. *Nat Genet* 2009;**41**:118–124.

39. Kehrer-Sawatzki, H., *et al.* Mutation and expression analysis of the KRIT1 gene associated with cerebral cavernous malformations. *Acta Neuropathol* 2002;**104**:231–240.

40. Gault, J., Shenkar, R., Recksiek, P. & Awad, I. A. Biallelic somatic and germ line CCM1 truncating mutations in a cerebral cavernous malformation lesion. *Stroke* 2005;**36**:872–874.

41. Gault, J., Awad, I. A., Recksiek, P., *et al.* Cerebral cavernous malformations: somatic mutations in vascular endothelial cells. *Neurosurgery* 2009;**65**:138–144; discussion 144–145.

42. Akers, A. L., Johnson, E., Steinberg, G. K., Zabramski, J. M. & Marchuk, D. A. Biallelic somatic and germline mutations in cerebral cavernous malformations (CCMs): evidence for a two-hit mechanism of CCM pathogenesis. *Hum Mol Genet* 2009;**18**:919–930.

43. Pagenstecher, A., Stahl, S., Sure, U. & Felbor, U. A two-hit mechanism causes cerebral cavernous malformations: complete inactivation of CCM1, CCM2 or CCM3 in affected endothelial cells. *Hum Mol Genet* 2009;**18**:911–918.

44. Gianfrancesco, F., Esposito, T., Penco, S., *et al.* ZPLD1 gene is disrupted in a patient with balanced translocation that exhibits cerebral cavernous malformations. *Neuroscience* 2008;**155**:345–349.

45. Biesecker, L. G. Exome sequencing makes medical genomics a reality. *Nat Genet* 2010;**42**:13–14.

Molecular biology of cerebral cavernous malformation

Jun Zhang

Hereditary CCMs have been found to be caused by a loss-of-function mutation in one of three CCM genes: KRIT1 (CCM1), MGC4607 (malcavernin, CCM2), and PDCD10 (CCM3). Mutations seen with KRIT1 in pedigrees with CCM1 were the first to be found [1–4]. Subsequently, MGC4607, a phosphotyrosine-binding protein, was identified linked to the CCM2 locus [5], and mutations in PDCD10, an apoptotic protein, was identified in cases linked to the CCM3 locus [6]. Current genetic data suggest that mutation within any of three defined CCM genes is required for the initiation and progression of cerebral cavernous malformations [7].

The interlaced CCM complex anchors the endothelial cell performance

Interaction among three CCM genes to form a CCM complex

To date, researchers have established that all three CCM genes interact with each other and form a CCM complex [8–11]. While the precise pathophysiology connecting the CCM protein complex to microvascular malformation remains elusive, the complex's critical importance is evidenced by the observation that at least one of three CCM genes is disrupted in most human CCMs. Expression studies demonstrated that three CCM proteins significantly parallel the expression pattern in the various neuronal cell layers of the brain at several time points during development, thereby recognizing a role for these CCM proteins during the angiogenesis process and suggesting their possible coordinated involvement in the same cellular signal pathway that is important for neurovascular development [12,13].

Through our yeast-two hybrid experiments, among all the krit1-interacting positive colonies, we found that MGC4607 is second numerically behind icap1α [14]. We have defined that MGC4607 indeed binds to krit1 via two (2nd or 3rd) NPXY motifs in the middle of krit1 compared to the first NPXY motif of the N-terminal krit1 binding to icap1α [15]. MGC4607 has been predicted to be a PTB protein [5]. Although mutational studies have demonstrated that each of two NPXY motifs is sufficient for MGC4607 binding, two NPXY motifs would significantly enhance the interaction. The redundancy of the NPXY motif might illustrate the physiological importance of this interaction [11,14]. The interaction between MGC4607 and PDCD10 was also defined through affinity pull-down with mass spectrometry, yeast two-hybrid analysis and co-immunoprecipation experiments [9,10].

Each of CCM genes interacts with their respective cellular partners

Partial truncated CCM1 gene was originally identified through its interaction with the Ras-family GTPase krev1/rap1a in a two-hybrid screen as krit1 (Krev Interaction Trapped 1), inferring a potential role in GTPase signaling cascades [16]. Surprisingly, by two-hybrid analysis and co-immunoprecipation, we demonstrated that full-length krit1 fails to interact with rap1a but shows strong interaction with integrin cytoplasmic domain-associated protein-1α (icap1α) [15,17]. Icap1α binds to a NPXY motif in the cytoplasmic domain of β1 integrin [18,19]. The NPXY motif is a well-known binding substrate for phosphotyrosine binding domain (PTB) proteins, and icap1α has been proven to be a PTB protein [20]. We have shown that, like the cytoplasmic C-terminal region of β1 integrin, the N-terminus of krit1 contains a conserved and functionally important NPXY motif that plays a crucial role in the interaction with icap1α. Mutational

Cavernous Malformations of the Nervous System, ed. Daniele Rigamonti. Published by Cambridge University Press.
© Cambridge University Press 2011.

studies demonstrated that the Asn and Tyr residues of the NPXY motif are critical for icap1α binding. Also, like the β1 integrin cytoplasmic domain, krit1 only interacts with icap1α (a full-length 200 amino acid protein) but not with icap1β, a shorter alternatively spliced (internally truncated) isoform protein of 150 amino acids with much less cellular abundance [15]. Interestingly, full-length krit1 was further reported to interact with rap1a through its FERM domain [21]. Another report indicated that full-length krit1 prefers to interact with rap1a-GTP, an active form of rap1a small GTPase. However, the same paper also found that krit1 interacts with tubulin as well [22], which is another controversial interaction for krit1. Krit1 was primarily reported to interact with tubulin [23]. However, the antibody used for krit1 recognized a protein of the same size as tubulin; furthermore, the krit1 construct was a truncated form, making this interaction spurious [22,8]. Clearly further investigation is needed to address these questions. Recently, krit1 has also been reported to interact with sorting nexin, SNX17, further indicating its extremely important role in β1 integrin signaling [24].

MGC4607 was reported to interact with cellular factors, Rac, Mekk3, and Mkk3 directly [9,25,26]. Interestingly, both icap1α and tubulin were also pulled-down through affinity capture–mass spectrometry experiments using MGC4607 as bait [9,26]. However, this pull-down is highly likely through their directly binding to krit1, and then a krit1–MGC4607 interaction. Cellular factors EF1A1 and RIN2 were also pulled-down in this affinity capture–mass spectrometry experiment. Further experimental data are certainly needed to confirm whether they directly interact with MGC4607 or not.

Currently, PDCD10 has been found to interact with the most cellular factors. PDCD10 was found to interact with Ste20-related kinase MST4, its relative members of the germinal center kinase III family, STK25 and STK24, and FAP1 through yeast two-hybrid analysis followed by co-immunoprecipitation [10,27] and affinity pull-down with mass spectrometry assay [28–30]. By analyzing a large multiprotein assembly, termed the striatin-interacting phosphatase and kinase (STRIPAK) complex, a large group of cellular factors potentially interacting with PDCD10 were identified. These factors include the cytoskeletal protein cortactin interacting proteins, CTTNBP2 and CTTNBP2NL (CTTNBP2 N-terminal like), the sarcolemmal membrane-associated protein, SLMAP, and

its related coiled-coil proteins suppressor, SIKE and FGFR1OP2; serine/threonine protein phosphatase subunits, PPP2CA, PPP2R1A, and PPP2R1B, the striatins, STRN, STRN3, and STRN4, striatins associated protein MOB3, and two novel proteins STRIP1 and STRIP2 [29,30]. However, whether any of them directly binds to PDCD10 or simply to the CCM complex remains to be determined.

The interlaced interaction among CCM proteins and their cellular partners is illustrated in Fig. 5.1.

Current understanding of cellular functions of CCM genes

Molecular biology of krit1

Among the three CCM genes, the 84 kDa full-length CCM1 protein was the first identified and is the most studied. The originally identified krit1 (Krev Interaction Trapped 1) gene was a partial clone [30]. During the cloning of the murine krit1 cDNA, we identified previously missed 5′ coding exons that extend the amino terminus by 207 amino acids [4]. Subsequent studies revealed that these exons are also utilized in other vertebrates including humans [31,32]. This novel N-terminal extension contains an NPXY motif that is used to interact with icap1α and a putative nuclear localization signal sequence (NLS) [4]. Two additional NPXY motifs were found in the center of krit1, which is used to interact with MGC4607 [11,14,24,33]. Multiple ankyrin repeats are also found in the center of krit1. Such domains can be seen in actin-associated proteins and suggest interaction with the cytoskeleton. In its C-terminus, krit1 contains a putative nuclear export signal sequence (NES) and a FERM domain that is often seen in proteins associated with the cytoplasmic aspect of the cell membrane. Such motifs might be predicted in a protein found in a focal adhesion plaque formed by the clustering of integrins on the intracellular surface (Fig. 5.2).

Krit1-mediated integrin β1 signaling in in vitro endothelial cell models

To further evaluate whether integrin β1 and krit1 bind to the same site in icap1α, and perhaps compete for this binding site, we determined whether induced expression of krit1 could diminish the interaction between icap1α and integrin β1 in a yeast cell system. After induced expression of krit1 using a methionine-responsive promoter, we observed decreased expression of β-galactosidase, an indirect measure of the

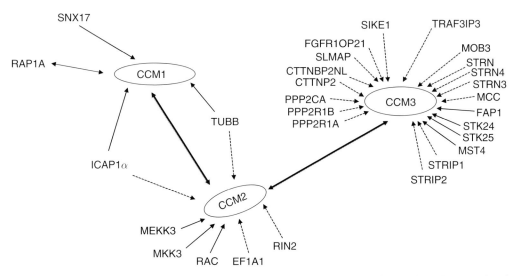

Figure 5.1. CCM interacting complex. The schematic diagram summarizes the proposed networks and CCM interlaced complex formed by three CCM genes based on our current knowledge. Solid arrow lines indicate the confirmed gene-specific interactions. Dashed arrow lines indicate potential interactions based on the affinity pull-down/MS analysis; however, further experiments are needed to confirm whether the detected interaction is direct or not.

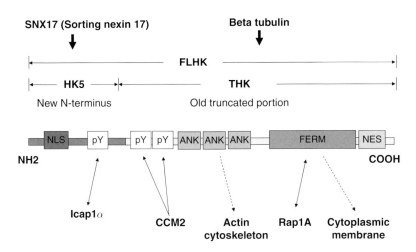

Figure 5.2. The domains and their functions of the CCM1 gene. The schematic diagram summarizes the domains and functions of full-length krit1 based on our current knowledge. Solid arrow lines indicate the confirmed interactions with a specific domain. Dashed arrow lines indicate proposed interactions based on the domain's well-known functions. Arrowheads indicate the confirmed interactions with an undefined binding site. See color plate section.

extent of interaction between icap1α and β1 integrin. These data suggested that sequestering icap1α by krit1 might normally downregulate β1 integrin-mediated signaling. In this view, a decrease in krit1 (as occurs in CCMs) would allow excessive icap1α-mediated signaling, resulting in altered angiogenesis [15].

Interestingly, we further found that icap1α protein is dramatically decreased after siRNA-mediated silencing of krit1 expression in mammalian cells; however, no decrease was found in icap1α mRNA levels. Likewise, similar phenomena were also observed in MGC4607 upon depletion of krit1. These data suggest

that krit1 could stabilize both icap1α and MGC4607, and thus modulate regulation of β1-integrin-mediated signal transduction through its interaction with them from different domains [34].

Our in vitro data demonstrate that depleting either krit1 or icap1α significantly inhibits endothelial cell proliferation, following our results that depletion of krit1 significantly decreases endothelial cell number [34]. We then assessed the function of MAP kinase signaling cascades that influence cell proliferation and are known to be regulated by β1 integrin [35]. Three major MAP kinase pathways were further examined.

We found that depletion of either krit1 or icap1α inhibits phosphorylation of factors along the ERK-MAP kinase pathway but not along the JNK kinase and p38 MAP kinase pathways. Therefore, it is posited that β1-integrin regulates the ERK-MAP kinase pathway via focal adhesion kinase (FAK), with subsequent regulation of the downstream RAF, MEK1, and ERK kinases [34].

To further understand the cellular mechanism underlying the concordant effects of krit1 and icap1α depletion on the ERK-MAP kinase pathway, we studied the subcellular localization of both proteins, and found that krit1 distributes in both the cytoplasm and nucleus, although it is predominantly expressed in the cytoplasm. This result is consistent with our previous finding of a strong putative nuclear localization signal in the N-terminus of krit1. By comparison, we found that icap1α is highly concentrated in the nucleus, but distributed in the cytoplasm as well. We then showed that both krit1 and icap1α further accumulate in the nucleus upon treatment with leptomycin B, a specific inhibitor of Crm1-mediated nuclear export. These data document that despite discordant predominant localization at steady state, both proteins shuttle between the nucleus and the cytoplasm [34].

A decrease in cell number could be the result of decreased cell proliferation, increased cell death, or a combination of both [34]. We further demonstrated that depletion of krit1 significantly inhibits endothelial survival, resulting in significantly increased apoptosis in endothelial cells. Since integrin-linked kinase is a major regulator of cell survival in β1 integrin signaling, the phosphorylation status of ILK was next examined, and found to be dramatically decreased upon depletion of either krit1 or icap1α. β1-Integrin regulates the AKT1-BAD signaling pathway via ILK. We further demonstrated that depletion of either krit1 or icap1α inhibits phosphorylation in the AKT1-BAD cascade. Dephosphorylation of pBAD initiates activation of caspases and cleavage of PARP, which leads to cell apoptosis [14].

Next, our cell invasion assay revealed that silencing of krit1 significantly impairs cell motility [14]. This finding associates with decreased steady state abundance of Rac1-GTP, a known positive regulator of cell motility [36,37].

In summary, krit1 modulates endothelial cell performance through its regulation of β1-integrin signaling pathways, in which β1-integrin regulates endothelial cell

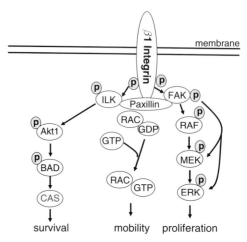

Figure 5.3. Schematic summary of the krit1-mediated β1-integrin signaling through the multiple interactions of its cytoplasmic domain, at the site of the docking protein paxillin, with focal adhesion kinase (FAK), which ultimately regulates ERK kinase activity in the MAP kinase cascade, Rac1 GTPase, and integrin linked kinase (ILK), which regulates the AKT1-mediated survival signal pathway.

proliferation through the FAK-ERK-MAP kinase signaling pathway, cell survival via the ILK-AKT1-BAD signaling pathway, and cell motility through the Rac1-GTP pathway (Fig. 5.3).

Our initial hypothesis that krit1 functions as a sponge for icap1α was based on the knowledge that the cytoplasmic tails of β1-integrin and krit1 compete for binding of icap1α through their common NPXY motifs. In this model, depletion of krit1 would lead to excess icap1α in the cytoplasm available to interact with β1-integrin, and enhanced β1-integrin signaling. This model suggests that depletion of icap1α or krit1 should have discordant effects on β1-integrin signaling, specifically a relative abrogation and accentuation, respectively [15]. Contrary to prediction, however, our in vitro RNAi experiments demonstrate apparent cooperation between krit1 and icap1α. Depletion of either leads to decreased β1-integrin signal transduction. Given this new information, the observed patterns of subcellular localization for krit1 and icap1α might have significant biological implications. Several previous reports documented icap1α's localization to the cell membrane and emphasized its membrane-associated functions [38,39]. And one report further suggested that icap1α is primarily localized in the nucleus [39]. We also found clear evidence of nuclear localization [34,40]. More significantly, our data suggest that krit1 may cargo icap1α in or out of the nucleus and target the protein to the cell membrane,

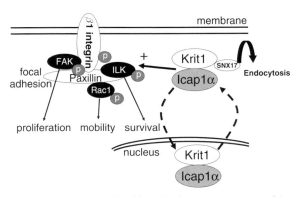

Figure 5.4. Current model of krit1 shuttling icap1a in or out of the nucleus and mediating recruitment of icap1a to focal adhesions is strongly supported by the concordant effects of krit1 and icap1a depletion on β1-integrin-mediated signaling events. Recruitment of excessive krit1 by SNX17 to endocytosis indicates the precise cellular regulatory mechanism of krit1 abundance around focal adhesions and the essential role of krit1 in the regulation of β1-integrin-mediated signaling events.

thus titrating icap1α's regulation of β1-integrin (Fig. 5.4). This model is in keeping with the apparent complementary effect suggested by our RNAi experiments. Our new model invokes krit1-mediated compartmentalization of icap1α in the regulated homeostasis of focal adhesions and in the maintenance of β1-integrin signaling (Fig. 5.4). Our finding that depletion of either krit1 or icap1α decreases β1 integrin signaling is most consistent with krit1-mediated recruitment of icap1α to focal adhesions. In this view, CCM manifests a relative failure of recruitment of certain signal regulatory proteins (such as icap1α) with a consequent reduction in β1-integrin-mediated events (Fig. 5.4) [7].

Following our hypothesis, we found that krit1-independent targeting of icap1 to the cell membrane through myristylation greatly enhances multiple β1-integrin signaling cascades [40]. Furthermore, following cellular fractionation, icap1α can be detected in both the cytoplasm and nucleus. Krit1 depletion leads to a decrease in icap1α levels in the cytoplasm and, surprisingly, no icap1α can be detected in the nuclear fraction [34]. This suggests that icap1α is stabilized by krit1 and may be dependent on it for nuclear shuttling. Confocal immunohistochemistry confirmed both a reduction in the abundance and nuclear localization of icap1α upon depletion of krit1 [34]. Another report demonstrated that kri1, a nematode ortholog of krit1, promotes the nuclear localization of the transcription factor in the intestine (DAF-16) in response to the lipophilic hormone signaling [41].

Participation of krit1 in endothelial cell junction in in vitro endothelial cell models

Krit1 was also found to be colocalized and physically associated with endothelial cell junctional proteins through its FERM domain. Furthermore, the interaction between krit1 junctional proteins is regulated by rap1 [22]. This study also reported that rap1 increases KRIT-1 targeting to endothelial cell–cell junctions where it suppresses stress fibers and stabilizes junctional integrity [22]. Our in vitro data on human endothelial cell experiments also showed that the adherent junction of cultured endothelial cells is perturbed upon depletion of krit1 [40].

Molecular biology of MGC4607

MGC4607 modulates endothelial cell performance via regulating p38 MAPK kinase activation

MGC4607 has been found to organize a complex consisting of the small GTPase Rac, MEKK3, and MKK3 for the activation of p38MAPK. Depletion of MGC4607 completely abrogates sorbitol-induced p38 activation, indicating the importance of MGC4607 for the activation of p38 [26]. The protein p38 is well known for its critical role in gene transcription regulation and post-translational modification of cytoskeletal remodeling proteins [9,25,26]. Therefore, MGC4607 plays a pivotal role in endothelial cell performance through modulating gene transcription and post-translational modification upon interpreting the signals supplied from its upstream targets.

MGC4607 plays a crucial role for differentiation and survival of neuronal cells

It has also been reported that MGC4607 is a key mediator of TrkA-dependent cell death in pediatric neuroblastic tumors [42]. In this study, both the PTB and Karet domains of MGC4607 were found to be required for TrkA-dependent cell death, such that the PTB domain determines the binding specificity, and the Karet domain leads to death signal pathways [42]. TrkA receptors are well known for promoting neuronal cell survival. However, in some neuroblastic tumors, TrkA activation can instead induce apoptosis [43]. Downregulation of MGC4607 in neuroblastoma cells attenuates TrkA-dependent death [42], suggesting that MGC4607 is a distinctive type of tumor suppressor that modulates tyrosine kinase signaling [43]. These data demonstrate that MGC4607 might play an alternative role in different cell types.

Molecular biology of PDCD10

Among the three CCM genes, the molecular property and cellular function of 25 kDa PDCD10 protein is the smallest and the least defined. PDCD10 was originally identified through an induced apoptosis in a premyeloid cell line [18]. Immunohistochemical data showed that PDCD10 protein was expressed in the neurovascular unit. However, its expression is weak in venous structures within cortical, subcortical, and brainstem tissue. In the vasculature, PDCD10 protein is strongly expressed in arterial endothelium but weakly or not at all in venous endothelium of extracerebral tissue [44].

PDCD10 is involved in cell survival signaling

PDCD10 is initially identified from the apoptotic premyeloid cells, indicating its potential role in apoptosis [18]. In in vitro cell culture systems, PDCD10 was reported to induce apoptosis through p38 – caspase3 apoptotic signaling [45]. However, a more detailed description of the molecular and cellular signaling pathways for PDCD10-mediated apoptosis is needed to better understand its mechanism in cellular function.

PDCD10 is involved in cell proliferation signaling

PDCD10 was found to bind MST4 [27], a Ste20-related kinase that has been proved to mediate cell growth and transformation via modulating the ERK pathway [46]. Therefore, the current data strongly suggest that, like krit1, PDCD10 might modulate the endothelial cell performance and toward angiogenesis through its involvement in the regulation of both cell proliferation and cell survival.

PDCD10 is the downstream target in unspecified cellular signaling

It has been reported that PDCD10 directly binds to serine/threonine kinase 24 and 25 respectively (STK24 and STK25), but PDCD10 can only be phosphorylated by STK25. PDCD10 also interacts with the phosphatase domain of Fas-associated phosphatase-1, FAP-1, and is dephosphorylated by the C-terminal catalytic domain of FAP-1 [10]. Apparently, the upstream cellular factors modulate the activity of PDCD10 through the mechanism of phosphorylation/dephosphorylation by STK25 and FAP1. Whether this phosphorylation/dephosphorylation of PDCD10 in its signaling pathway is associated with the regulation of either cell survival or cell proliferation is still unknown. Therefore, the signal pathways upon PDCD10 activation and inactivation

via phosphorylation/dephosphorylation need to be further explored.

Animal CCM models unveil more functional role for CCM genes

Recently more attention has been directed toward the roles played by the CCM complex in vasculogenesis or angiogenesis in animal models.

The molecular and developmental roles of Ccm1 and Ccm2 in the animal model

In contrast to humans, major cardiovascular defects have been implicated in animal models with Ccm1 and Ccm2 mutations [47–49]. Enlarged heart chambers and major blood vessel changes were described in Ccm1 (*santa, san*) and Ccm2 (*valentine, vtn*) mutant zebrafish lines, respectively [47–50]. It has been postulated that both Ccm1 and Ccm2 regulate the concentric growth of myocardium without changing the fate of cardiomyocyte or endothelial cells [49]. In mice, Ccm1 knockouts were reported to induce dilatation of heart chambers and large arteries (aorta) and to preferentially narrow certain arteries, leading to the hypothesis that Ccm1 is essential for vasculogenesis – the *de novo* formation of the blood vessel backbone. Associated heart defects were presumed secondary to vascular malformation [51]. Two studies in zebrafish embryos posited that Ccm1 and Ccm2 mutations cause the dilatation of major vessels (especially primitive veins) and the progressive thinning of endothelial cells lining these primitive vessels [50,52]. While one of the two studies reported significantly increased endothelial cells in the primitive vessels of Ccm1 mutants [52], the other emphasized that the endothelial cell number or contacts in these primitive vessels remained constant [50]. Nevertheless, both studies agreed that Ccm1 proteins regulate the genesis of vascular endothelial cells, particularly vascular tubular formation during vasculogenesis, further supporting the perturbed vasculogenesis hypothesis found in mouse models [50–52]. Two recent studies in mouse and zebrafish emphasized defective endothelial association and barrier function, or excessive dysfunctional sprouting which leads to vessel enlargement in the primitive vessels of Ccm2 mutants [53,54]. How these observations relate to the human condition remains to be answered [7].

Our in vitro cellular data show that induced loss of krit1 expression initiates down-regulation of β1-

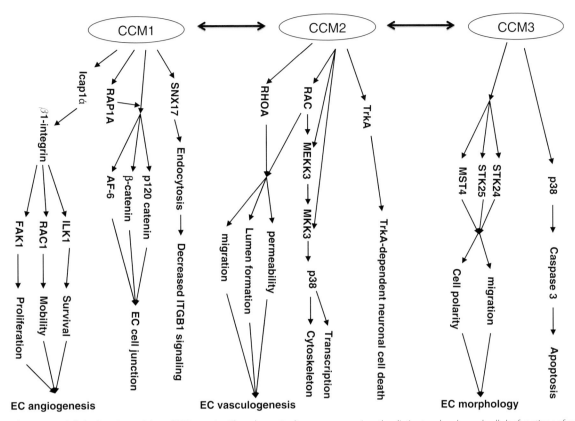

Figure 5.5. Cellular functions of three CCM proteins. The schematic diagram summarizes the distinct molecular and cellular functions of each of three CCM gene products based on our current knowledge.

integrin signaling via the ILK pathway, resulting in decreased survival of cultured endothelial cells. It is difficult to reconcile how loss of endothelial cellular survival or increased apoptosis culminates in the abnormal venous sinusoids seen in Ccms. However, we found that Ccm1 (*san*) zebrafish have more enhanced apoptosis within the vasculature, leading to perturbed vasculogenesis/angiogenesis. These animal data further validate our previous belief that krit1 protein is involved in endothelial cell survival [55]. Altered expression of vascular endothelial cell receptors (tie2 and flk1) within the vasculature in *san/vtn* zebrafish has been reported, indicating the involvement of endothelial cells in the pathogenesis of Ccm mutant zebrafish [52]. We postulate that the primary phenotype of abnormal circulation observed in Ccm1/2 (*san/vtn*) zebrafish might result from perturbed vasculature, which is caused by increased apoptosis within vascular endothelial cells. These data let us believe that krit1-icap1-β1-integrin signaling may play

essential roles in all cell types in vertebrate cellular development, while Ccm interlaced complex (krit1-MGC4607-PDCD10) and their modulated β1-integrin signal pathway may have a significant effect on microvascular endothelial cell performance in vivo. In this view, low Ccm gene-expressing vascular endothelial cells may fail to maintain the balance of proliferation and apoptosis, then ultimately undergo dramatic loss of endothelial cells, and lead to destruction of microvasculature [7].

The molecular and developmental roles of CCM3

A recent report demonstrates that a cardiovascular phenotype identical to Ccm1 and Ccm2 zebrafish was observed after morpholino combined knockdown of PDCD10 zebrafish ortholog, Ccm3a and Ccm3b [56]. This Ccm1/2 zebrafish cardiovascular phenotype was further recapitulated by morpholino-induced in-frame skipping of the exon encoding the STK25 and MST4 binding site of zebrafish Ccm3a if Ccm3b was repressed in parallel, indicating that simply blocking the interaction between PDCD10 and either STK25 or MST4 could lead to the in vivo Ccm1/2 zebrafish phenotype [56]. However, the preliminary morpholino knockdown data of Ccm3 zebrafish from our lab and others (John Mably, personal communication) indicate that although there are some similarities, the phenotype of Ccm3 zebrafish is distinguishable from that of Ccm1/2 zebrafish, further emphasizing the need for further work in the Ccm3 animal model.

Summary

Recently, a plethora of data has been generated regarding each of three CCM genes' cellular function and molecular roles during signal transduction and pathogenesis (Fig. 5.5). The challenges we are facing now are to address the following two questions: (1) how do we link all these seemingly isolated events together to form a vivid signaling network; (2) and how do we determine the direction that information flows among the CCM complex during the cellular signal transduction? An understanding of the molecular etiology of CCMs is essential for new technologies and concepts in clinical application. Dissection of the pathogenetic sequence of CCMs at the molecular and cellular level will certainly provide opportunities for improving diagnostic practices and for developing new therapeutic strategies. Elucidation of molecular and cellular etiologies of CCMs would not only shed light onto the mechanism of abnormal blood vessel genesis, angiogenesis, and progression that predisposes patients to stroke, but more importantly this information would provide patient benefit.

References

1. Laberge-le Couteulx, S., Jung, H. H., *et al.* Truncating mutations in CCM1, encoding KRIT1, cause hereditarycavernous angiomas. *Nat Genet* 1999;**23**:189–193.

2. Sahoo, T., Johnson, E. W., *et al.* Mutations in the gene encoding KRIT1, a Krev-1/rap1a binding protein, cause cerebral cavernous malformations (CCM1). *Hum Mol Genet* 1999;**8**:2325–2333.

3. Eerola, I., Plate, K. H., *et al.* KRIT1 is mutated in hyperkeratotic cutaneous capillary-venous malformation associated with cerebral capillary malformation. *Hum Mol Genet* 2000;**9**:1351–1355.

4. Zhang, J., Clatterbuck, R. E., *et al.* Cloning of the murine Krit1 cDNA reveals novel mammalian 5' coding exons. *Genomics* 2000;**70**:392–395.

5. Liquori, C. L., Berg, M. J., *et al.* Mutations in a gene encoding a novel protein containing a phosphotyrosine-binding domain cause type 2 cerebral cavernous malformations. *Am J Hum Genet* 2003;**73**:1459–1464.

6. Bergametti, F., Denier, C., *et al.* Mutations within the programmed cell death 10 gene cause cerebral cavernous malformations. *Am J Hum Genet* 2005;**76**:42–51.

7. Batra, S., Lin, D., *et al.* Cavernous malformations: natural history, diagnosis and treatment. *Nat Rev Neurol* 2009;659–670.

8. Zawistowski, J. S., Stalheim, L., *et al.* CCM1 and CCM2 protein interactions in cell signaling: implications for cerebral cavernous malformations pathogenesis. *Hum Mol Genet* 2005;**14**:2521–2531.

9. Hilder, T. L., Malone, M. H., *et al.* Proteomic identification of the cerebral cavernous malformation signaling complex. *J Proteome Res* 2007;**6**:4343–4355.

10. Voss, K., Stahl, S., *et al.* CCM3 interacts with CCM2 indicating common pathogenesis for cerebral cavernous malformations. *Neurogenetics* 2007;**8**:249–256.

11. Zhang, J., Rigamonti, D., *et al.* Interaction between krit1 and malcavernin: implications for the pathogenesis of cerebral cavernous malformations. *Neurosurgery* 2007;**60**:353–359; discussion 359.

12. Marcos Toledano, M. M., Portilla Cuenca, J. C., *et al.* [Pseudo-emesis gravidarum caused by complicated cerebral venous angioma]. *Neurologia* 2006;**21**:92–95.

13. Seker, A., Pricola, K. L., *et al.* CCM2 expression parallels that of CCM1. *Stroke* 2006;**37**:518–523.

14. Zhang, J., Basu, S., *et al.* Pathogenesis of cerebral cavernous malformation: Depletion of Krit1 leads to perturbation of 1 integrin-mediated endothelial cell mobility and survival. *Am J Hum Genet* 2004;suppl: S222.

15. Zhang, J., Clatterbuck, R. E., *et al.* Interaction between krit1 and icap1alpha infers perturbation of integrin beta1-mediated angiogenesis in the pathogenesis of cerebral cavernous malformation. *Hum Mol Genet* 2001;**10**:2953–2960.

16. Serebriiskii, I., Estojak, J., *et al.* Association of Krev-1/rap1a with Krit1, a novel ankyrin repeat-containing protein encoded by a gene mapping to 7q21–22. *Oncogene* 1997;**15**:1043–1049.

17. Zawistowski, J. S., Serebriiskii, I. G., *et al.* KRIT1 association with the integrin-binding protein ICAP-1: a new direction in the elucidation of cerebral cavernous malformations (CCM1) pathogenesis. *Hum Mol Genet* 2002;**11**:389–396.

18. Wang, Y. G., Liu, H. T., *et al.* cDNA cloning and expression of an apoptosis-related gene, human TFAR-15 gene. *Science in China C Life Sci* 1999;:331–336.

19. Kim, D. G., Choe, W. J., *et al.* Radiosurgery of intracranial cavernous malformations. *Acta Neurochir (Wien)* 2002;**144**:869–878; discussion 878.

20. Chang, D. D., Wong, C., *et al.* ICAP-1, a novel beta1 integrin cytoplasmic domain-associated protein, binds to a conserved and functionally important NPXY sequence motif of beta1 integrin. *J Cell Biol* 1997;**138**:1149–1157.

21. Glading, A., Han, J., *et al.* KRIT-1/CCM1 is a Rap1 effector that regulates endothelial cell cell junctions. *J Cell Biol* 2007;**179**:247–254.

22. Beraud-Dufour, S., Gautier, R., *et al.* Krit 1 interactions with microtubules and membranes are regulated by Rap1 and integrin cytoplasmic domain associated protein-1. *FEBS J* 2007;**274**:5518–5532.

23. Gunel, M., Laurans, M. S., *et al.* KRIT1, a gene mutated in cerebral cavernous malformation, encodes a microtubule-associated protein. *Proc Natl Acad Sci USA* 2002;**99**:10677–10682.

24. Czubayko, M., Knauth, P., *et al.* Sorting nexin 17, a non-self-assembling and a PtdIns(3)P high class affinity protein, interacts with the cerebral cavernous malformation related protein KRIT1. *Biochem Biophys Res Commun* 2006;**345**:1264–1272.

25. Uhlik, M. T., Abell, A. N., *et al.* Rac-MEKK3-MKK3 scaffolding for p38 MAPK activation during hyperosmotic shock. *Nat Cell Biol* 2003;**5**:1104–1110.

26. Hilder, T. L., Malone, M. H., *et al.* Hyperosmotic induction of mitogen-activated protein kinase scaffolding. *Methods Enzymol* 2007;**428**:297–312.

27. Ma, X., Zhao, H., *et al.* PDCD10 interacts with Ste20-related kinase MST4 to promote cell growth and transformation via modulation of the ERK pathway. *Mol Biol Cell* 2007;**18**:1965–1978.

28. Rual, J. F., Venkatesan, K., *et al.* Towards a proteome-scale map of the human protein-protein interaction network. *Nature* 2005;**437**:1173–1178.

29. Ewing, R. M., Chu, P., *et al.* Large-scale mapping of human protein-protein interactions by mass spectrometry. *Mol Syst Biol* 2007;**3**:89.

30. Goudreault, M., D'Ambrosio, L. M., *et al.* A PP2A phosphatase high density interaction network identifies a novel striatin-interacting phosphatase and kinase complex linked to the cerebral cavernous malformation 3 (CCM3) protein. *Mol Cell Proteomics* 2009;**8**:157–171.

31. Eerola, I., McIntyre, B., *et al.* Identification of eight novel 5′-exons in cerebral capillary malformation gene-1 (CCM1) encoding KRIT1. *Biochim Biophys Acta* 2001;**1517**:464–467.

32. Sahoo, T., Goenaga-Diaz, E., *et al.* Computational and experimental analyses reveal previously undetected coding exons of the KRIT1 (CCM1) gene. *Genomics* 2001;**71**:123–126.

33. Zawistowski, J. S., Uhlik, M. T., *et al.* Interaction of the Cerebral Cavernous Malformations type 1 and 2 gene products. *Am J Hum Genet* 2004;suppl:S60.

34. Zhang, J., Basu, S., *et al.* krit1 modulates beta1-integrin-mediated endothelial cell proliferation. *Neurosurgery* 2008;**63**:571–578; discussion 578.

35. Schlaepfer, D. D. & Hunter, T. Focal adhesion kinase overexpression enhances ras-dependent integrin signaling to ERK2/mitogen-activated protein kinase through interactions with and activation of c-Src. *J Biol Chem* 1997;**272**:13189–13195.

36. Arthur, W. T., Noren, N. K., *et al.* Regulation of Rho family GTPases by cell-cell and cell-matrix adhesion. *Biol Res* 2002;**35**:239–246.

37. Davis, G. E., Bayless, K. J., *et al.* Molecular basis of endothelial cell morphogenesis in three-dimensional extracellular matrices. *Anat Rec* 2002;**268**:252–275.

38. Degani, S., Balzac, F., *et al.* The integrin cytoplasmic domain-associated protein ICAP-1 binds and regulates Rho family GTPases during cell spreading. *J Cell Biol* 2002;**156**:377–388.

39. Bouvard, D., Vignoud, L., *et al.* Disruption of focal adhesions by integrin cytoplasmic domain-associated protein-1 alpha. *J Biol Chem* 2003;**278**:6567–6574.

40. Zhang, J., Clatterbuck, R. E., *et al.* New insight of the molecular pathogenesis of CCM. *The 1st international workshop on the pathogenesis of cerebral cavernous malformation*. Duke, North Carolina, 2005.

41. Bahary, N., Goishi, K., *et al.* Duplicate VegfA genes and orthologues of the KDR receptor tyrosine kinase family mediate vascular development in the zebrafish. *Blood* 2007;**110**:3627–3636.

42. Harel, L., Costa, B., *et al.* CCM2 mediates death signaling by the TrkA receptor tyrosine kinase. *Neuron* 2009;**63**:585–591.

43. Gruber-Olipitz, M. & Segal, R. A. Live or let die: CCM2 provides the link. *Neuron* 2009;**63**:559–560.

44. Tanriover, G., Boylan, A. J., *et al.* PDCD10, the gene mutated in cerebral cavernous malformation 3, is expressed in the neurovascular unit. *Neurosurgery* 2008;**62**:930–938; discussion 938.

45. Chen, L., Tanriover, G., *et al.* Apoptotic functions of PDCD10/CCM3, the gene mutated in cerebral cavernous malformation 3. *Stroke* 2009;**40**:1474–1481.

46. Lin, J. L., Chen, H. C., *et al.* MST4, a new Ste20-related kinase that mediates cell growth and transformation via modulating ERK pathway. *Oncogene* 2001;**20**:6559–6569.

47. Chen, J. N., Haffter, P., *et al.* Mutations affecting the cardiovascular system and other internal organs in zebrafish. *Development* 1996;**123**:293–302.

48. Stainier, D. Y., Fouquet, B., *et al.* Mutations affecting the formation and function of the cardiovascular system in the zebrafish embryo. *Development* 1996;**123**:285–292.

49. Mably, J. D., Chuang, L. P., *et al.* Santa and valentine pattern concentric growth of cardiac myocardium in the zebrafish. *Development* 2006;**133**:3139–3146.

50. Hogan, B. M., Bussmann, J., *et al.* Ccm1 cell autonomously regulates endothelial cellular morphogenesis and vascular tubulogenesis in zebrafish. *Hum Mol Genet* 2008;**17**:2424–2432.

51. Whitehead, K. J., Plummer, N. W., *et al.* Ccm1 is required for arterial morphogenesis: implications for the etiology of human cavernous malformations. *Development* 2004;**131**:1437–1448.

52. Jin, S.-W., Herzog, W., *et al.* A transgene-assisted genetic screen identifies essential regulators of vascular development in vertebrate embryos. *Dev Biol* 2007;**307**:29–42.

53. Kleaveland, B., Zheng, X., *et al.* Regulation of cardiovascular development and integrity by the heart of glass-cerebral cavernous malformation protein pathway. *Nat Med* 2009;**15**:169–176.

54. Whitehead, K. J., Chan, A. C., *et al.* The cerebral cavernous malformation signaling pathway promotes vascular integrity via Rho GTPases. *Nat Med* 2009;**15**:177–184.

55. Liu, H. L., Rigamonti, D., *et al.* CCM1 plays essential role in b-integrin-mediated endothelial cell integrity. *Translational Stroke Res* 2010.

56. Voss, K., Stahl, S., *et al.* Functional analyses of human and zebrafish 18-amino acid in-frame deletion pave the way for domain mapping of the cerebral cavernous malformation 3 protein. *Hum Mutat* 2009;**30**:1003–1011.

Cavernous malformations and radiation

Eugenio Pozzati and Nicola Acciarri

Cavernous malformations and radiation

Cavernous malformations (CM), or cavernomas, have been generally considered congenital vascular lesions and occur in two distinct forms, sporadic and familial: patients with the familial form usually have multiple lesions and those with the sporadic form have a single lesion. However, an increasing number of *de novo* CMs has been reported, suggesting a different mechanism of induction: these CMs represent an etiologic spectrum and encompass single and multiple lesions which occur in patients without apparent familiarity and mainly attributable to the cumulative effects of host and external agents (irradiation, infection, iatrogen seeding, hemodynamic and hormonal factors) [1–13].

Cavernomas represent primary malformations made up of abnormal vessels formed in response to a "noxa" occurring both during embryogenesis and in one's lifetime. Besides a genetic origin, cavernomas may represent a "convergent" vascular disease consisting of a labyrinthic aggregate of endothelial-lined channels resulting from angiogenesis activation in response to chronic hemorrhages, thrombosis and recanalization events, preferentially in a hypertensive venous milieau [4].

The concept of an "acquired" cavernoma arose when this lesion occurred in patients with previous normal MR imaging. Probably, MR imaging does not cover all the spectrum of the disease: at an early stage of their development, CMs do represent a discrete telangiectatic abnormality which may be "MRI occult" and may appear only later as a *de novo* lesion, generally after an "original" bleed [4].

It has been shown that therapeutic irradiation of the brain and spinal cord (cranio-spinal, whole brain, local field and focused), besides its early effects on the cerebral vasculature (fibrinoid necrosis of the vascular walls, endothelial injury and proliferation of capillary telangiectasia), plays a role in the delayed genesis of a vascular entity mimicking a CM, unaccompanied by other manifestations of radiation damage [14–23]. This acquired vascular lesion occurs in an otherwise normal brain and is not a typical CM, but instead a pathological variant deranged by irradiation. Since the first descriptions at the end of the eighties [1,4,5], many cases have been reported and now post-irradiation CMs constitute the best-known group of *de novo* non-familial lesions, although they remain rare and the precise prevalence is poorly understood. In a recent review of the post-irradiation CMs [24], the mean age at diagnosis was 11.7 years, the mean radiation dose was 60.45 Gy and the mean latency interval between radiotherapy and cavernoma development was 8.9 years (range 5 months to 41 years). The majority of post-irradiation CMs appeared in children irradiated before 10 years and were not dose-dependent. In adults, a more precise correlation between a radiation dose > 30 Gy and a shorter latency to development of cavernomas may exist [26,27].

Post-irradiation CMs have generally occurred in young people treated for a great variety of intracranial neoplasms (medulloblastoma in particular) and blood malignancies, mainly in childhood owing to the greater deleterious effect of radiation on the developing nervous system and its vasculature [14].

In one retrospective study, children with a medulloblastoma who received whole-brain radiation therapy had a 4.8% incidence rate of CM development occurring on average 5.5 years after irradiation [25–27]. Their incidence increased over time and at 10 years was 43% of irradiated cases in one series:

Cavernous Malformations of the Nervous System, ed. Daniele Rigamonti. Published by Cambridge University Press.
© Cambridge University Press 2011.

fortunately, most cavernomas followed a benign course and did not require operation [28].

In infancy, cranio-spinal irradiation for acute lymphocytic leukemia (ALL), performed in order to prevent CNS diffusion, plays a preponderant role in the formation of *de novo* cerebral CMs and constitutes the third most common malignancy associated with their induction [24–27].

Multiple CMs are found in about one-third of cases and are more likely to occur in patients who were irradiated at a younger age [25–28]: they may have a different latency in the same individual, with new lesions occurring at different times even several years apart, and careful MR imaging follow-up is necessary, particularly in children receiving whole-brain irradiation. There is no significant difference in the frequency of CMs between the group of irradiated patients that did and the group that did not undergo chemotherapy: only one report refers to the possible occurrence of a CM associated with chemotherapy [23].

De novo formation of CMs may also occur after radiation of the spinal cord and lumbar roots, both after cranio-spinal and after selective radiation for spinal or abdominal tumors [29,30]. The few reported cases were children under 16 years when first irradiated. In patients with malignant intracranial neoplasms undergoing cranio-spinal irradiation or with a past history of cancer and radiotherapy, radiation-induced spinal cavernomas should be differentiated from spinal seeding of the original tumor in order to avoid inappropriate treatment. Recently, a syndrome of very late postradiation lumbosacral radiculopathy with spinal root cavernomas mimicking carcinomatous meningitis has been described [31].

The complex pathogenesis of post-irradiation CMs is still debated and may range between direct *de novo* induction and triggering of a pre-existent, albeit occult, vascular lesion [4,5,15] considering that CM and telangiectasia may represent a spectrum within a single pathological entity and that endothelial cells which are the predominant cellular component of CMs seem poorly differentiated when compared to other cerebrovascular malformations and more radiosensitive [32,33].

The role of altered angiogenesis in the behavior of CMs has been widely investigated and seems particularly relevant in the subgroup of radiation-induced lesions: a complex disturbance involving vascular growth factors and a number of structural and matrix proteins contributes to the formation and growth of these lesions [34–36]. A release of vascular endothelial growth factor (VEGF) promoted by irradiation and expressed mostly in children plays a key role in the induction of CMs [15,17,19]. Among its effects and besides neoangiogenesis, VEGF may cause loss of tight junctions and fenestration of the endothelial cells and may promote the hemorrhage and growth of a pre-existent radiologically occult CM.

As suggested by Okeda and Shibata [37], radiation may particularly affect the endothelium of veins, producing a veno-occlusive disease with subsequent development of venous hypertension and promotion of ischemia, microhemorrhages, and angiogenic factor production: these vascular changes may compact and originate a lesion with the overall effect of mimicking a vascular malformation.

On this basis, Gaensler *et al.* [14] suggested that radiation of the brain may induce a telangiectasia consisting of ectatic venules and capillaries which may represent collateralization of venous drainage from areas of post-irradiation congestion or occlusion. Some reports of post-irradiation CM formed at the site of a venous angioma (or DVA) confirm this mechanism [11,23] and suggest that irradiation of a region containing a venous anomaly may be at major risk of developing a *de novo* cavernoma.

Otherwise, Larson *et al.* [15] have suggested that radiation may promote a proliferative endothelial pathway causing a pre-existent capillary telangiectasia to evolve into a CM.

Alternatively, irradiation may trigger a genetic or other type of latent predisposition: CMs can arise as a result of radiation-induced mutation in the KRIT1 pathway, a "second hit" in an area of genetically predisposed vascular tissue [38]. However, none of the cases of post-irradiation CMs displayed a family history as well as at the sites with high familial occurrence of the disease, as if a different type of host predisposition might be operative in these patients. Some relationship with latent hereditary hemorrhagic telangiectasia (HHT) has been suggested [39,40] considering that brain irradiation may interfere with its vascular genetic aberration and induce an erratic proliferative endothelial vasculopathy.

Clinical features of post-irradiation CMs are often related to the onset of a moderate cerebral hemorrhage and include epilepsy, headache, vomiting, and focal neurological signs: some patients may remain asymptomatic during the course of the disease. Massive intracerebral bleeding is rare. An increased risk of hemorrhage is generally reported in radiation-induced

CMs compared with spontaneous lesions: intracerebral bleeding appears to be associated with post-irradiation CMs in 25% to 50% of the cases with a risk of hemorrhage varying from 3.6 to 6.7% per year [20,21,24,26,27]. Surgical intervention was required in about half of patients presenting with intracranial hemorrhage [24].

We have also found hemorrhagic accrual in the first 2 years in three cases with recurrent bleeding: these findings may be extended to the overall subgroup of *de novo* CMs and reinforce the recent observation of clustering hemorrhages in the first years after presentation [41]. This bleeding pattern adapts well to relative clinical instability of the lesion after its formation and to the progressive quiescence related to the acquisition of a stable histological structure.

Post-irradiation CMs initially reflect a prevalent "fragile" endothelial structure lacking the typical aging changes and often assume a lacy (or "en dentelles") configuration characterized by closely packed sinusoids with scarce fibrous tissue [42] associated with telangiectatic foci and a thrombosed venous drainage. Some inhibition of fibrous proliferation may characterize post-irradiation CMs and differentiate the evolution of this subgroup from its spontaneous counterpart.

Regarding other histopathological differences between congenital and post-irradiation CMs, Challa *et al.* [43] believe that the presence of small amounts of neural parenchyma may help differentiate post-irradiation from true cavernous angiomas and probably reveals a relatively recent formation of the lesion, well before substitution of intervening neural tissue by progressive reactive fibrosis and gliosis. This conformation may increase the interfacing brain-cavernoma and the interaction with vascular growth factors expressed in the adjacent brain [44,45]. This "microenvironment" may represent a structural distinction in the central nervous tissue, which may predispose to different lesion activity.

The appearance of a new or hemorrhagic cerebral lesion after remote radiotherapy may raise some problems of differential diagnosis with tumor recurrence or metastasis [26,27]: at onset, the MR imaging may be not readily consistent with the classic appearance of a CM, as indicated in the classification of Zabramski *et al.* [46], but further MR imaging generally displays a clue to the underlying CM and therefore histological confirmation is generally not necessary. Irradiation may promote cyst formation in relation to increased permeability, osmotic properties and alterations of the blood–brain barrier in the nascent malformation. Fluid levels related to sedimentation of red blood cells may represent the equivalent of a rebleed in a resolving hematoma, similar to the hemorrhagic events in chronic subdural hematomas, and possible expression of an altered fibrinolytic system stemming from irradiation [47].

Besides whole brain irradiation, some correlation between focused irradiation and cavernoma induction within the thin perilesional irradiated field may also be considered. Although the benefits of radiosurgery for CMs have not been clearly demonstrated and a discussion of this treatment is beyond the scope of this chapter, some comments on the radiation damage of this procedure may be useful. Radiation injury after radiosurgery is located in brain tissue 1 mm to 10 mm from the lesion border and appears higher in CMs compared with that associated with AVMs [32]. For CMs receiving radiosurgery in the subset of the familial/multiple form of the disease, the risk of radiation-induced growth of a CM may be greater in view of potential radiation-induced mutation in an area of genetically predisposed vascular tissue. In one of our patients with multiple cavernomas, we have found a *de novo* lesion adjacent to an expanding CM of the caudate nucleus irradiated with a gamma knife 3 years earlier: the new lesion had hemorrhagic presentation and cystic expansion [3,4]. Recently, a similar case of chronic encapsulated hematoma secondary to a *de novo* plurihemorrhagic cavernoma after radiosurgery for a cerebral AVM has been reported [48]. A further case of cavernoma induction 10 years after gamma knife for a vestibular schwannoma has recently been described [49]: the area of cavernoma induction had been exposed to 7 Gy, which was much lower than expected and suggests that cavernomas can occur in the brain after a low dose of irradiation.

The vast field of cerebral exposure to radiation encompasses not only therapeutic but also diagnostic irradiation. Recent data show that brain exposure during fluoroscopy for endovascular treatments can reach clinically significant levels, comparable to the mean dose of 1.5 Gy estimated to increase the relative risk of inducing meningiomas, gliomas, and nerve sheath tumors [50]. In the cadaver, the scalp doses recorded after 120 minutes of fluoroscopy were 1.71 Gy. A peak dose of 1.38 Gy corresponding to a fluoroscopy time of 95.3 minutes for an endovascular treatment of an AVM was recorded in an in vivo study performed by Lekovic *et al.* [50]. This emerging aspect of radiation damage is represented by the prolonged exposure of the brain to fluoroscopy during multiple endovascular procedures, particularly for complex cerebral AVMs. Based on a case we have recently encountered, we question whether these endovascular procedures sometimes associated with radiosurgery are enough to trigger the formation of CMs.

Case report

This 35-year-old woman with epileptic seizures secondary to a large left sided parieto-occipital AVM underwent three endovascular procedures with n-BCA in 1994 resulting in a partial occlusion of the malformation. At that time, MRI performed in Switzerland did not demonstrate adjunctive lesions. In April 2008, after an intracerebral bleed, she was admitted to our hospital and underwent two endovascular procedures with Onyx on the residual malformation over a 2 month period. Control MRI in June demonstrated the presence of a cavernous malformation in the opposite parietal lobe. Total obliteration of the AVM was not achieved and further treatment with Cyberknife was performed on the residual AVM in November 2008. MRI in May 2009 showed the formation of a second cavernous malformation adjacent to the left AVM: both cavernomas were asymptomatic and no treatment was performed.

Although we cannot calculate the total dosimetry of five endovascular procedures, one radiosurgical treatment and countless cerebral angiograms and CT scans performed over a 15 year period in this case, a dose of at least 7 Gy corresponding to the multiple endovascular procedures (excluding radiosurgery) may be presumptively anticipated at the time of appearance of the first CM on the basis of the dosimetry in Lekovic's report [50]. The spontaneous association of AVMs and CMs is very unusual: the cumulative effects of repeat fluoroscopy and radiosurgery may have contributed to the triggering of multiple de novo CMs in our case with an AVM.

Findings in our 19 cases

We have reviewed our experience between 1980 and 2008 with 19 cases of post-irradiation CMs: six craniospinal or whole-brain, 12 local field, and one focused irradiation. Irradiation was performed for brain tumors in 13 cases (three oligodendrogliomas, three cerebral or cerebellar astrocytomas, two medulloblastomas, two invasive pituitary adenomas, one giant cell tumor, two

pineal dysgerminomas), cavernous angioma in one and lymphoma or ALL in four children: in one patient, *de novo* formation of a temporal cavernoma occurred after radiation therapy of a rhinopharyngeal carcinoma. The radiation dose varied from 800 to 5400 cGy. All lesions were within the radiation ports. No dose-response relationship was observed. The time interval between irradiation and the detection of the CM varied from 3 to 18 years (mean 8.1 years). The ratio of females to males was 12:7, 12 patients were < 16 years old when first irradiated, the mean age at diagnosis of the CM was 25.6 years (range, 10 to 51 years) and at irradiation was 15.8 years (range, 2.5 to 43 years). Two patients had multiple CMs developing at different times after the initial irradiation and one also had induction of a different lesion (meningioma).

Eight patients presented with acute symptoms due to hemorrhage (headache, vomiting, focal signs), four with seizures (one with hemorrhage) and seven were asymptomatic (one with hemorrhage) when the lesion was detected. The initial MRI was that of a hemorrhagic Type I lesion in 11 cases, Type III in three, and Type II in four (one patient had only CT scanning). Cystic changes with fluid levels occurred in five cases. The Type II lesion, which represents the typical aspect of a CM with its reticulated appearance and black ring, occurred in a minority of post-irradiation cases, as if some derangement of the usual sequence of progression to a more organized fibro-endothelial structure could be aborted. Type I lesions changed to Type III in four patients treated conservatively while one Type III lesion changed to Type I in one patient (8). Six patients were operated on 2 years after symptoms began (two had recurrent bleeding before surgery) and 13 are undergoing radiological and clinical monitoring. Recurrent hemorrhage did not occur in six unoperated cases during the observation period at a mean interval of 5.1 years (range, 10 months to 12 years).

An additional observation in line with some "fragility" of *de novo* CMs regards their surgical appearance: contrary to the compact conglomeration of congenital forms, new lesions tended to be elusive and the surgical specimens often consisted of faint endothelial spaces and hemorrhagic material.

In our series, three adult patients with post-irradiation cavernomas had low-grade oligodendrogliomas (ODG): one of them also became pregnant 1 year before the formation of the *de novo* CM and 6 years after irradiation (Fig. 6.1a,b). VEGF over-expression in ODG is a predictive factor for tumor progression [51]. It is possible that

(a)　　　　　　　　　　(b)

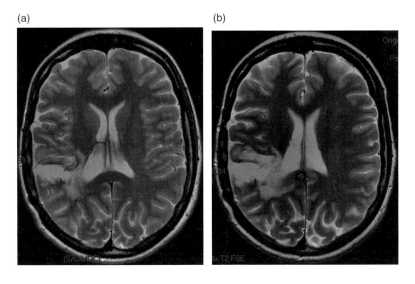

Figure 6.1. This 36 year-old woman underwent resection of a right pararolandic oligodendroglioma grade II in 2002, followed by 50 Gy WBRT. At that time and in the following years, the callosal region remained normal (a, performed in 2008). In 2008 the patient got pregnant and was delivered of a child. (b) An axial T2W MR image obtained in 2009 demonstrated an asymptomatic splenial cavernoma and some recurrence of the tumor deep in the parietal lobe and callosal region . Cumulative risk factors (irradiation, hormones, tumoral growth factors) may contribute to the formation of radiation-induced CMs.

the cumulative effects of tumoral VEGF and irradiation may be responsible for an increased incidence of cavernoma formation in the subgroup of long-standing ODG patients and that the *de novo* malformation may represent an early indicator of tumoral progression even before the visible recurrence of the tumor.

Conclusions

In conclusion, although post-irradiation CMs certainly represent a subset of lesions with an aggressive natural history in terms of hemorrhagic presentation, a prolonged follow-up indicates that several patients remain asymptomatic or have self-limiting courses and some presumed over-offensive stance of their clinical behavior has recently been mitigated. Surgical resection is recommended only in clinically aggressive malformations with hemorrhagic course and growth propensity. Cumulative host risk factors (growth factors, hormones, hemodynamics, genetics) seem to facilitate the formation of post-irradiation CMs. The appearance of CMs after low-dose irradiation in patients undergoing radiosurgery for a variety of intracranial lesions and extensive fluoroscopy during complex endovascular procedures amplifies the spectrum of possible radio-induced cavernous malformations.

References

1. Pozzati, E., Giuliani, G., Nuzzo, G., *et al.* The growth of cerebral cavernous angiomas. *Neurosurgery* 1989;**25**:92–97.

2. Pozzati, E., Acciarri, N., Tognetti, F., *et al.* Growth, subsequent bleeding, and de novo appearance of cerebral cavernous angiomas. *Neurosurgery* 1996;**38**:662–669.

3. Pozzati, E., Giangaspero, F., Marliani, F., *et al.* Occult cerebrovascular malformations after irradiation. *Neurosurgery* 1996;**39**:677–684.

4. Pozzati, E. Cavernous malformations as dynamic lesions: de novo formation, radiologic changes and radiation induced forms. In R. Spetzler and G. Lanzino, eds., *Cavernous Malformations of the Brain and Spinal Cord* (New York: Thieme, 2005), pp. 30–40.

5. Wilson, C. B. Cryptic cerebrovascular malformations. *Clin Neurosurg* 1992;**38**:49–84.

6. Detwiler, P. W., Porter, R. W., Zabramski, J. M., *et al.* De novo formation of a central nervous system cavernous malformation: implication for predicting risk of hemorrhage: case report and review of the literature. *J Neurosurg* 1997;**87**:629–632.

7. Sure, U., Butz, N., Schlegel, J., *et al.* Endothelial proliferation, neoangiogenesis and potential de novo generation of cerebrovascular malformations. *J Neurosurg* 2001;**96**:972–977.

8. Fender, L. J., Lenthall, R. K. & Jaspan, T. De novo development of presumed cavernomas following resolution of E. coli empyemas. *Neuroradiology* 2000;**42**:778–780.

9. Ogilvy, C., Moayeri, N. & Golden, J. A. Appearance of a cavernous hemangioma in the cerebral cortex after biopsy of a deeper lesion. *Neurosurgery* 1993;**33**:303–309.

10. Ludemann, W., Ellerkamp, V., Stan, A., *et al.* De novo development of cavernous malformation of the brain:

significance of factors with paracrine and endocrine activity: case report. *Neurosurgery* 2002;**50**:646–650.

11. Maeder, P., Gudinchet, F., Meuli, R., *et al.* Development of cavernous malformation of the brain. *AJNR* 1998;**19**:1141–1143.

12. Ciricillo, S. F., Dillon, W. P., Fink, M. E., *et al.* Progression of multiple occult vascular malformations associated with anomalous venous drainage. Case report. *J Neurosurg* 1994;**81**:477–481.

13. Dillon, W. Cryptic vascular malformations: controversies in terminology, diagnosis, pathophysiology and treatment. *AJNR* 1997;**18**:1839–1846.

14. Gaensler, E. H. L., Dillon, W. P., Edwards, M. S. B., *et al.* Radiation-induced telangiectasia in brain simulates cryptic vascular malformations. *Radiology* 1994;**193**:629–636.

15. Larson, J. J., Ball, W. S., Bove, K. E., *et al.* Formation of intracerebral cavernous malformations after irradiation treatment for central nervous system neoplasia in children. *J Neurosurg* 1998;**88**:51–56.

16. Valk, P. E. & Dillon, W. P. Radiation injury of the brain *AJNR* 1991; **12**:45–62.

17. Ball, W. S., Prenger, E. C. & Ballard, E. T. Neurotoxicity of radio/chemitherapy in children: pathologic and MR correlation. *AJNR* 1992;**13**:761–766.

18. Pouissant, T. Y., Siffert, J., Barnes, P. D., *et al.* Hemorrhagic vasculopathy after treatment of central nervous system neoplasia in childhood: diagnosis and follow-up. *AJNR* 1995;**16**:693–699.

19. Koike, S., Aida, N., Hata, M., *et al.* Asymptomatic radiation induced telangiectasia in children after cranial irradiation: frequency, latency, and dose relation. *Radiology* 2004;**230**:93–99.

20. Heckl, S., Aschoff, A. & Kunze, S. Radiation-induced cavernous hemangiomas of the brain. A late effect predominantly in children. *Cancer* 2002;**94**:3285–3291.

21. Strenger, V., Sovinz, P., Lackner, H., *et al.* Intracerebral cavernous hemangioma after cranial irradiation in childhood. Incidence and risk factors. *Strahlenther Onkol* 2008;**184**:276–280.

22. Detwiler, P. W., Porter, R. W., Zabramski, J. M. & Spetzler, R. F. Origin of de novo central nervous system cavernomas. *J Neurosurg* (Letter), 1998;**88**:616–617.

23. Brunken, M., Sagehorn, S., Leppien, A., *et al.* De novo formation of a cavernoma in association with a preformed venous malformation during immunosuppressive treatment. *Zentralbl Neurochir* 1999;**60**:81–85.

24. Nimjee, S. M., Powers, C. J. & Bulsara, K. R. Review of the literature on de novo formation of cavernous malformations of the central nervous system after radiation therapy. *Neurosurg Focus* 2006;**21**:1–6.

25. Baumgartner, J. E., Ater, J. L., Ha, C. S., *et al.* Pathologically proven cavernous angiomas of the brain following radiation therapy for pediatric brain tumors. *Pediatr Neurosurg* 2003;**39**:201–207.

26. Burn, S., Gunny, R., Phipps, K., *et al.* Incidence of cavernoma development in children after radiotherapy for brain tumors. *J. Neurosurg (Pediatrics)* 2007;**106**:379–383.

27. Jain, R., Robertson, P. L., Gandhi, D., *et al.* Radiation-induced cavernomas of the brain. *AJNR* 2005;**26**:1158–1162.

28. Lew, S., Morgan, J., Psaty, E., *et al.* Cumulative incidence of radiation-induced cavernomas in long-term survivors of medulloblastoma. *J Neurosurg (Pediatrics)* 2006;**104**:103–107.

29. Maraire, J. N., Abdulrauf, I., Berger, S., *et al.* De novo development of a cavernous malformation of the spinal cord following spinal axis radiation. *J Neurosurg* 1999;**90**:234–238.

30. Yoshino, M., Morita, A., Shibahara, J., *et al.* Radiation-induced spinal cord cavernous malformation, case report. *J Neurosurg (Pediatrics)* 2005;**102**:101–104.

31. Ducray, F., Guillevin, R., Psimaras, D., *et al.* Postradiation lumbosacral radiculopathy with spinal root cavernomas mimicking carcinomatous meningitis. *Neuro Oncol* 2008;**10**:1035–1039.

32. Clatterbuck, E., Eberhart, G., Crain, B., *et al.* Ultrastructural and immunocytochemical evidence that an incompetent blood-brain barrier is related to the pathophysiology of cavernous malformations. *J Neurol Neurosurg Psychiatry* 2001;**71**:188–192.

33. Tu, J., Stoodley, M. A., Morgan, M. K., *et al.* Different responses of cavernous malformations and arteriovenous malformations to radiosurgery. *J Clin Neurosci* 2009;**16**:945–949.

34. Rothbart, D., Awad, I. A., Lee, J., *et al.* Expression of angiogenic factors and structural proteins in central nervous system vascular malformations. *Neurosurgery* 1996;**38**:915–925.

35. Kilic, T., Pamir, N., Kullu, S., *et al.* Expression of structural proteins and angiogenic factors in cerebrovascular anomalies. *Neurosurgery* 2000;**46**:1179–1192.

36. Wong, J. H., Awad, I. A. & Kim, J. H. Ultrastructural pathological features of cerebrovascular malformations: a preliminary report. *Neurosurgery* 2000;**46**:1454–1459.

37. Okeda, R. & Shibata, T. Radiation encephalopathy: an autopsy case and some comments on the pathogenesis of delayed radionecrosis of the central nervous system. *Acta Pathol Jpn* 1973;**23**:868–883.

38. Jabbour, P. M., Gault, J., Shenkar, R., *et al.* Molecular biology of cerebral cavernous malformations. In G. Lanzino and R. Spetzler, eds., *Cavernous Malformations of the Brain and Spinal Cord* (New York: Thieme, 2007), pp. 11–21.

39. Robinson, J. R., Brown, A. P. & Spetzler, R. F. Occult malformation with anomalous venous drainage. *J Neurosurg* (Letter) 1995;**82**:311–312.

40. Marchuk, D., Srinivasan, S., Squire, T., *et al.* Vascular morphogenesis: tales of two syndromes. *Hum Mol Gen* 2003;**12**:97–112.

41. Barker, F. G., Amin-Hanjani, S., Butler, W. E., *et al.* Temporal clustering of hemorrhages from untreated cavernous malformations of the central nervous system. *Neurosurgery* 2001;**49**:15–24.

42. Lechevalier, B. Etude neuro-pathologique des cavernomes. *Neurochirurgie* 1989;**35**:78–81.

43. Challa, V., Moody, D. & Brown, W. Vascular malformations of the central nervous system. *J Neuropathol Exp Neurol* 1995;**54**:609–621.

44. Porter, P. J., Willinsky, R. A., Harper, W., *et al.* Cerebral cavernous malformations: natural history and prognosis after clinical deterioration with or without hemorrhage. *J Neurosurg* 1997;**87**:190–197.

45. Clatterbuck, R. E., Moriarity, J. L., Elmaci, I., *et al.* Dynamic nature of cavernous malformations: a prospective magnetic resonance imaging study with volumetric analysis. *J Neurosurg* 2000;**93**:981–986.

46. Zabramski, J. M., Wascher, T. M., Spetzler, R. F., *et al.* The natural history of familial cavernous malformations: results of an ongoing study. *J Neurosurg* 1994;**80**:422–432.

47. Frim, D. M., Zec, N., Golden, J., *et al.* Immunohistochemically identifiable tissue plasminogen activator in cavernous angioma: mechanism for rehemorrhage and lesion growth. *Pediatr Neurosurg* 1996;**25**:137–142.

48. Motegi, H., Kuroda, S., Ishii, N., *et al.* De novo formation of cavernoma after radiosurgery for adult cerebral arteriovenous malformation. Case report. *Neurol Med Chir (Tokio)* 2008;**48**:397–400.

49. Sasagawa, Y., Akai, T., Itou, S., *et al.* Gamma knife radiosurgery-induced cavernous hemangioma: case report. *Neurosurgery* 2009;**64**: E1006–E1007.

50. Lekovic, G. P., Kim, L. J., Gonzales, L. F., *et al.* Radiation exposure during endovascular procedures. *Neurosurgery* 2008;**63**:81–86.

51. Quon, H., Hasbini, A., Cougnard, J., *et al.* Assessment of tumor angiogenesis as a prognostic factor of survival in patients with oligodendroglioma. *J Neurooncol* 2009 (Epub ahead of print).

Neuroimaging of cavernous malformations

Doris D. M. Lin and Wael Abdalla

Introduction

Cavernous malformations (CMs), also known as cavernous hemangiomas, cavernomas and cavernous angiomas, can be classified as arteriovenous malformations (AVM) without shunt, and represent the most common type of angiographically occult vascular malformations [1–4]. These lesions are not generally detected on angiograms because of very slow flow or spontaneous thrombosis, and include AVM with thrombosed arteries, small venous angiomas and capillary telangiectasia [2,5]. They can be, however, best evaluated by magnetic resonance imaging (MRI) and demonstrate characteristic features. Cavernous malformation can occur anywhere in the central nervous system, but most frequently in the cerebrum. In this chapter, the imaging findings of cranial and spinal cavernous malformations will be presented, with emphasis on MRI and its various sequences that are particularly sensitive for detection.

Neuroimaging modalities and their roles in evaluating CMs

CT is less sensitive than MRI in detection of CMs, especially in small lesions under 1 cm [6]. CT would, however, show at least one lesion in a child with symptoms [7]. A non-complicated CM may be detected as small as 1 cm, depending on its attenuation. The CT appearance is often nonspecific, presenting as a well circumscribed, slightly hyperattenuated mass relative to the brain parenchyma but similar in attenuation to that of vessels (Fig. 7.1a), with no or mild enhancement following intravenous administration of iodinated contrast medium. Occasionally a CM can be calcified particularly when it is larger (Fig. 7.1b,c), in which case the differential diagnosis may include granulomatous infection, inflammatory disease, hamartoma,

treated neoplasm or vascular calcifications. Mostly CT is useful in evaluating CMs complicated by acute hemorrhage, which may appear as a well defined, hyperdense area with no or mild perilesional edema (Fig. 7.2) compared to hematomas due to other etiologies. Large hematomas, about 4–5 cm, are more common in children than adults. The CM may be seen located eccentrically in the hematoma, displaying a density different from that of the hematoma [7]. CT would also be a reasonable tool for following a patient with a known diagnosis of CM – for assessment of hemorrhage during acute symptoms and subsequent evolution of hematoma. Another utility of CT may be in the evaluation of osseous structures of the skull base for posterior fossa and, particularly, brainstem CMs. Large lesions may, over time, cause remodeling of adjacent bones.

On angiography, CMs are avascular masses, with no dilated arterial feeders, early venous draining, or parenchymal vascular staining. Mass effect may be evident only if the CM is large enough. Arteriography plays little, if any, role in the diagnosis of CM. Angiography is, however, indicated for the evaluation of unusual-appearing lesions and acute intraparenchymal hematomas, when the underlying etiology is uncertain by MRI or CT. Finally, it may also be useful to characterize concomitant vascular malformations. Venous angioma, or developmental venous anomaly (DVA), occurs at a high frequency, of up to about 30% of cases, in association with CM [8,9]. While small DVAs are also angiographically occult, DVAs can rarely be arterialized or associated with AVM, and accompany CMs in mixed vascular malformations [10]. The presence of arteriovenous shunting would be best delineated by conventional angiography. Figure 7.3 shows an example of a small CM that is associated with a rather prominent DVA nearby, prompting angiographic evaluation to exclude an AVM.

Cavernous Malformations of the Nervous System, ed. Daniele Rigamonti. Published by Cambridge University Press.

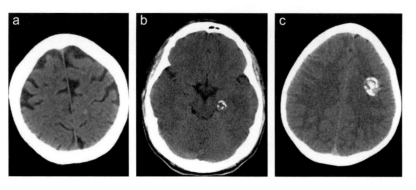

Figure 7.1. Appearance of cavernous malformations on non-contrast head CT: (a) a 3-mm slightly hyper-attenuated lesion in the high left parietal white matter; (b) a 1-cm left medial temporal lobe lesion with peripheral egg-shell like calcification; (c) a 2 × 3 cm left frontal white matter mass with heavy dystrophic calcification. Note that none of these lesions is associated with any vasogenic edema or significant mass effect.

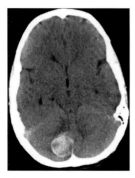

Figure 7.2. Acute hemorrhage due to a cavernous malformation in an 11-year-old boy. Axial non-contrast CT shows a spherical hematoma in the medial right cerebellum.

Conventional X-ray of the skull plays no role in the diagnostic evaluation, and usually shows no abnormality particularly in children. However, associated or secondary findings such as calcification [7], widening or erosion of the sella turcica, erosion of the sphenoid bone or petrous apex may be found [11–14].

MR sequences and hardware

MRI is the most sensitive and specific imaging modality for the diagnosis and characterization of cerebral CMs [15]. It is more sensitive and specific compared to CT particularly in multiple small sized CMs [16]. T1-weighted (T1W) spin-echo and T2W fast spin-echo MR images provide morphological delineation, and are also useful to estimate the age of the blood products associated with these lesions [7]. T2*W (or hemosiderin-sensitive) gradient-echo sequences are very sensitive to paramagnetic susceptibility effect associated with hemorrhagic byproducts including hemosiderin, and are therefore the best sequences for detecting small

lesions (Fig. 7.4) [7]. T2*W gradient-echo MRI is considered to be the sequence of choice for the diagnosis of the familial type of cerebral CMs, which often present as multiple small intracerebral lesions that can be inconspicuous on conventional spin-echo sequences (Fig. 7.5) [17–19]. Based on the same principle, but acquired at a high resolution as a 3D slab, is the pulse sequence dubbed "susceptibility-weighted imaging" (SWI), also known as "high-resolution blood-oxygenation level dependent venography" (HRBV) [20]. SWI can delineate the margins of lesions better than a conventional T2* gradient-echo sequence, and may provide a means of detecting both patent and thrombosed vessels [20]. Because of its high resolution, this sequence also delineates the peripherally located CMs better. It allows detection of smaller sized CMs with greater confidence, therefore providing earlier diagnosis of the familial type disease, and helps confirm whether *de novo* lesions are indeed new, or simply the enlargement of the tiny pre-existing lesions [19,21].

High magnetic field strength (3.0 tesla (T)) MRI systems are becoming widely used in clinical practice. MRI at 3.0 T provides greater resolution of CM lesions compared to images acquired at a conventional (i.e. 1.5 T or lower) magnetic strength [22]. The general imaging characteristics of CMs are the same at 3.0 T as 1.5 T, but the sinusoidal spaces are even better depicted on T1 and T2W images at 3.0 T (see Fig. 7.6). There is also greater sensitivity of detection using the T2*W sequence at the higher field, since the magnetic susceptibility effect increases linearly with field strength. A combination of high field scanner and the SWI pulse sequence, therefore, at present offers the best methodology for the detection and morphological characterization of CMs [22,23].

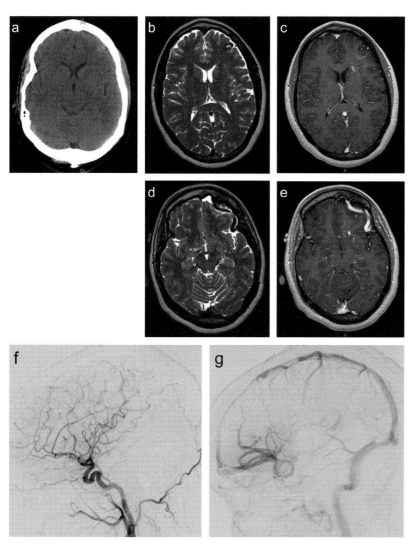

Figure 7.3. (a–e) Cavernous malformation associated with a large developmental venous anomaly (DVA). (a) Non-contrast head CT shows a small ovoid, slightly hyper-attenuated lesion in the left frontal lobe near the cortex. (b) The same lesion on T2W MRI shows the characteristic appearance of CM with a hyperintense core and dark rim. (c) On T1W image after Gd-DTPA contrast, the CM does not show any significant enhancement other than perhaps a punctate area centrally. There is, however, curvilinear contrast enhancement adjacent to the CM extending through the left frontal white matter near the left frontal horn. (d) At a higher image slice, a curvilinear flow void consistent with a large venous structure courses along the left fontal lobe. (e) Contrast-enhanced T1W image shows avid enhancement within the venous structure, as well as smaller areas of enhancement in the left frontal white matter in a typical appearance of "caput medusae", representing a DVA with a large draining vein. (f, g) Developmental venous anomaly shown on cerebral angiography. (f) Lateral view of digital subtraction angiography following left common carotid injection shows normal appearance of intracranial arteries during the arterial phase; there is no anomalous arterioveous shunting. (g) During the delayed venous phase of the same injection, a prominent draining vein is depicted in the inferior frontal region, compatible with a DVA.

Histopathology and imaging correlation

CMs represent masses of dilated sinusoidal vascular spaces and are composed of tightly packed, variable-sized vessels, which lack elastic fibers and muscles in their walls, but are lined by a single layer of endothelial cells and lack a true capsule. On gross examination, they have a multilobular appearance similar to mulberries. They are not associated with any large arterial feeders or draining veins, and there is no intervening brain tissue. Typically the intralesional vessels are thrombosed, and over time there is organization of the thrombus and calcification, with surrounding hemosiderin deposits due to chronic and repeated hemorrhage.

The histopathological features of CMs correlate nicely with findings on MRI. There are two key features in CMs: the presence of intra- or perilesional hemosiderin deposits on T2W sequences, and morphology indicative of blood products within the lesion [7]. T1W and T2W images show a typical CM as a slightly lobular lesion often with a reticulated appearance, namely, many small rounded compartments representing sinusoidal spaces that contain blood of different ages [24]. The lesion typically shows hypo- to isointense signal and occasionally mixed hyperintensity due to methemoglobin on T1W images, and hyperintense signal on T2W. There is no surrounding edema or significant mass effect. The margin of the lesion is dark on T2W images due to hemosiderin deposition. The T2 hypointense rim is the most characteristic, nearly pathognomonic, imaging feature for a CM, and may at times be quite extensive in the surrounding brain parenchyma, reflecting hemosiderin stain from previous, repeated hemorrhage (Fig. 7.7). As the

intralesional vascular spaces may be thrombosed with different degrees of reorganization, the CM demonstrates variable contrast enhancement ranging from none to moderate. It has been reported that delayed MRI performed 1 hour after intravenous contrast injection reveals enhancement of most CMs, except for areas of hemorrhage and hemosiderin deposition [25].

Typical MR appearance of cerebral CMs

Based on pathological correlation and MR signal characteristics, Zabramski *et al.* [26] classified CMs into four types. Type I lesions have a core of T1 hyperintensity reflecting the presence of methemoglobin; on T2W scan these lesions may demonstrate a hypointense rim surrounding a core of either hyperintensity (reflecting methemoglobin) or hypointensity (indicating aged blood products of hemosiderin and ferritin), as depicted in Fig. 7.8. These MR signal characteristics correspond to subacute hemorrhage surrounded by hemosiderin-laden macrophages and gliotic reaction on histopathology. Type II lesions, most frequently encountered with a characteristic MR appearance, demonstrate a reticulated core of mixed signal intensity on both T1 and T2W images, lined by a T2 dark rim (see Fig. 7.6). Pathologically these lesions correspond to loculated areas of hemorrhage and thrombosis of varying stage, surrounded by gliosis and hemosiderin-stained brain tissue. Type III lesions are iso- or hypointense on T1W images, and dark on T2W images with additional perilesional T2 hypointensity, related to chronic hemorrhage with hemosiderin staining within and around the lesion (Fig. 7.9). Type IV lesions are generally inconspicuous on T1 or T2W images, but are best depicted as a punctuate area of dark signal on gradient-echo

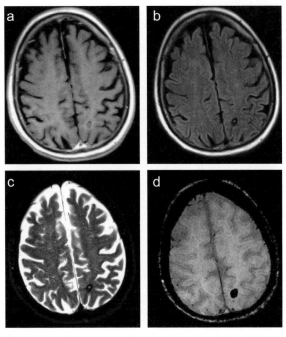

Figure 7.4. CM in various MR pulse sequences. (a) Axial T1W image shows a small (subcentimeter) lesion in the left high parietal white matter, iso- to slightly hypointense relative to the adjacent brain parenchyma. (b) Axial FLAIR and (c) T2W images show the lesion containing a hyperintense core and peripheral dark rim due to hemosiderin. There is no surrounding vasogenic edema. (d) Hemosiderin-sensitive gradient-echo or susceptibility-weighted image shows a larger area of dark signal due to "blooming" or susceptibility artifact. The same lesion on CT is shown in Fig. 7.1a.

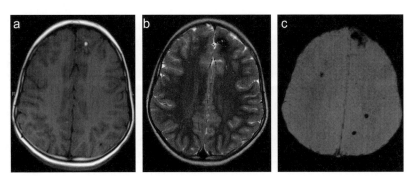

Figure 7.5. Hemosiderin-sensitive or T2*W gradient-echo MRI is more sensitive in depicting small cavernous malformations than conventional T1 or T2-weighted images. Eight-year-old boy who has multiple cavernous malformations; (a) T1W image shows a punctate hyperintensity in the medial left frontal lobe in the subcortical region. (b) The same lesion is better shown on T2W image with tiny reticulated hyperintensity centrally and dark signal peripherally. (c) T2*W gradient-echo image shows, in addition to the left medial frontal CM, several punctate dark lesions scattered in the bilateral centrum semiovale.

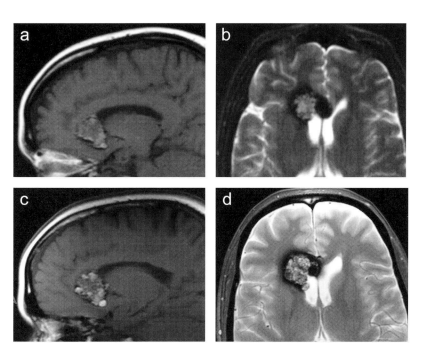

Figure 7.6. Zabramski type II cavernous malformation shown on MRI obtained at 1.5 T (a, b) and 3.0 T (c, d). (a) T1W shows a characteristic appearance of a multilobular, reticulated CM with mixed T1 signal intensity; (b) on T2W, the CM displays a central core with mixed signal intensity and a reticulated appearance, with a T2 dark rim. The reticulated sinusoidal spaces are more distinctly demonstrated at 3.0 T on both (c) T1W and (d) T2W images.

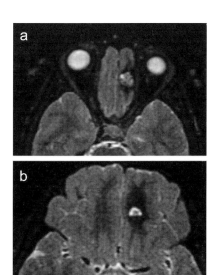

Figure 7.7. Prominent hemosiderin stain can be seen in the parenchyma adjacent to a CM. (a, b) Two consecutive axial T2W images show a CM in the left gyrus rectus.

sequences, and correspond to CMs and telangiectasies on histopathology (Fig. 7.10) [26,27]. Most type IV lesions are stable over time, but a small subset of these may progress into type I and type II lesions [28].

Other associated vascular malformations may be present, the most common of which is venous angioma or DVA (Fig. 7.11), and, occasionally, capillary telangiectasia. Rarely is there an associated venous malformation with arteriovenous shunting or AVM [10,27]. Concomitant occurrence of capillary telangiectasia, CM, and DVA in the brainstem in an individual has been described, suggesting that these may represent lesions along a spectrum of the same pathological process, perhaps arising from a disrupted pattern of local capillary-venous formation during development [29].

The pathogenesis of CM is the subject of discussion. Since the primordial vascular plexus, which is also lined by a single layer of endothelial cells, closely resembles a CM, it is postulated that CM may arise from failure of normal differentiation of the embryonic vascular plexus. Some authors also suggest dysplasia of the angioblastic mesoderm, and others consider CMs as hamartomatous lesions. Neuroimaging follow-up of CM cases suggested that they arise from the distal vascular radicles of a venous angioma, perhaps explained by a physiological mechanism related to venous hypertension [1,30]. The occurrence of mixed vascular malformations in association with CMs has led to a number of hypotheses of common pathogenesis, or possible causation and evolution among the different types of vascular lesions [10]. These associated vascular malformations tend to be

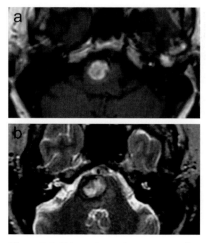

Figure 7.8. Zabramski type I cavernous malformation. (a) T1W image shows a circumscribed hyperintense lesion in the right pons. (b) On T2W the lesion is heterogeneously hyperintense with a dark rim, surrounded by minimal edema.

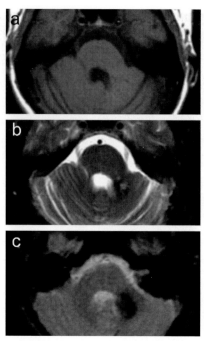

Figure 7.9. Zabramski type III CM in the left middle cerebellar peduncle. (a) The lesion is isointense to the adjacent brain parenchyma and therefore inconspicuous on T1W. (b) T2W shows a hyperintense core and dark rim. (c) More exaggerated dark signal is seen on the T2*W gradient-echo image.

angiographically occult (except for rare cases of associated AVM) and are best depicted on contrast enhanced MR examinations.

Atypical MR appearance of cerebral CMs

CMs may have atypical appearance, most often related to complication of hemorrhage. When small, a CM simply shows a punctate dark area, best detected on T2*W images (see Figs. 7.4 and 7.5) and may be inconspicuous on conventional images. Unless there is recent or acute hemorrhage, a CM is not accompanied by vasogenic edema or significant mass effect. Very rarely, CMs present as cystic lesions (Fig. 7.12) often accompanied by a characteristic angiomatous nodule demonstrating a reticulated mixed signal intensity region along the cystic wall [31,32]. This reticulated heterogeneous signal (particularly evident on T2W images) is, again, archetypal of CMs [24], while the cystic portion is probably formed as a result of slow, local hemorrhage within the sinusoids.

Acute hemorrhagic lesions

Upon acute or recent hemorrhage the appearance may be distorted, making it more challenging to diagnose with certainty. Symptomatic CM (Fig. 7.13) frequently shows a large sharply marginated, spherical, acute or subacute hematoma with the cavernomatous lesion within demonstrating the characteristic signals [7]. However, in the presence of acute or subacute hematoma, the causative underlying lesion may be related to vascular malformations that commonly include both AVM and cavernous malformation, in addition to other etiologies. Evidence of multiple episodes of repeated bleeding, a characteristic hemosiderin ring, and encapsulation favors a CM, while the presence of mass effect, single-aged blood product and expansile hemorrhage favors an AVM [33]. Perilesional edema is a variable feature; the presence of edema was thought by some authors to favor AVM rather than CMs [33], while others believed that edema was not infrequent with CMs with recent hemorrhage [34]. The variable appearance most likely depends on the acuity of bleeding.

Differential diagnosis

Slightly hyperdense lesions on CT that may simulate the appearance of a CM can also be due to either AVMs or dense neoplasms such as meningioma or lymphoma. In the presence of calcification, granulomatous infection, inflammatory disease, hamartoma, treated neoplasm or vascular calcification might all be considered in the differential diagnosis.

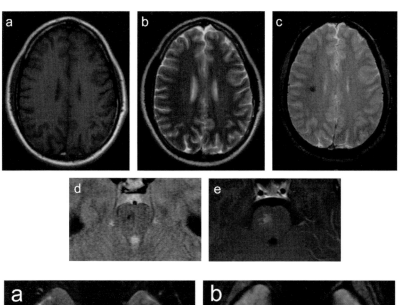

Figure 7.10. Zabramski type IV CM and a typical capillary telangiectasia on MRI. (a) T1W image fails to demonstrate any lesion. (b) T2W image vaguely shows a punctate hypointensity in the mid right corona radiata. This lesion is best demonstrated as an area of signal loss on (c) T2*W gradient-echo image. A typical capillary telangiectasia of a different case is shown in the right paramedian pons as a mild hypointensity on the T2W (d) and a blush of contrast enhancement on T1W after Gd-DTPA injection (e).

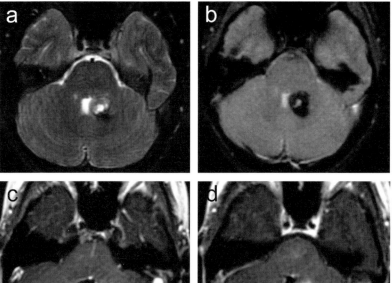

Figure 7.11. MR appearance of a CM associated with venous angioma and capillary telangiectasia. (a) T2W image shows a CM in the left middle cerebellar peduncle slightly indenting the fourth ventricular wall. The lesion "blooms" on T2*W image, shown in (b). (c, d) Post Gd-DTPA T1W images show enhancement in the left middle cerebellar peduncle and additional patchy and linear enhancement in the mid pons, characteristic of venous angiomas and capillary telangiectasia.

An acute hematoma may be caused by other vascular malformations (including AVM, arteriovenous fistula (AVF), aneurysm, or capillary telangiectasia), hypertensive or amyloid angiopathy, or underlying neoplasm. Finally, multiple hemosiderin deposits in brain parenchyma, best shown on SWI, can be related to various processes including radiation telangiectasia, treated metastases, previous traumatic brain injury, hypertension and amyloid angiopathy [35].

Size, distribution and location of cerebral CMs

In both adults and children, 80% of CMs are located supratentorially, the frontal lobe being most frequently involved, followed by the temporal and parietal lobes. The lesions are usually cortical-based or within the subcortical white matter, and relatively rare in the basal ganglia, hypothalamus or ventricular

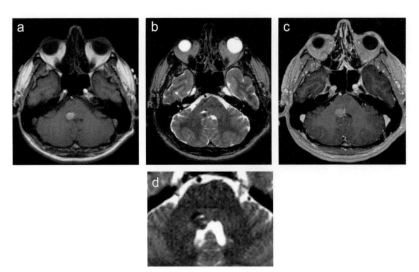

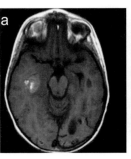

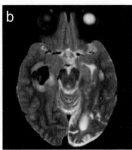

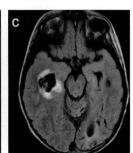

Figure 7.12. Cystic-appearing CM. (a) A circumscribed lesion in the right dorsal pons on T1W image. There is a suggestion of fluid-fluid level within the lesion containing slightly different signal intensities. This feature is better depicted on (b) T2W, with a hyperintense signal in the non-dependent portion and hypointense signal in the dependent portion of the lesion. (c) Post Gd-DTPA T1W does not show significant contrast enhancement. (d) T2W, magnified view of the lesion shows heterogeneous signal characteristic of the angiomatous portion of a CM.

Figure 7.13. Acute hemorrhage due to a right temporal CM on MRI. The hematoma shows mixed iso- and hyper-intensities on T1W image (a), and dark signal on T2W (b) and FLAIR (c) images, reflecting intracellular methemoglobin blood products. The hematoma is associated with mild vasogenic edema. These images were obtained from a 6-year-old boy with AML and anaplastic astrocytoma who underwent surgery, radiation, and chemotherapy and developed multiple cavernous malformations 2 years after radiation. Note also there is left temporal and occipital encephalomalacia related to previous treatment.

system. About 20% of all lesions are located infratentorially, affecting the brainstem more commonly in children than adults, and most frequently involving the pons. The familial type of cavernous malformation tends to present as multiple lesions at the infratentorial location at younger age, although sporadic cases may also display a similar picture [36–40].

Intraventricular CMs are rare, accounting for 2–10% of patients with cerebral cavernomas [41]. These patients may present with headaches, nausea and vomiting, cranial nerve deficits and hydrocephalus, but not typically epilepsy. In a series of 12 patients with intraventricular CMs, more than half of them were found to present acutely related to hemorrhage. The "true" intraventricular CMs are lesions attached to the ependyma or choroid plexus without extension beyond the ventricular wall. Because of their location and appearance, intraventricular CMs may mimic choroid plexus papilloma, intraventricular meningioma or ependymoma.

Occasionally CMs are found in the cavernous sinus, either intracavernous (arising from components of the cavernous sinus) or extracavernous (arising from surrounding tissue) in location [13]. In contrast to cerebral CMs, lesions in the cavernous sinus do not have a pathognomonic appearance on MRI [42]. Cavernous sinus CM may grow into a dumbbell-shaped mass occupying the middle cranial fossa and parasellar region [43]. Usually it is hypo- to isointense on T1W images and hyperintense on T2W images, with homogeneous enhancement after Gd-DTPA contrast administration [42]. Because of the location and enhancement pattern, differential diagnoses include cavernous sinus meningioma and schwannoma. Special care should be taken not to misdiagnose a CM in this location for a meningioma (a much more common lesion), since complete resection of a CM is difficult and there is an increased surgical risk of severe bleeding and injury of adjacent neurovascular structures [14,44–46]. Identification of a cavernous sinus CM would, therefore, call for a different surgical strategy and special precautions.

CMs are dynamic lesions and undergo change in response to repeated hemorrhage. They tend to vary in number and size with time [47]. With increasing age the number of CMs can increase, and this is best documented on T2* and SWI sequences [20]. CM lesions have been reported to range in size from 0.1 to 9 cm [48]. CMs tend to be larger in children, with an average size of 6.7 cm, while in adults the average size is 2–3 cm. The larger size in children is probably related to the tendency for bleeding and cyst formation [7].

Genetics and pathogenesis

Central nervous system CMs may occur sporadically or, in 20% of cases, have a familial link [49]. In the former, the affected individual more often has only one CM, although in about 33% of cases multiple lesions can be detected. In contrast, 75% of patients with the familial type have multiple CMs, although the presence of only a single lesion does not exclude the possibility of having other members of the family affected. The familial type is inherited as an autosomal dominant disorder and the gene has been localized in Hispanic Americans to the long arm of chromosome 7, with a high degree of penetrance and genetic heterogeneity [50–52]. The gene encodes CCM 1 (cerebral cavernous malformation), also known as KRIT1 (Krev interaction-trapped 1 protein) [52]. Two other loci are mapped to the short arm of chromosome 7 (encoding CCM2), and the long arm of chromosome 3 (CCM3), respectively. A high incidence of familial occurrence is observed in individuals of Mexican-American descent [52], and it is suggested that there may be a link between cerebral CMs and Spanish ancestry [53].

Usually, neither the familial nor the sporadic type is associated with other pathological entities; however, there has been one case report of CM, probably incidental, in a patient with neurofibromatosis type I [7]. Aside from genetic susceptibility, cranial radiation is supported by growing literature to be a predisposing factor in cerebral CM, particularly in patients who have received radiation therapy during childhood [54–56]. The postulated mechanism is that radiation induces vascular endothelial hyperplasia with hyalinization and fibrinoid necrosis of the vessel

wall, resulting in vascular thrombosis, exudation and hemorrhage [57,58]. Vascular proliferative lesions manifesting as capillary telangiectasia and CMs probably occur as a physiological response to this veno-occlusive vasculopathy [57,59].

Capillary telangiectasia and CMs may be sequential, variant manifestations of the same pathological process [24,60]. In adults, since CMs frequently develop at the distal radical vein of a venous malformation, DVA or venous angioma is postulated to be a promoting factor (in contradistinction, DVA is rarely associated with CMs in children) [1]. In several series, DVA and CMs are found concurrently in about 36% of cases [19,21].

Spinal cavernous malformations

Spinal CMs are less common than intracerebral CMs [61], and are estimated to account for 3–16% of all spinal vascular malformations [62]. Similar to intracerebral CMs, they are well circumscribed, dark blue or brown colored in gross morphology, and consist of abnormally dilated vascular spaces lined by endothelium without any intervening neural tissue [62,63]. In descending frequency of occurrence, they may be located in the extradural, intramedullary, and intradural extramedullary compartments, and extremely rarely in the intradural extramedullary space [62]. Most extramedullary CMs are encapsulated, while many of the intramedullary variety are devoid of a true capsule [62–64]. Extradural CMs represent 4% of all spinal epidural tumors [62] and 5–12% of intraspinal vascular abnormalities [65]. They are usually located posterolaterally to the cord and may extend to the neural foramina, at times with an extraspinal component [66,67]. The most common extradural CMs are due to extension from vertebral hemangiomas, although they can also occur without such association [68].

Demographics

The thoracic region is the most common location for spinal CMs [69], followed by the cervical and then the lumbar region [62,67]. Cauda equina is the least frequent site of occurrence, but the most common location for intradural extramedullary CMs [63,64]. Overall there is slight male predominance or near equal occurrence of M:F = 11:9 [61]; however, intramedullary CMs show a female predominance of M:F = 1:2 [62,70,71]. In intradural extramedullary CMs the

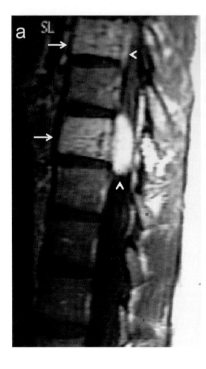
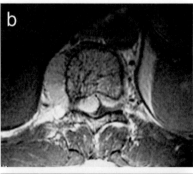
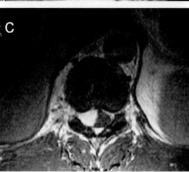

Figure 7.14. Extradural hemangiomas associated with a vertebral hemangioma. (a) Post Gd-DTPA sagittal T1W image of the spine at the thoracolumbar junction shows two vertebral hemangiomata (arrows) with contrast enhancement and coarse trabeculation. Associated, avidly enhancing soft tissue masses are present in the extradural space (arrowheads). (b, c) Post Gd-DTPA axial T1W images through the lower lesion (at the level of L1) show soft tissue masses in the right perivertebral region and anterior epidural compartment, causing compression of the thecal sac.

M:F ratio is 2:1 [62,64,72], and extradural CMs also show male predominance [67,73]. Most individuals present during the age of 25 to 55 years [61,67,71].

MR appearance

MRI is the most reliable method for diagnosis of spinal CMs [62,73]. Depending on location, whether intradural or extradural, spinal CMs have a different appearance. A typical extradural spinal CM appears as a lobulated and well-circumscribed mass, homogeneously isointense relative to the cord on T1W images, hyperintense on T2W images but slightly less than the signal intensity of CSF. It shows uniform enhancement after Gd-DTPA administration [67,68,74–76] (Fig. 7.14). A distinct line of hypointensity on T1 and T2W images has been reported segregating extradural CM from the cord [77]. Differential diagnosis for extradural CMs may include angiolipomas (which also contain fatty elements), vascular malformation extending from vertebrae, lymphoma, and metastases.

Intradural CMs have an appearance akin to the intracerebral lesions, and typically show T2 hypointensity with high signal intensity spots, most likely due to chronic hemorrhagic products of various stages [68,70,78] (Fig. 7.15). Hematomyelia may be a complication and can be best depicted by T2*W

gradient-echo sequences (Fig. 7.16). Intramedullary neoplasms such as ependymomas (which frequently contain hemorrhagic blood products) and hemorrhagic metastases may mimic spinal CMs. Similar to cerebral lesions, an uncomplicated intramedullary CM is well circumscribed and not associated with vasogenic edema. Figure 7.17 illustrates an example in which there is a lesion characteristic of a CM, but accompanied by extensive cord edema. Further evaluation with spinal angiography showed an AVM at the same site, suggesting that the lesion represented a spinal CM–AVM complex or possibly an AVM associated with hemorrhage that simulates a CM.

Clinical presentation

Presenting symptoms of spinal CMs vary according to lesion rate of progression and anatomic location, and may be acute, subacute, or chronic [61]. Most commonly, the presentation is in the form of slowly progressive radiculopathy (in cervical and lumbar regions) or spinal cord compressive symptoms [61]. There may be intermittent symptoms with periods of remission [67,70,78], likely explained by episodes of small bleedings within the CMs [71]. For example, one case of spinal CM was initially diagnosed as intermittent claudication [79]. Acute presentation

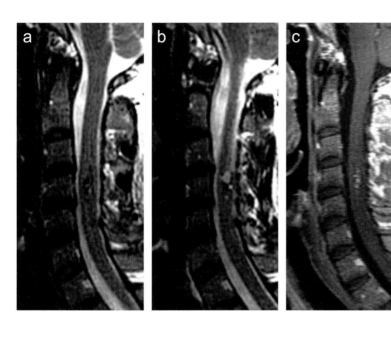

Figure 7.15. MR appearance of intramedullary spinal CM. (a, b) Sagittal T2W images of the cervical spine show a mutilobular lesion within the C4 cord. The lesion has a reticulated appearance containing a hyperintense core with peripheral hypointensity. There is no associated cord edema. (c) Post Gd-DTPA T1W image shows some patchy enhancement within the lesion.

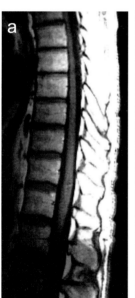
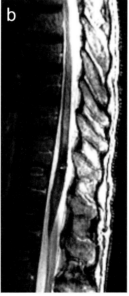
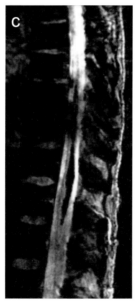

Figure 7.16. Hematomyelia associated with intramedullary CM. (a) Sagittal T1W image shows a small intramedullary lesion at the thoracolumbar junction, mostly iso- to minimally hyperintense relative to the adjacent cord parenchyma, making it rather inconspicuous. It is better seen on (b), a T2W image with a small hyperintense center and surrounding dark signal. (c) T2*W gradient-echo image shows much more extensive loss of signal along the dorsal surface of the cord cephalad and caudally, reflecting hemosiderin stain from previous, probably repeated, hemorrhage related to the spinal CM.

may be incited by occlusion or thrombosis resulting in an abrupt increase in CM size [71,79], or acute hemorrhage including formation of extradural hematoma [73,80], hematomyelia, and subarachnoid hemorrhage [64,72,81]. A case report suggested acute presentation precipitated by trauma, which led to micro-bleeding within the CM [82]. Local tenderness may be present [64,83]. Some authors reported association between spinal CMs and vascular skin dysplasia [62,84,85].

Other neuroimaging modalities

Imaging modalities other than MRI may reveal mass lesions, but they are not diagnostic for spinal CMs [70,78,86,87]. On plain radiograph, an extradural

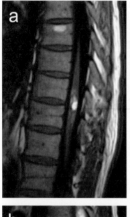

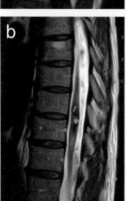

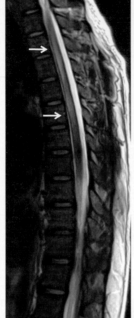

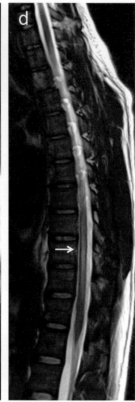

Figure 7.17. Unusual case of CM-like lesion associated with extensive cord edema. (a) T1W and (b) T2W sagittal images show an intramedullary lesion within the mid-thoracic cord with features compatible with a CM that has recently bled (containing T1 and T2 hyperintense methemoglobin blood products, typically seen in a Zabramski type I lesion). However, there is a long segment of T2 hyperintensity (arrows) suggestive of vasogenic edema in the cord proximally (c) and caudally (d). The atypical appearance prompted the performance of a spinal angiogram, which revealed an AVM at the site of the lesion.

spinal CM may cause widening of the intervertebral foramina or erosion of the pedicle [70,78,87]. On myelography, extradural CM almost always reveals complete blockade of the contrast column [69,73], while intramedullary CM may be apparent only if the lesion causes sufficient cord enlargement [62,70,78].

Angiography in general shows no abnormality; however, in two case reports abnormalities were documented on angiograms [79]. In one case of extradural cervical CMs, spinal angiogram revealed a normal-appearing anterior spinal artery forming anastomosis with muscular arterial branches extending from the cervical to the upper thoracic region, denoting the hypervascular nature of the epidural lesion, and delineating its location, which was confirmed intraoperatively [79].

Computed tomography may demonstrate CM as a well-defined mass that is isodense to spinal cord and muscles [75,76,86]. CMs may also show contrast enhancement [77].

References

1. Dillon, W. P. Cryptic vascular malformations: controversies in terminology, diagnosis, pathophysiology, and treatment. *AJNR Am J Neuroradiol* 1997;**18**:1839–1846.

2. McCormick, W. F., Hardman, J. M. & Boulter, T. R. Vascular malformations ("angiomas") of the brain, with special reference to those occurring in the posterior fossa. *J Neurosurg* 1968;**28**:241–251.

3. McCormick, W. F. & Nofzinger, J. D. "Cryptic" vascular malformations of the central nervous system. *J Neurosurg* 1966;**24**:865–875.

4. Roberson, G. H., Kase, C. S. & Wolpow, E. R. Telangiectases and cavernous angiomas of the brainstem: "cryptic" vascular malformations. Report of a case. *Neuroradiology* 1974;**8**:83–89.

5. McCormick, W. F. The pathology of vascular ("arteriovenous") malformations. *J Neurosurg* 1966;**24**:807–816.

6. Kaard, H. P., Khangure, M. S. & Waring, P. Extraaxial parasellar cavernous hemangioma. *AJNR Am J Neuroradiol* 1990;**11**:1259–1261.

7. Mottolese, C., *et al.* Central nervous system cavernomas in the pediatric age group. *Neurosurg Rev* 2001;**24**:55–71; discussion 72–73.

8. Pinker, K., *et al.* Are cerebral cavernomas truly nonenhancing lesions and thereby distinguishable

from arteriovenous malformations? MRI findings and histopathological correlation. *Magn Reson Imaging* 2006;**24**:631–637.

9. Rabinov, J. D. Diagnostic imaging of angiographically occult vascular malformations. *Neurosurg Clin N Am* 1999;**10**:419–432.

10. Awad, I. A., *et al.* Mixed vascular malformations of the brain: clinical and pathogenetic considerations. *Neurosurgery* 1993;**33**:179–188; discussion 188.

11. Fehlings, M. G. & Tucker, W. S. Cavernous hemangioma of Meckel's cave. Case report. *J Neurosurg* 1988;**68**:645–647.

12. Sawamura, Y. & de Tribolet, N. Cavernous hemangioma in the cavernous sinus: case report. *Neurosurgery* 1990;**26**:126–128.

13. Sepehrnia, A., *et al.* Cavernous angioma of the cavernous sinus: case report. *Neurosurgery* 1990;**27**:151–154; discussion 154–155.

14. Simard, J. M., *et al.* Cavernous angioma: a review of 126 collected and 12 new clinical cases. *Neurosurgery* 1986;**18**:162–172.

15. Bradac, G. B., *et al.* Cavernous sinus meningiomas: an MRI study. *Neuroradiology* 1987;**29**:578–581.

16. Perl, J. & Ross J. Diagnostic imaging of cavernous malformations. In I. A. Awad and D. L. Barrow, eds., *Cavernous Malformations* (Park Ridge: AANS Publications Committee, 1993), pp. 37–48.

17. Brunereau, L., *et al.* Familial form of cerebral cavernous malformations: evaluation of gradient-spin-echo (GRASE) imaging in lesion detection and characterization at 1.5 T. *Neuroradiology* 2001;**43**:973–979.

18. Labauge, P., *et al.* Prospective follow-up of 33 asymptomatic patients with familial cerebral cavernous malformations. *Neurology* 2001;**57**:1825–1828.

19. Lehnhardt, F. G., *et al.* Value of gradient-echo magnetic resonance imaging in the diagnosis of familial cerebral cavernous malformation. *Arch Neurol* 2005;**62**:653–658.

20. Lee, B. C., *et al.* MR high-resolution blood oxygenation level-dependent venography of occult (low-flow) vascular lesions. *AJNR Am J Neuroradiol* 1999;**20**:1239–1242.

21. Martin, N. A., Wilson, C. B. & Stein, B. M. Venous and cavernous malformations. In C. B. Wilson and M. B. Stein, eds., *Intracranial Arteriovenous Malformations* (Baltimore, MD: Williams & Wilkins, 1984), pp. 234–245.

22. Schmitz, B. L., *et al.* Advantages and pitfalls in 3T MR brain imaging: a pictorial review. *AJNR Am J Neuroradiol* 2005;**26**:2229–2237.

23. Pinker, K., *et al.* Improved preoperative evaluation of cerebral cavernomas by high-field, high-resolution susceptibility-weighted magnetic resonance imaging at 3 Tesla: comparison with standard (1.5 T) magnetic resonance imaging and correlation with histopathological findings – preliminary results. *Invest Radiol* 2007;**42**:346–351.

24. Rigamonti, D., *et al.* The MRI appearance of cavernous malformations (angiomas). *J Neurosurg* 1987;**67**:518–524.

25. Thiex, R., *et al.* Giant cavernoma of the brain stem: value of delayed MR imaging after contrast injection. *Eur Radiol* 2003;**13**(Suppl 6):L219–225.

26. Zabramski, J. M., Henn, J. S. & Coons, S. Pathology of cerebral vascular malformations. *Neurosurg Clin N Am* 1999;**10**:395–410.

27. Rigamonti, D., *et al.* Cavernous malformations and capillary telangiectasia: a spectrum within a single pathological entity. *Neurosurgery* 1991;**28**:60–64.

28. Clatterbuck, R. E., Elmaci, I. & Rigamonti, D. The nature and fate of punctate (type IV) cavernous malformations. *Neurosurgery* 2001;**49**:26–30; discussion 30–32.

29. Clatterbuck, R. E., Elmaci, I. & Rigamonti, D. The juxtaposition of a capillary telangiectasia, cavernous malformation, and developmental venous anomaly in the brainstem of a single patient: case report. *Neurosurgery* 2001;**49**:1246–1250.

30. Campeau, N. G. & Lane, J. I. De novo development of a lesion with the appearance of a cavernous malformation adjacent to an existing developmental venous anomaly. *AJNR Am J Neuroradiol* 2005;**26**:156–159.

31. Hatashita, S., Miyajima, M. & Koga, N. Cystic cavernous angioma – case report. *Neurol Med Chir (Tokyo)* 1991;**31**:414–416.

32. Kondziolka, D., Lunsford, L. D. & Kestle, J. R. The natural history of cerebral cavernous malformations. *J Neurosurg* 1995;**83**:820–824.

33. Vanefsky, M. A., *et al.* Correlation of magnetic resonance characteristics and histopathological type of angiographically occult vascular malformations. *Neurosurgery* 1999;**44**:1174–1180; discussion 1180–1181.

34. Willinsky, R., *et al.* Follow-up MR of intracranial cavernomas. The relationship between haemorrhagic events and morphology. *Interv Neuroradiol* 1996;**2**:127–135.

35. Batra, S., *et al.* Cavernous malformations: natural history, diagnosis and treatment. *Nat Rev Neurol* 2009;**5**:659–670.

36. Cavalheiro, S. B. F. Cavernous hemangiomas. In D. R. C. Choux, A. D. Hockley and M. L. Walker, eds., *Pediatric Neurosurgery* (London: Churchill Livingstone, 1999), pp. 691–701.

37. Edwards, M. S., Baumgartner, J. E. & Wilson, C. B. Cavernous and other cryptic vascular malformations in the pediatric age group. In I. A. Awad and D. L. Barrow, eds., *Cavernous Malformations* (Park Ridge: AANS Publications Committee, 1993), pp. 163–183, 185–186.

38. Mazza, C., *et al.* Cerebral cavernous malformations (cavernomas) in the pediatric age-group. *Childs Nerv Syst* 1991;**7**:139–146.

39. Scott, R. M. Brain stem cavernous angiomas in children. *Pediatr Neurosurg* 1990;**16**:281–286.

40. Scott, R. M., *et al.* Cavernous angiomas of the central nervous system in children. *J Neurosurg* 1992;**76**:38–46.

41. Kivelev, J., *et al.* Intraventricular cerebral cavernomas: a series of 12 patients and review of the literature. *J Neurosurg* 2010;**112**:140–149.

42. Mendonca, J. L., *et al.* Cavernous angioma of the cavernous sinus: imaging findings. *Arq Neuropsiquiatr* 2004;**62**:1004–1007.

43. Sohn, C. H., *et al.* Characteristic MR imaging findings of cavernous hemangiomas in the cavernous sinus. *AJNR Am J Neuroradiol* 2003;**24**:1148–1151.

44. Goel, A. & Nadkarni, T. D. Cavernous haemangioma in the cavernous sinus. *Br J Neurosurg* 1995;**9**:77–80.

45. Kawai, K., *et al.* Extracerebral cavernous hemangioma of the middle fossa. *Surg Neurol* 1978;**9**:19–25.

46. Ueki, K., *et al.* Cavernous angioma of the middle fossa: a case report and characteristic MRI findings. *Radiat Med* 1993;**11**:31–35.

47. Pozzati, E., *et al.* Growth, subsequent bleeding, and de novo appearance of cerebral cavernous angiomas. *Neurosurgery* 1996;**38**:662–669; discussion 669–670.

48. Maraire, J. N. & Awad, I. A. Intracranial cavernous malformations: lesion behavior and management strategies. *Neurosurgery* 1995;**37**:591–605.

49. Anson, J. A. & Spetzler, R. F. Surgical resection of intramedullary spinal cord cavernous malformations. *J Neurosurg* 1993;**78**:446–451.

50. Dubovsky, J., *et al.* A gene responsible for cavernous malformations of the brain maps to chromosome 7q. *Hum Mol Genet* 1995;**4**:453–458.

51. Gunel, M., *et al.* A founder mutation as a cause of cerebral cavernous malformation in Hispanic Americans. *New Engl J Med* 1996;**334**:946–951.

52. Sahoo, T., *et al.* Mutations in the gene encoding KRIT1, a Krev-1/rap1a binding protein, cause cerebral cavernous malformations (CCM1). *Hum Mol Genet* 1999;**8**:2325–2333.

53. Garcia-Moreno, J. M., *et al.* [Familial cerebral cavernomatosis associated with cutaneous angiomas]. *Rev Neurol* 1998;**27**:484–490.

54. Brühl, K., *et al.* Cerebral cavernomas and telangiectasias as secondary disease following acute lymphatic leukaemia and cranial irradiation. *Neuroradiology* 1995;**37**:S54.

55. Jain, R., *et al.*, Radiation-induced cavernomas of the brain. *AJNR Am J Neuroradiol* 2005;**26**:1158–1162.

56. Nimjee, S. M., Powers, C. J. & Bulsara, K. R. Review of the literature on de novo formation of cavernous malformations of the central nervous system after radiation therapy. *Neurosurg Focus* 2006;**21**:e4.

57. Okeda, R. & Shibata, T. Radiation encephalopathy – an autopsy case and some comments on the pathogenesis of delayed radionecrosis of central nervous system. *Acta Pathol Jpn* 1973;**23**:867–883.

58. Poussaint, T. Y., *et al.* Hemorrhagic vasculopathy after treatment of central nervous system neoplasia in childhood: diagnosis and follow-up. *AJNR Am J Neuroradiol* 1995;**16**:693–699.

59. Gaensler, E. H., *et al.* Radiation-induced telangiectasia in the brain simulates cryptic vascular malformations at MR imaging. *Radiology* 1994;**193**:629–636.

60. Larson, J. J., *et al.* Formation of intracerebral cavernous malformations after radiation treatment for central nervous system neoplasia in children. *J Neurosurg* 1998;**88**:51–56

61. Appiah, G. A., Knuckey, N. W. & Robbins, P. D. Extradural spinal cavernous haemangioma: case report and review of the literature. *J Clin Neurosci* 2001;**8**:176–179.

62. Sharma, R., Rout, D. & Radhakrishnan, V. V. Intradural spinal cavernomas. *Br J Neurosurg* 1992;**6**:351–356.

63. Rao, G. P., *et al.* Spinal intradural extramedullary cavernous angiomas: report of four cases and review of the literature. *Br J Neurosurg* 1997;**11**:228–232.

64. Duke, B. J., Levy, A. S. & Lillehei, K. O. Cavernous angiomas of the cauda equina: case report and review of the literature. *Surg Neurol* 1998;**50**:442–445.

65. El Mostarchid, B., *et al.* Intramedullary cavernous angioma. Two case-reports. *Joint Bone Spine* 2003;**70**:538–540.

66. Fukushima, M., *et al.* Dumbbell-shaped spinal extradural hemangioma. *Arch Orthop Trauma Surg* 1987;**106**:394–396.

67. Graziani, N., *et al.* Cavernous angiomas and arteriovenous malformations of the spinal epidural space: report of 11 cases. *Neurosurgery* 1994;**35**:856–863; discussion 863–864.

68. Isla, A., *et al.* Spinal epidural hemangiomas. *J Neurosurg Sci* 1993;**37**:39–42.

69. Lopate, G., Black, J. T. & Grubb, R. L. Jr. Cavernous hemangioma of the spinal cord: report of 2 unusual cases. *Neurology* 1990;**40**:1791–1793.

70. Fontaine, S., *et al.* Cavernous hemangiomas of the spinal cord: MR imaging. *Radiology* 1988;**166**:839–841.

71. Ogilvy, C. S., Louis, D. N. & Ojemann, R. G. Intramedullary cavernous angiomas of the spinal cord: clinical presentation, pathological features, and surgical management. *Neurosurgery* 1992;**31**:219–229; discussion 229–230.

72. Bruni, P., *et al.* Subarachnoid hemorrhage from cavernous angioma of the cauda equina: case report. *Surg Neurol* 1994;**41**:226–229.

73. Hillman, J. & Bynke, O. Solitary extradural cavernous hemangiomas in the spinal canal. Report of five cases. *Surg Neurol* 1991;**36**:19–24.

74. Decker, R. E., San Augustin, W. & Epstein, J. A. Spinal epidural venous angioma causing foraminal enlargement and erosion of vertebral body. Case report. *J Neurosurg* 1978;**49**:605–606.

75. Harrington, J. F., Jr., Khan, A. & Grunnet, M. Spinal epidural cavernous angioma presenting as a lumbar radiculopathy with analysis of magnetic resonance imaging characteristics: case report. *Neurosurgery* 1995;**36**:581–584.

76. Zevgaridis, D., *et al.* Spinal epidural cavernous hemangiomas. Report of three cases and review of the literature. *J Neurosurg* 1998;**88**:903–908.

77. Enomoto, H. & Goto, H. Spinal epidural cavernous angioma. MRI finding. *Neuroradiology* 1991;**33**:462.

78. Cosgrove, G. R., *et al.* Cavernous angiomas of the spinal cord. *J Neurosurg* 1988;**68**:31–36.

79. Padovani, R., *et al.* Extrathecal cavernous hemangioma. *Surg Neurol* 1982;**18**:463–465.

80. Kubo, Y., Nishiura, I. & Koyama, T. [Repeated transient paraparesis due to solitary spinal epidural arterio-venous malformation. A case report.] *No Shinkei Geka* 1984;**12**:857–862.

81. Heimberger, K., *et al.* Spinal cavernous haemangioma (intradural-extramedullary) underlying repeated subarachnoid haemorrhage. *J Neurol* 1982;**226**:289–293.

82. Richardson, R. R. & Cerullo, L. J. Spinal epidural cavernous hemangioma. *Surg Neurol* 1979;**12**:266–268.

83. Ueda, S., *et al.* Cavernous angioma of the cauda equina producing subarachnoid hemorrhage. Case report. *J Neurosurg* 1987;**66**:134–136.

84. Johnston, L. M. Epidural haemangioma with compression of spinal cord. *JAMA* 1938;**110**:119–122.

85. Kaplan, A. Acute spinal cord compression following haemorrhage within extradural neoplasm. *Am J Surg* 1942;**57**:450.

86. Lee, J. P., *et al.* Spinal extradural cavernous hemangioma. *Surg Neurol* 1990;**34**:345–351.

87. Morioka, T., *et al.* Dumbbell-shaped spinal epidural cavernous angioma. *Surg Neurol* 1986;**25**:142–144.

Clinical features and medical management of cavernous malformations

Michel J. Berg and Tegan Vay

Introduction

Cavernous malformations (CMs) can occur anywhere in the Central Nervous System (CNS) and account for 5–13% of all intracerebral vascular lesions [1]. The prevalence of CMs was 0.4% in a large autopsy study and ranged from 0.4% to 0.6% in prospective cohort studies with equal frequency in males and females [1–3]. CMs are characterized by clusters of vascular caverns lined by a single endothelial cell layer filled with blood or thrombus with no intervening brain parenchyma. They are often multilobulated with lobules separated by a dysmorphic collagen matrix [4]. The immature vessel wall with impaired endothelial cell tight junctions and lack of smooth muscle contributes to the tendency of CMs to microhemorrhage and, less frequently, to develop clinically evident larger hemorrhages.

CMs can be asymptomatic, typically identified as an incidental MRI finding, or diagnosed after a patient presents with CM-induced symptoms, which are most commonly seizures, focal neurological deficits, or headache [5]. In a small percentage, skin and retinal angiomas can be present [6]. This chapter will discuss the clinical presentation, ongoing symptomatology, medical management, and psychosocial aspects of CNS cavernous malformations.

Clinical features

Seizures are the most common clinical manifestation of cavernous malformations followed by focal neurological deficits and headaches [2]. Both microhemorrhages and clinically evident large hemorrhages from CMs can cause these symptoms.

Seizures

The spaces between the vascular caverns in CMs contain no functional neural tissue so CMs are not intrinsically epileptogenic. The brittle nature of the vessel wall and the defects of inter-endothelial cell tight junctions, however, allow leakage of blood into the surrounding brain parenchyma. This microhemorrhage classically results in a surrounding ring of deposited hemosiderin and associated gliosis [7]. Epilepsy may be the result of oxidative damage in the neural tissue surrounding the CM due to iron radicals released from the degrading hemoglobin. Subsequently, the seizures themselves can cause additional permanent remote epileptogenic alterations. This remote effect has important implications for the management of cerebral CMs as resection is more likely to "cure" epilepsy in CMs with recently developed seizures. Older lesions with a longer history of recurrent seizures may have permanent remote damage and resection of CMs with longer standing epilepsy has a lower statistical likelihood of improving seizure frequency and severity [8].

All seizures associated with CMs have a focal onset. The seizures can be exclusively simple partial (auras) with no impairment of consciousness with the symptoms expressed referable to the function of the brain at the location of the CM. Seizures arising in the frontal lobes with motor components often affect physical function (simple partial seizures with impairment) and generally affect quality-of-life. Simple partial seizures arising in sensory regions can be without impairment, and when these are the only seizure type may minimally affect quality-of-life. As with any focal seizure, the hypersynchronous neuronal activity can propagate through a variety of pathways and transition to a complex partial seizure and further secondarily generalize into a convulsion. CMs in the temporal lobe and limbic system more commonly develop complex components with impairment of consciousness and sometimes also secondarily generalize. In patients

Cavernous Malformations of the Nervous System, ed. Daniele Rigamonti. Published by Cambridge University Press.
© Cambridge University Press 2011.

with multiple CMs, only one of the CMs is usually associated with the seizure focus. However, identification of the responsible CM can be elusive, even with video-EEG long-term monitoring with intracranial electrodes. There are some patients where several CMs, typically located in close proximity, are involved in a seizure circuit.

Headache

New-onset headache or abrupt change in a chronic headache pattern is a common presenting symptom of CM [9]. In more than one fourth of patients, headache is the only symptom [5]. The headache can be focal and have migrainous features with or without an aura and associated nausea, vomiting, photophobia, and phonophobia. Chronic daily headache can also occur. CM-induced chronic headache disorders can be disabling and a challenge to successfully treat. In a patient with known CM, a headache that is particularly severe, or a headache that occurs in a patient without habitual headaches, raises the concern of a significant CM hemorrhage and may warrant neuroimaging.

Focal neurological deficits

Focal neurological deficits can be acute due to an abrupt hemorrhage or can appear as a slowly developing process related to mass effect from recurrent small hemorrhages and the associated surrounding edema. The majority of CMs located in the cerebral hemispheres are not symptomatic due their relatively small size or location in non-eloquent brain regions. However, when located in or near eloquent cerebral brain regions, in the brainstem, or in the spinal cord, enlargement of an existing CM or development of a de novo CM can result in clinical signs or symptoms.

A wide variety of focal neurological deficits have been reported with CMs with the signs and symptoms directly related to the location of the CM. CMs have been described in almost every compartment associated with the CNS including cranial nerve traverses, intraventricular locations, and abutting meningeal surfaces. CMs can arise within the internal auditory canal causing sensorineural hearing loss and facial symptoms [10]. CMs causing vision loss may arise within the occipital lobe [11] or within the optic nerve, chiasm, or tract [12]. The resulting visual deficits can be correctable with prompt surgery [13]. CMs arising within the ventricles, especially near the foramen of Monro or the floor of the third ventricle, can

present with obstructive hydrocephalus [14]. CMs in the ventricular system tend to have more rapid growth and more symptoms of mass effect. An aggressive surgical treatment approach should be considered in patients presenting with hydrocephalus due to ventricular associated CMs [15].

Cavernous malformations of the spinal cord are less frequent, accounting for 5–12% of spinal vascular abnormalities [16]. They can be epidural, intradural, or intramedullary. Spinal CMs present with focal neurological symptoms that depend on the location within the spinal canal or cord. These symptoms range from slow spinal compression to acute decline associated with rapidly developing hematomyelia. The natural history of spinal CMs is not well understood, but as a group spinal cord CMs tend to present with slow, progressive deterioration [17,18]. Surgical treatment is the definitive therapy for these lesions and radiotherapy should be reserved for inoperative patients [17]. CMs are histologically and immunohistochemically identical regardless of where in the CNS they arise; however, CMs involving the dura have been reported to be more vascular than intramedullary lesions [18].

Hemorrhage

Hemorrhage is the underlying mechanism for the transition of asymptomatic to symptomatic CMs in most cases. Hemorrhage can also be asymptomatic and only detected on neuroimaging. The amount of bleeding is usually small, but can be large, depending on the size and location. Although rare, a CM hemorrhage can result in death through a variety of mechanisms including mass effect and seizures.

Estimates of MRI-detectable rates of recent hemorrhage range from 0.25% to 6% per lesion per year; however, only a portion of these have clinical manifestations. All CMs, except the punctate-sized "type-4" evident on GRE and SWI MRI, presumptively have had intermittent microhemorrhages [1]. After a first clinically evident hemorrhage, there is as high as a 30 to 40% annual risk of recurrent hemorrhage into the same CM (although not necessarily symptomatic) [19,20].

The likelihood of clinical symptoms and disability is higher for CMs located in the brainstem [21]. While there are similar rates of radiographically detectable hemorrhage in both cerebral and brainstem lesions, rates of symptomatic hemorrhages are significantly higher for brainstem lesions due to the increased density of eloquent tissue in the brainstem [22]. The rate of clinical disability developing after hemorrhage increases with increasing age, infratentorial location, and previous hemorrhage.

Diagnosis

Deciding on the diagnosis of lesions consistent with CMs on neuroimaging is a commonly encountered clinical challenge. There is overlap in the differential diagnoses that needs to be considered in patients with the sporadic form with a single CM and those with the familial form with multiple CMs.

The differential diagnosis for abnormalities consistent with CMs includes most types of CNS lesions associated with hemorrhage. Medium and large-sized mixed-signal round or spherical abnormalities on T1 and T2 MRI with a surrounding rim of low signal on T2 images can occur in any lesion with past hemorrhage including contusions or hemorrhagic tumors. Features that help differentiate these diagnoses include the degree of surrounding edema, the hemosiderin rim, and interior heterogeneity. Most tumors have substantial associated edema, especially those that are metastatic. Additionally, the hypointense rim characteristic of CMs is usually not present in tumors [23]. Since contusions are typically due to a single event, the central region is usually more homogeneous in a contusion compared to a CM and contusions are typically located in the periphery of the cerebral hemispheres. Small thrombosed AVMs can be difficult to distinguish from CMs; however, if there is subarachnoid or intraventricular hemorrhage, AVM is more likely [24].

Vascular malformations of the brain are classified into four groups based on pathological features: arteriovenous malformation, cavernous malformation, developmental venous anomalies (DVAs), and capillary telangiectasia [25]. Except for CMs, these other vascular lesions typically enhance with contrast on MRI and usually are visible on contrast angiography although small capillary telangiectasias and DVAs can be angiographically occult. CMs enhance less frequently and are usually not visible on conventional contrast angiography (i.e. angiographically occult). About one-half of single sporadic CMs have an associated vascular lesion (either a DVA or a capillary telangiectasia). Care must be taken not to misinterpret a DVA (venous angioma) associated with a CM as a draining vein from a small thrombosed AVM and vice versa.

In patients with the familial form of CM, multiple punctate lesions that are only visualized with T2 gradient-echo (GRE) or susceptibility-weighted imaging (SWI) MRI are often present. These are thought to be precursor CMs ("type 4 lesions"). These lesions have the same MRI signal characteristics as microhemorrhages present in chronic hypertension, intracerebral hemorrhage, ischemic cerebrovascular disease, cerebral amyloid angiopathy (CAA), and cerebral autosomal dominant arteriopathy with subcortical infarcts and leukoencephalopathy (CADASIL) [26]. In CM the microhemorrhages are typically distributed throughout the brain whereas in CAA, ischemic cerebrovascular disease, and CADASIL they tend to be located within the cerebral hemisphere white matter. In chronic hypertension and intracerebral hemorrhage the microhemorrhages typically are located within the deeper brain structures including the basal ganglia, diencephalon, and pons. Also, in these other conditions, concurrent periventricular white matter high T2 signal lesions are typically present (e.g. small vessel disease).

Despite the difficulties in establishing a definitive diagnosis using MRI alone, lesions confirmed on pathological analysis correlate to MRI appearance in 80 to 100% of patients [27].

History, physical exam

Serial histories and physical exams are the mainstay in the management of people with CMs since these lesions are chronic and often evolve. A careful history of symptoms can help to determine the likelihood that a CM may be present in a potentially affected individual. Symptoms including seizures, headaches, and focal neurological deficits should be sought. Patients who present with these symptoms in conjunction with a family history of CM are likely to have the familial form of the disease. History is also important in determining the level of risk of symptomatic hemorrhage in a patient with known CMs. Asymptomatic lesions are less likely to bleed than lesions that have been active in the past.

About one-half of symptomatic CMs are sporadic, presenting in people with no family history of cavernous lesions or somatic mutation in one of the CCM genes [28]. Mutations in three genes have thus far been implicated in predisposition to CMs (see chapter 4 on genetics). In the familial form of CM, about 90% of affected patients have multiple CMs on brain MRI, 5% have one CM and 5% have no detectable CMs [6]. Penetrance increases with age. Patients with mutations in the CCM3 gene tend to present earlier in life (childhood or teen years) and CCM3 is thought to have a more severe phenotype [29].

CMs are generally diagnosed with MRI, but a careful physical exam, including a complete neurological exam, is important to assess for focal or generalized neurological deficits. In a patient with known CMs it is important to follow serial neurological examinations as a new focal deficit can be the first indication of an expanding lesion. About 10% of patients with CM gene mutations have cutaneous angiomas and about 5% have retinal angiomas [6]. CMs in other organ systems, besides skin and retina, are reported so rarely that it is likely these associations are coincidental.

Cutaneous manifestations of CM

At least three distinct cutaneous vascular malformation phenotypes occur in about 10% of people with familial CM [30]. Hyperkeratotic cutaneous capillary venous malformations (HCCVM) represent about 40% of the cutaneous lesions. These are purplish-crimson colored, irregularly shaped small papules (3–10 mm diameter) or larger macules (up to 7 cm diameter) with overlying hyperkeratotic epidermis. Sometimes HCCVMs occur in clusters. These lesions are composed of dilated capillaries and venous channels in the dermis and hypodermis with hyperkeratotic epidermis. Surgical removal of these lesions is sometimes followed by local recurrence [31]. In most cases HCCVM is associated with mutations in the CCM1 (KRIT1) gene [32].

About one-third of the cutaneous lesions identified in people with familial CM are capillary malformations and one-fifth are venous malformations [30]. Most patients with these manifestations also have CCM1 (KRIT1) gene mutations. The venous malformations can be late-onset, tiny bluish, soft, cutaneous papules located mainly on the face, arm, and abdomen [33].

Retinal manifestations of CM

Retinal angiomas associated with familial CM are rarely symptomatic. These are present in about 5% of people with familial CM [34]. These lesions are usually unilateral and stable; retinal hemorrhage or visual impairment is rare. Retinal angiomas are associated with mutations in all three CCM genes [34].

Neuroimaging

CT scans are relatively insensitive for diagnosing CMs as most CMs are occult on CT. However, sometimes CT reveals calcification within CMs that is not visible on MRI. CT is the preferred study to assess for acute hemorrhage. The low sensitivity makes CT a poor choice for diagnosing and following suspected CMs.

CMs are classified among the angiographically occult vascular malformations. Many of the characteristics of CMs, including their narrow caliber, low flow nature, and propensity to thrombosis, make conventional angiography an ineffective radiological tool for CM detection [35]. While most CMs are angiographically occult, occasional lesions will appear as an avascular mass, minimal vascular abnormality, a late blush, or with signs of neovascularization on angiography [5].

High-field-strength MRI is the diagnostic study of choice to visualize CMs [36]. CMs can typically be seen on T1, T2, gradient-recalled echo (GRE) and susceptibility-weighted (SWI) MRI. MRI with T1, T2-weighted and T2-GRE sequences is the gold standard for imaging CMs. Susceptibility-weighted imaging (SWI) may be the most sensitive sequence for imaging small lesions in familial CM, but is a newer technique and is potentially confounded by the prominent appearance of venous structures [37]. Lower-field-strength MRIs are less sensitive to the susceptibility effects that reveal CMs; care must be taken when comparing CMs from MRIs with different field strengths as more CMs may be visible in the same patient with higher-field-strength MRI [38].

Classifying CMs based on the MRI patterns has potential clinical implications. CMs can be divided into four distinct types based on their appearance on different MRI sequences [39]:

> Type I lesions have a hyperintense core on T1-weighted images and a hypointense rim with hemosiderin deposits evident on T2-weighted images. The high T1 signal in the core is due to methemoglobin and is indicative of subacute hemorrhage weeks to months old.
>
> Type II lesions have a mixed-signal reticulated core on both T1 and T2-weighted images and a hypointense rim on T2 images. These lesions consist of areas of hemorrhage and thrombosis of varying ages with blood present in several stages of degradation. There is gliotic brain tissue with hemosiderin deposits surrounding the lesion.
>
> Type III CMs are present on T2-weighted and GRE or SWI sequences. Type III lesions appear as an iso- or hypointense area of signal and typically represent chronic lesions with past hemorrhage that has resolved with hemosiderin staining. These are often present in patients with the familial form and are often asymptomatic.

Type IV CMs appear as hypointense punctuate foci similar in appearance to capillary telangiectasias and microhemorrhages and are only seen on GRE or SWI images [1,39].

The clinical importance of this classification is based on the presumption that both type I and II lesions are in an "active" state and have the highest tendency to rebleed and produce recurrent symptoms [1], whereas type III lesions may have hemorrhaged in the remote past, but are not necessarily at increased risk of hemorrhage and type IV lesions are precursor lesions and infrequently expand. However, type III and IV lesions are not always benign and must hemorrhage, albeit rarely, to convert to type I and type II lesions.

Most CMs do not enhance with contrast, but occasionally some contrast enhancement is present. The meaning of contrast enhancement is not clear, and whether contrast-enhancing CMs are more or less prone to future hemorrhage is not known. Care should be taken to not confuse a contrast-enhancing DVA or capillary telangiectasia associated with a CM as contrast enhancement of the CM itself. Additionally, care should be taken not to confuse high signal on T1 images due to particulate calcium or methemoglobin as enhancement. It is not known whether calcified CMs are more or less likely to hemorrhage.

Unfortunately there is no imaging modality or imaging pattern demonstrated to directly predict the likely future "activity" of a CM. Tagged-RBC SPECT has been proposed as a test that could predict "activity" based on the timing of delayed accumulation of the radiotracer in the CM and may warrant further investigation [40].

Testing asymptomatic family members for CM

In a patient recently diagnosed with CM, the presence of multiple lesions on MRI or a positive family history of seizures or strokes at a young age (especially brain hemorrhages) raises the possibility of familial CM. Headache disorders are so common in the general population that they are usually not very helpful in identifying other potentially affected family members.

Although there is no current medical therapy that is proven to prevent the development or expansion of CMs, it makes good sense to avoid certain drugs and activities that could increase the probability of CM expression in someone at risk for developing CMs (discussed below). Thus, the authors believe that it is often appropriate to determine whether family members are at risk for CMs. However, such testing has a number of psychological and social implications.

Using brain MRIs to screen for CMs in at-risk family members in a pedigree with suspected familial CM has variable diagnostic accuracy as familial CM expression is age dependent [29,41]. A child (or young adult) may have a normal brain MRI yet still develop symptomatic CMs at a later age. Thus, although highly sensitive for CMs, MRI is not necessarily the best or only test that should be performed.

Genetic mutation testing can be considered in all at-risk members of families suspected of harboring a CM gene mutation. However, at the current time clinical testing only detects mutations in about 85% of familial cases. In the United States, enactment of the Genetic Information Nondiscrimination Act of 2008 protects US citizens from discrimination in health insurance coverage and employment based on genetic information [42]. Unfortunately, this act does not prohibit the use of the genetic information in assessing eligibility or costs of life, disability, and long-term care insurance. Similarly, an MRI scan that reveals CMs could have insurance repercussions.

Learning that one has asymptomatic CMs or a genetic mutation that can lead to significant morbidity later in life may result in significant psychosocial stress with wide variations in different people. Thus, prior to screening MRI or genetic testing in asymptomatic family members, individuals should discuss these issues with their physicians and weigh the psychological, social, and financial implications of learning that they are at risk for developing symptomatic CMs.

The diagnosis of familial CM (even if made in only one individual due to multiple CMs on neuroimaging or identification of a causative CCM1, 2, or 3 gene mutation) can have psychological effects on the patient's family members, including those who are asymptomatic as, until tested, there is uncertainty whether they are also affected by CMs. No specific studies have been conducted on the psychological impact of genetic testing in CM families but research from families with other heritable conditions may apply. Each of the family members needs to arrive at their own decision about testing, but it is reasonable to encourage that testing be considered. A negative result can provide significant relief for unaffected family members. A positive result might cause transient distress, but it enables the affected individual to initiate appropriate preventative care and monitoring [43].

For people who are likely to be a member of a family with familial CM, referral to a genetics clinic may be appropriate. These clinics are practiced in helping family members understand the consequences of genetic testing and can guide each family member in making an informed decision about whether or not to undergo testing [44].

Medical management of cavernous malformations

A term that has been applied to CMs is "expectant management". This strategy encompasses regular clinical follow-up to evaluate for new signs and symptoms and sequential MRIs to assess for CM evolution [45]. This approach is indicated for patients with multiple and surgically inaccessible CMs.

For a patient with a single surgically accessible CM, especially one that has been symptomatic, resection should be considered early in the course as it can be "curative" [5,46–48]. Younger patients with accessible lesions and no significant co-morbid conditions are typically the best candidates for resection. The decision between resecting and following long-term a CM that is surgically accessible needs to involve balancing the surgical risks against the likelihood of the CM becoming symptomatic along with the psychological burden incurred by the patient who may be troubled by the thought that there is a brain lesion that could become symptomatic at any time. Deciding against the operation can result in decades of follow-up with an ever-present risk that the CM could become symptomatic [5].

For patients with multiple CMs, surgery is usually not a curative option. In such patients a symptomatic, surgically accessible CM can be considered for resection but typically the asymptomatic lesions are left in place [8]. In these patients the remaining CMs should be monitored over the long term even after the symptomatic lesion is surgically removed and symptoms resolve.

Medical management is the mainstay of treatment in patients with multiple CMs or single CMs where surgical treatment is not feasible due to location or patient choice. Unfortunately, there are no available randomized controlled trial data to guide us with most of the basic medical management issues. The following medical management recommendations are largely based on expert opinion. In many situations, the usual standards of care apply with special modifications taking into account the pathological features of CMs, particularly their hemorrhagic and epileptogenic propensities.

Frequency of follow-up examinations and neuroimaging

There are no formal guidelines for the timing of examination or imaging follow-up [49]. A rational strategy consists of annual complete neurological examinations and MRI scans with appropriate sequences (including T2-GRE) for initial follow-up [1,41]. If symptoms occur in the interim, an urgent evaluation may be indicated. After a CM becomes symptomatic, more frequent evaluations, perhaps every 3 to 6 months or more often should be considered. If the CM remains stable and no new lesions are found on MRI over several years, it is reasonable to extend the interval between MRIs, but not to stop neuroimaging altogether. Serial (e.g. annual) neurological examinations should be continued indefinitely.

Large-scale, prospective trials are needed to clarify treatment outcomes and allow formulation of medical management guidelines. This effort may be aided by a recent attempt to standardize definitions of CNS hemorrhage [50]. Similarly, it is important that there is a standardized approach to MRI reporting of CMs including lesion size, location, imaging parameters, associated vascular anomalies, and chronological changes. The goal of standardized systems for defining and reporting CMs is to develop a valid evidence base to guide CM management.

Hemorrhage risk factors

Almost all care providers of people with CM recommend avoidance of agents that interfere with the coagulation cascade or platelet function. Thus, warfarin (Coumadin, others), heparin (and its various analogs and derivatives), aspirin, and non-steroidal anti-inflammatory drugs (NSAIDs) are universally discouraged, although not necessarily contraindicated in all circumstances (see below). In addition, alcohol, due to its antiplatelet effect, should be minimized or avoided.

Seizure risk factors

Activities and medications that lower the seizure threshold should be minimized in patients with CMs located within the cerebral hemispheres whether or not they have epilepsy. Patients with cerebral CMs should be advised to avoid excessive stressors, both physical and emotional. The physical stressors to avoid include over-tired states, excessive (or any) alcohol consumption, and illegal drug use (especially cocaine and other vasoactive and activating agents). When ill, especially with fever (which in some people substantially lowers the seizure threshold), around the clock acetaminophen for 1–3 days should be considered. (Aspirin and NSAIDs should be avoided due to their antiplatelet properties.)

Patients with CMs and epilepsy should be treated with the spectrum of anti-epileptic drugs (AEDs) used for focal seizures. Choosing a specific drug is beyond the scope of this discussion. When a patient's seizures are refractory to medication it is important to reassess medication compliance, dosing, and possible drug interactions [51].

In patients with medically refractory epilepsy, surgical excision of the causative CM results in seizure control, with or without ongoing AEDs, in the majority (50–91%) [5,48]. The probability of achieving seizure control is highest if all grossly abnormal brain tissue surrounding the CM is resected. Resection of noncontiguous epileptogenic tissue should only be undertaken if patients have severe refractory epilepsy or if previous lesionectomy was unsuccessful in managing symptoms [8].

Headache and other pain syndromes

The safest analgesic in patients with CM is acetaminophen. Narcotics do not have added risks in patients with CM, but there is always the concern of iatrogenic addiction in all patients given narcotics. Aspirin and non-steroidal anti-inflammatory drugs (NSAIDs) possibly increase the risk of hemorrhage given that they cause impaired platelet function [52]. Tramadol lowers the seizure threshold and should not be used in patients with cerebral CMs. The Cox-2 inhibiters, such as celecoxib, have unknown risks and benefits in CM. Theoretically Cox-2 inhibitors should be safe from the standpoint of hemorrhage risk and probably should be used before NSAIDs if necessary.

Acute migraine treatment with triptans and ergots probably has low risk. These agents act on serotonin and adrenergic receptors especially in smooth muscle to produce vasoconstriction and other effects [53]. Since smooth muscle is not present in CMs and given that CMs are relatively isolated from arterial hemodynamic changes, there is likely little effect of these agents on the CMs. However, the influence of these drugs on CMs through effects on the associated venous circulation and on receptors within the CM

not associated with muscle is not known. The authors know of numerous patients with CM and severe migraine headaches treated with oral, intranasal, and injectable forms of triptans without incident.

Treatment with migraine prophylactic drugs should be considered for those with frequent or severe headaches and can include beta and calcium channel blockers, antidepressants, antiepileptic drugs, and the wide variety of less frequently used migraine prophylactic agents. The antidepressants that have a greater tendency to lower seizure threshold, including bupropion and amitriptyline, should be avoided in patients with cerebral CMs, if possible. Valproic acid is generally safe as long as the patient does not develop decreases in fibrinogen or platelet levels that sometimes occur with this drug. If valproic acid is used, fibrinogen and platelet levels should be periodically monitored especially shortly after initiating therapy.

Neuropathic-mediated chronic pain can be successfully treated in some patients with certain AEDs, including carbamazepine, gabapentin, topiramate, and pregabalin. These drugs have no special concerns in patients with CM. Low-dose tricyclic antidepressants can also be effective but the precautions inherent from the seizure threshold-lowering effect, especially of amitriptyline, need to be considered.

Other co-morbid conditions

Medical management of other conditions in CM patients should take into account the heightened risk of hemorrhage and seizures. As discussed above, anticoagulant and anti-platelet drugs should be avoided if possible. Drugs that lower the seizure threshold should be avoided in patients with CMs in their cerebral hemispheres [54]. A suggested list of drugs to avoid is provided in Table 8.1. None of these medications is absolutely contraindicated.

Difficult medical management decisions

See Chapter 19.

Potentially beneficial medications

There is no known medical therapy that decreases the likelihood of symptomatic transformation or impedes the development of CMs. It is not known whether drugs with pro-thrombotic properties such as estrogens and Cox-2 inhibitors, which slightly increase the risk of

Table 8.1 Suggested drugs to avoid in people with cavernous malformations

Category	Examples
Anticoagulants	Warfarin, heparin and its analogs and derivatives
Anti-platelet agents	Aspirin, NSAIDs, clopidogrel, ticlopidine, cilostazol, dipyridamole and others
Seizure threshold-lowering medications	Fluoroquinolone antibiotics (ciprofloxacin, norfloxacin, levofloxacin, moxifloxacin, others) Tramadol Bupropion, amitriptyline Clozapine Diphenhydramine many others
Alcohol	(due to antiplatelet and seizure threshold-lowering effects)
Cocaine and other activating agents	(due to vasoactive and seizure threshold-lowering effects)

NSAIDs, non-steroidal anti-inflammatory drugs.

myocardial infarction and stroke in the general population, are paradoxically beneficial in people with CMs.

Although hereditary hemorrhagic telangiectasia (HHT), also known as Osler-Weber-Rendu syndrome, is clearly a different disease than CM, the presence of angiogenesis and recurrent hemorrhage in both conditions suggests that overlapping therapies may eventually be discovered. Thus, it is reasonable to note the therapies that have potential for success in HHT. HHT is an autosomal dominant disease with localized angiogenesis leading to formation of telangiectasias and arteriovenous malformations in many locations including the nose, mouth, skin, conjunctivae, gastrointestinal tract, liver, lungs, and brain. Recurrent epistaxis and gastrointestinal blood loss causing anemia are common symptoms and offer a readily accessible means of measuring therapy outcomes.

Numerous medical therapies have been attempted in HHT. There are case reports, case series, and small randomized studies that have indicated positive responses to a variety of treatments in HHT. Favorable results in HHT have been reported with a variety of hormones including combinations of estrogen, testosterone, progesterone and the anti-estrogen, tamoxifen [55–58]. Similarly, positive results in HHT have also been reported with the anti-fibrinolytic agents aminocaproic acid and tranexamic acid [59,60] and the anti-angiogenic agents, thalidomide and bevacizumab (a vascular endothelial growth factor (VEGF) inhibitor) [61,62]. There is a single case report of involution of HHT after 12 months of treatment with alpha-interferon for hepatitis

C infection [63]. At this time, however, none of these therapies is proven or standard for HHT, but many deserve further study. It is reasonable to contemplate that eventually similar studies can be considered for CM although assessing outcomes is more difficult in CM than HHT.

It has recently been proposed that lipid-lowering drugs in the statin class may be beneficial in CM. In a mouse model with a mutation in the CCM2 gene homolog, simvastatin prevented endothelial cell barrier disruption, presumably by inhibiting the Rho GTPase signaling pathway, which is known to be activated by the CCM2 mutation [64]. Similarly, other Rho-kinase inhibitors including fasudil, which moderates angiogenesis and vascular abnormalities in a number of animal models, have been proposed as a potential treatment for CM [65]. However, none of these drugs has undergone human trials in CM.

Assuming a treatment has benefits in humans based on theoretical or animal data is fraught with peril. Some patients with CM may feel desperate and encourage well-meaning physicians to institute therapies based on theory or animal data. The authors strongly recommend that patients with CM not be treated with any of these agents as a primary treatment for CM until data from appropriately performed randomized controlled trials are available. Patients with CM can be encouraged to seek out such trials.

The conclusion must be that there are no proven beneficial drug treatments for CM at this time. However, use of approved drugs including estrogens,

Cox-2 inhibitors, and statins in patients with CM who have appropriate indications based on other co-morbid conditions is reasonable. There is no reason to suspect that these drugs carry elevated risks in patients with CM beyond those that are present in the general population.

Pregnancy

CMs occur in women with childbearing potential, making management in pregnancy an important issue. The two major areas of concern are the effects of pregnancy on CMs and the implications of the mother's condition on the child.

Controversy exists regarding the effects of pregnancy on CMs. There are case reports associating enlargement of CMs, symptomatic hemorrhage, and increased frequency of seizures in pregnant patients with CMs [48,66]. The hormonal state present in pregnancy promoting vascular endothelial proliferation has been proposed as a potential mechanism to explain an increased risk of hemorrhage in CMs during pregnancy [48]. Proliferation of the brittle and immature endothelium of CM vessels may result in a "leakier" CM with greater propensity to bleed and enlarge. Micro or macro-hemorrhages could also result in seizures. However, in the authors' experience, most CMs do not change during pregnancy.

Given that there is a potential risk of symptomatic transformation of CMs during pregnancy a woman with a CM in a surgically amenable location may opt to have it removed prior to a planned pregnancy [1]. Prior to a planned pregnancy, an MRI should be performed, even if the patient has been asymptomatic, as a baseline study [41]. The behavior of CMs during pregnancy and the post-partum period needs further systematic research before we can best advise women considering pregnancy [67].

The effects of the mother's condition on the child relates to heredity and teratogenicity. Almost all people with multiple CMs and some with single CMs have a causative gene mutation. The three known CM genes are autosomal dominant but penetrance is incomplete and the exact hereditary risk is unknown although it is likely close to 50% [29]. If either potential parent has CM the possibility that a heritable mutation is present and may be passed to the child may influence decisions regarding pregnancy. Discussion with a genetics counselor and perhaps gene testing prior to conception may be valuable. Patients can be advised about the possibility of using in vitro fertilization with pre-implantation genetic testing and implantation of only non-affected blastocysts if the patient does not want to risk passing on the mutated gene [68]. However, this is a costly approach that limits availability to many.

Females of childbearing potential with both CM and epilepsy require special consideration. The choice of AEDs in this situation is complex and is based on both epilepsy and teratogenic considerations. The teratogenic potential of the newer AEDs is not completely known. All of the older AEDs carry a substantial risk of teratogenicity. The teratogenic risks need to be balanced against the risks to mother and fetus incurred by repeated seizures. Generally, if a woman has an unplanned pregnancy the AEDs should not be altered because of the increased risk of seizures during AED changes, which outweigh the risk of teratogenicity. Additionally, the teratogenic risk is likely to be present only in the early first trimester before the pregnancy is recognized.

Prior to a planned pregnancy, the AED choice has numerous caveats. Polytherapy should be avoided if possible in women of reproductive age and all drugs should be given at the lowest effective dose. During pregnancy absolute dosages of many AEDs need to be increased to maintain effective AED levels due to increased clearance [69]. Currently lamotrigine is often considered a good AED option during pregnancy as it is effective in a broad range of seizure types and thus far has low teratogenic potential. However, lamotrigine needs to be initiated slowly (over months due to the risk of severe rash) and, during pregnancy, lamotrigine levels need to be frequently monitored (monthly or more). Lamotrigine doses often have to be increased by a factor of two or more because of substantially increased lamotrigine clearance during pregnancy.

Recommendations for activity restrictions in patients with CMs

Tables 8.2 and 8.3 give the authors' perspective about behaviors that probably do not and those that potentially do increase the risk of hemorrhage of CMs. These restrictions are adapted from the Angioma Alliance (www.angiomaalliance.com). The rationale for these positions is also given below.

Flying

Modern aircraft, when at cruising altitudes of 30,000 or more feet above sea level, are pressurized to the equivalent pressure of about 7000 feet above sea level (which is a few hundred feet lower than Mexico City). At lower flying altitudes, the cabin pressurization may be higher and closer to that at sea level. The United States Federal Aviation Administration (FAA) regulations require that commercial airlines be pressurized to a pressure no lower than that present at 8000 feet above sea level. During normal commercial flights the pressure changes are gradual (but not as gradual as driving or walking up a mountain). Flying in modern aircraft in a major commercial airline probably poses minimal risk for people with CMs (as long as there is not a depressurization incident during the flight, which is rare). However, there are a few anecdotal reports of CMs becoming symptomatic during a flight or within a few days after flying; it is unknown whether these events are coincidental or in some way related to flying.

Other activities with probable little risk

Moderate exercise (including sexual intercourse) and straining during a bowel movement (Valsalva maneuver) cause minimal physiological effects and thus are not likely to pose a significant risk for people with CMs.

Table 8.2 Situations with unknown but probably minimal risks in people with CMs

Flying on commercial airlines
Moderate exercise (jogging, dancing, hiking, golf, bowling, etc.)
Valsalva maneuver – moderate (e.g. straining during a bowel movement)
Sexual intercourse

Extreme mountain climbing

Mountain climbing to extreme altitudes (e.g. above 8000 feet) and smoking are two activities that can result in relative hypoxia. With mountain climbing there is also a risk of acute mountain sickness with cerebral edema at high elevations. Although there is no direct evidence that CMs worsen with hypoxia, there is ample evidence that hypoxia causes physiological changes, including changes in vascular endothelial growth factor (VEGF), which is important in angiogenesis and regulation of vascular permeability and thus could potentially activate CM changes [70].

The amount of oxygen available from the air falls with elevation. Although air at high altitude still contains 21% oxygen, the lower barometric pressure results in less available oxygen. Hyperventilation is expected at high altitude, reducing carbon dioxide and resulting in a respiratory alkalosis and nocturnal periodic breathing patterns. Altitude diuresis occurs due to osmotic center reset resulting in hemoconcentration. These and other physiological changes associated with high altitudes may pose additional risks to CM stability.

Smoking

Smoking of tobacco (and marijuana for that matter) is not good for health for many reasons. In addition to the increased risk of atherosclerosis (stroke, peripheral vascular disease, and heart attack) smoking causes relative hypoxia, limiting the amount of oxygen available to the body's cells, which potentially could promote CM worsening. Tobacco-specific chemical compounds modulate the expression of large numbers

Table 8.3 Situations that possibly pose increased risk for people with CMs

Extreme mountain climbing (e.g. above 10,000 feet)
Smoking (tobacco and marijuana)
Water activities – unaccompanied (if seizures present or with cerebral CMs)
Scuba diving
Contact sports (due to risk of head trauma – boxing, tackle football, soccer, etc.)
Strenuous exercise (aggressive aerobic, power weightlifting); extreme Valsalva maneuver
Upside-down / inverted position
Skydiving; spelunking (caving); hang-gliding; surfing; windsurfing; solo private airplane flying – (if seizures present or with cerebral CMs)

of genes and nicotine has pro-angiogenic effects which may increase CM pathology.

Water activities

Swimming and other activities in water are not intrinsically more dangerous for someone with CM. However, if concurrent epilepsy is present, or if there is a cerebral CM placing the patient at increased risk for seizures, caution with water activities is advised. Having a seizure while in water can be fatal. People with active epilepsy should never be in water unless they are continuously directly observed by someone capable of moving them to safety in the event of a seizure. This includes taking baths (showers are safe as long as the drain works adequately and there is no accumulation of water in the tub).

Scuba diving

People with active epilepsy should not participate in scuba diving. Even those with longstanding fully controlled epilepsy are at increased risk while scuba diving. In part this risk is due to the use of sedative drugs, which include most of the AEDs. Sedation can cause nitrogen narcosis at unexpectedly shallow depths, which can lead to death, or require diving companions to participate in a rescue subjecting all involved to risks from an excessively rapid ascent.

Scuba diving may pose additional potential risks to people with CMs given the dramatic pressure and physiological changes.

Contact sports

It is not definitively known whether people with CMs are at greater risk from head injury compared to healthy controls. However, it makes sense that people with CMs should avoid activities that substantially increase the risk of head injury. These activities include the sports of boxing, tackle football, soccer, downhill skiing, aggressive biking, etc. The major risk from soccer is incurred in heading the ball; it is probably reasonably safe to play soccer as long as the person never heads the ball.

Caution should be taken with other sports where head injury can occur but is less likely. Helmets should be worn with any activity involving high speeds or heights including biking, baseball (when batting or running the bases), field hockey, lacrosse, horseback riding, climbing, skiing, snowboarding, skating, skateboarding, rollerblading, etc.

Strenuous exercise (aggressive aerobic, power weight lifting), extreme Valsalva maneuver

Strenuous exercising, power weightlifting and extreme Valsalva maneuvers with strong forcible exhalation against a closed airway can result in impaired central venous return causing a variety of physiological effects including elevated peripheral venous pressures especially in the valveless cerebrospinal venous system. Although there are no data that prove that CMs are at increased risk for hemorrhage or expansion with increased venous pressure, the authors have cared for patients who developed acute-onset symptoms associated with extreme Valsalva maneuvers. Sneezing against a closed glottis and violent coughing may also produce spike elevations in venous pressure. Patients with spinal and brainstem CMs may be particularly at risk for hemorrhage during these activities.

Hanging upside-down / inverted position

The upside-down position similarly results in decreased blood return from the cerebrospinal venous system with corresponding increased venous pressure. It seems careless to take a chance as the inverted position is rarely necessary. Usually the upside-down position involves children at play hanging on bars or floor inversion during specialized exercises. Thus, since these activities are not necessary, we recommend that people with CMs do not spend substantial periods of time (or any time) inverted.

Other potentially risky activities

The risk to people with CMs posed by skydiving, spelunking (caving), hang-gliding, surfing, windsurfing, solo private airplane flying, etc. relates to the possibility of having a seizure while involved in these activities. If epilepsy and cerebral CMs are not present, these activities probably do not need to be restricted.

Psychosocial aspects of CMs

The psychosocial impact of a diagnosis of a cavernous malformation must not be ignored. While the annual risk of hemorrhage is relatively low, the cumulative risk over several decades is not negligible and many patients suffer from a feeling of impending doom [5]. Patients with multiple CMs or a single CM in an inoperable location especially may experience significant fear and anxiety. This anxiety may further increase as new imaging methods (such as higher-field-strength MRIs and GRE and SWI sequences) show CMs for the first time that were not visualized on prior MRIs, requiring careful presentation of imaging results to patients [37,38,41]. Patients suffering substantial distress from worry related to CMs may benefit from counseling and other support systems such as the Angioma Alliance community forum available at: www.angiomaalliance.org.

References

1. Raychaudhuri, R., Batjer, H. H. & Awad, I. A. Intracranial cavernous angioma: a practical review of clinical and biological aspects. *Surg Neurol* 2005;**63**:319–328; discussion 328.

2. Kim, D. S., Park, Y. G., Choi, J. U., Chung, S. S. & Lee, K. C. An analysis of the natural history of cavernous malformations. *Surg Neurol* 1997;**48**:9–17; discussion 17–18.

3. Otten, P., Pizzolato, G. P., Rilliet, B. & Berney, J. 131 cases of cavernous angioma (cavernomas) of the CNS, discovered by retrospective analysis of 24,535 autopsies. [A propos de 131 cas d'angiomes caverneux (cavernomes) du s.n.c., reperes par l'analyse retrospective de 24 535 autopsies.] *Neuro-Chirurgie* 1989;**35**:82–83, 128–131.

4. Wong, J. H., Awad, I. A. & Kim, J. H. Ultrastructural pathological features of cerebrovascular malformations: A preliminary report. *Neurosurgery* 2000;**46**:1454–1459.

5. Maraire, J. N. & Awad, I. A. Intracranial cavernous malformations: Lesion behavior and management strategies. *Neurosurgery* 1995;**37**:591–605.

6. Labauge, P., Denier, C., Bergametti, F. & Tournier-Lasserve, E. Genetics of cavernous angiomas. *Lancet Neurol* 2007;**6**:237–244.

7. Kraemer, D. L. & Awad, I. A. Vascular malformations and epilepsy: Clinical considerations and basic mechanisms. *Epilepsia* 1994;**35**(Suppl 6):S30–43.

8. Awad, I. & Jabbour, P. Cerebral cavernous malformations and epilepsy. *Neurosurg Focus* 2006;**21**:e7.

9. Malik, S. N. & Young, W. B. Midbrain cavernous malformation causing migraine-like headache. *Cephalalgia* 2006;**26**:1016–1019.

10. Samii, M., Nakamura, M., Mirzai, S., Vorkapic, P. & Cervio, A. Cavernous angiomas within the internal auditory canal. *J Neurosurg* 2006;**105**:581–587.

11. Chicani, C. F., Miller, N. R. & Tamargo, R. J. Giant cavernous malformation of the occipital lobe. *J Neuro-Ophthalmol* 2003;**23**:151–153.

12. Hempelmann, R. G., Mater, E., Schroder, F. & Schon, R. Complete resection of a cavernous haemangioma of the optic nerve, the chiasm, and the optic tract. *Acta Neurochir* 2007;**149**:699–703; discussion 703.

13. Newman, H., Nevo, M., Constantini, S., Maimon, S. & Kesler, A. Chiasmal cavernoma: A rare cause of acute visual loss improved by prompt surgery. *Pediatr Neurosurg* 2008;**44**:414–417.

14. Chen, C. L., Leu, C. H., Jan, Y. J. & Shen, C. C. Intraventricular cavernous hemangioma at the foramen of Monro: Case report and literature review. *Clin Neurol Neurosurg* 2006;**108**:604–609.

15. Katayama, Y., Tsubokawa, T., Maeda, T. & Yamamoto, T. Surgical management of cavernous malformations of the third ventricle. *J Neurosurg* 1994;**80**:64–72.

16. Bakir, A., Savas, A., Yilmaz, E., *et al*. Spinal intradural-intramedullary cavernous malformation. Case report and literature review. *Pediatr Neurosurg* 2006;**42**:35–37.

17. Acciarri, N., Padovani, R., Giulioni, M. & Gaist, G. Surgical treatment of spinal cavernous angiomas. *J Neurosurg Sci* 1993;**37**:209–215.

18. Harrison, M. J., Eisenberg, M. B., Ullman, J. S., *et al*. Symptomatic cavernous malformations affecting the spine and spinal cord. *Neurosurgery* 1995;**37**:195–204; discussion 204–205.

19. Hauck, E. F., Barnett, S. L., White, J. A. & Samson, D. Symptomatic brainstem cavernomas. *Neurosurgery* 2009;**64**:61–70; discussion 70–71.

20. Porter, R. W., Detwiler, P. W., Spetzler, R. F., *et al*. Cavernous malformations of the brainstem: experience with 100 patients. *J Neurosurg* 1999;**90**:50–58.

21. Fritschi, J. A., Reulen, H. J., Spetzler, R. F. & Zabramski, J. M. Cavernous malformations of the brain stem. A review of 139 cases. *Acta Neurochir* 1994;**130**:35–46.

22. Kondziolka, D., Lunsford, L. D. & Kestle, J. R. The natural history of cerebral cavernous malformations. *J Neurosurg* 1995;**83**:820–824.

23. Sze, G., Krol, G., Olsen, W. L., *et al*. Hemorrhagic neoplasms: MR mimics of occult vascular malformations. *Am J Roentgenol* 1987;**149**:1223–1230.

24. Kucharczyk, W., Lemme-Pleghos, L., Uske, A., *et al*. Intracranial vascular malformations: MR and CT imaging. *Radiology* 1985;**156**:383–389.

25. Gault, J., Sarin, H., Awadallah, N. A., Shenkar, R. & Awad, I. A. Pathobiology of human cerebrovascular malformations: basic mechanisms and clinical relevance. *Neurosurgery* 2004;**55**:1–16; discussion 16–7.

26. Viswanathan, A. & Chabriat, H. Cerebral microhemorrhage. *Stroke* 2006;**37**:550–555.

27. Rigamonti, D., Drayer, B. P., Johnson, P. C., *et al.* The MRI appearance of cavernous malformations (angiomas). *J Neurosurg* 1987;**67**:518–524.

28. Del Curling, O., Jr, Kelly, D. L., Jr, Elster, A. D. & Craven, T. E. An analysis of the natural history of cavernous angiomas. *J Neurosurg* 1991;**75**:702–708.

29. Denier, C., Labauge, P., Bergametti, F., *et al.* Genotype-phenotype correlations in cerebral cavernous malformations patients. *Ann Neurol* 2006;**60**:550–556.

30. Sirvente, J., Enjolras, O., Wassef, M., Tournier-Lasserve, E. & Labauge, P. Frequency and phenotypes of cutaneous vascular malformations in a consecutive series of 417 patients with familial cerebral cavernous malformations. *J Eur Acad Dermatol* 2009;**23**:1066–1072.

31. Laberge-le Couteulx, S., Jung, H. H., Labauge, P., *et al.* Truncating mutations in CCM1, encoding KRIT1, cause hereditary cavernous angiomas. *Nat Genet* 1999;**23**:189–193.

32. Eerola, I., Plate, K. H., Spiegel, R., *et al.* KRIT1 is mutated in hyperkeratotic cutaneous capillary-venous malformation associated with cerebral capillary malformation. *Hum Mol Genet* 2000;**9**:1351–1355.

33. Toll, A., Parera, E., Gimenez-Arnau, A. M., *et al.* Cutaneous venous malformations in familial cerebral cavernomatosis caused by KRIT1 gene mutations. *Dermatology (Basel)* 2009;**218**:307–313.

34. Labauge, P., Krivosic, V., Denier, C., Tournier-Lasserve, E. & Gaudric, A. Frequency of retinal cavernomas in 60 patients with familial cerebral cavernomas: a clinical and genetic study. *Arch of Ophthalmol* 2006;**124**:885–886.

35. Lobato, R. D., Perez, C., Rivas, J. J. & Cordobes, F. Clinical, radiological, and pathological spectrum of angiographically occult intracranial vascular malformations. Analysis of 21 cases and review of the literature. *J Neurosurg* 1988;**68**:518–531.

36. Tomlinson, F. H., Houser, O. W., Scheithauer, B. W., *et al.* Angiographically occult vascular malformations: a correlative study of features on magnetic resonance imaging and histological examination. *Neurosurgery* 1994;**34**:792–799; discussion 799–800.

37. de Souza, J. M., Domingues, R. C., Cruz, L. C., Jr, *et al.* Susceptibility-weighted imaging for the evaluation of patients with familial cerebral cavernous malformations: a comparison with T2-weighted fast spin-echo and gradient-echo sequences. *American Journal of Neuroradiology* 2008;**29**:154–158.

38. Valanne, L. K., Ketonen, L. M. & Berg, M. J. Pseudoprogression of cerebral cavernous angiomas: The importance of proper magnetic resonance imaging technique. *J Neuroimaging* 1996;**6**:195–196.

39. Zabramski, J. M., Wascher, T. M., Spetzler, R. F., *et al.* The natural history of familial cavernous malformations: Results of an ongoing study. *J Neurosurg* 1994;**80**:422–432.

40. Berg, M. J., Cohn, F. S. & Ketonen, L. M. Detection of low flow blood in cerebral cavernous angiomas using tagged-RBC SPECT. *Neurology* 1994;**44**(suppl 2):408.

41. Lehnhardt, F. G., von Smekal, U., Ruckriem, B., *et al.* Value of gradient-echo magnetic resonance imaging in the diagnosis of familial cerebral cavernous malformation. *Arch Neurol* 2005;**62**:653–658.

42. Department of Health and Human Services 2009. "GINA" the genetic information nondiscrimination act of 2008: information for researchers and health care professionals. Retrieved 29 June 2010 from: http://www.genome.gov/Pages/PolicyEthics/GeneticDiscrimination/GINAInfoDoc.pdf.

43. Green, R. C., Roberts, J. S., Cupples, L. A., *et al.* Disclosure of APOE genotype for risk of Alzheimer's disease. *New Engl J Med* 2009;**361**:245–254.

44. Julian-Reynier, C., Welkenhuysen, M., Hagoel, L., Decruyenaere, M., Hopwood, P., & CRISCOM Working Group. Risk communication strategies: State of the art and effectiveness in the context of cancer genetic services. *Eur J Hum Genet* 2003;**11**:725–736.

45. Tarnaris, A., Fernandes, R. P. & Kitchen, N. D. Does conservative management for brain stem cavernomas have better long-term outcome? *Brit J Neurosurg* 2008;**22**:748–757.

46. Ojemann, R. G., Crowell, R. M. & Ogilvy, C. S. Management of cranial and spinal cavernous angiomas (honored guest lecture). *Clin Neurosurg* 1993;**40**:98–123.

47. LeDoux, M. S., Aronin, P. A. & Odrezin, G. T. Surgically treated cavernous angiomas of the brain stem: report of two cases and review of the literature. *Surg Neurol* 1991;**35**:395–399.

48. Robinson, J. R., Awad, I. A. & Little, J. R. Natural history of the cavernous angioma. *J Neurosurg* 1991;**75**:709–714.

49. Stapf, C. & Herve, D. From cavern-dwellers to cavernoma science: Towards a new philosophy of cerebral cavernous malformations. *Stroke* 2008;**39**:3129–3130.

50. Al-Shahi Salman, R., Berg, M. J., Morrison, L., Awad, I. A. & on behalf of the Angioma Alliance

Scientific Advisory Board. Hemorrhage from cavernous malformations of the brain: definition and reporting standards. *Stroke* 2008;**39**:3222–3230.

51. Dodick, D. W., Cascino, G. D. & Meyer, F. B. Vascular malformations and intractable epilepsy: outcome after surgical treatment. *Mayo Clin Proc* 1994;**69**:741–745.

52. Patrono, C., Baigent, C., Hirsh, J., Roth, G. & American College of Chest Physicians. Antiplatelet drugs: American college of chest physicians evidence-based clinical practice guidelines (8th edition). *Chest* 2008;**133**(6 Suppl):199S–233S.

53. Henkes, H., May, A., Kuhne, D., Berg-Dammer, E. & Diener, H. C. Sumatriptan: vasoactive effect on human dural vessels, demonstrated by subselective angiography. *Cephalalgia* 1996;**16**:224–230.

54. Pozzati, E., Zucchelli, M., Marliani, A. F. & Riccioli, L. A. Bleeding of a familial cerebral cavernous malformation after prophylactic anticoagulation therapy. case report. *Neurosurg Focus* 2006;**21**:e15.

55. Harrison, D. F. Use of estrogen in treatment of familial hemorrhagic telangiectasia. *Laryngoscope* 1982;**92**:314–320.

56. Van Cutsem, E., Rutgeerts, P., Geboes, K., Van Gompel F., & Vantrappen, G. Estrogen-progesterone treatment of Osler-Weber-Rendu disease. *J Clin Gastroenterol* 1988;**10**:676–679.

57. Vase, P. Estrogen treatment of hereditary hemorrhagic telangiectasia. A double-blind controlled clinical trial. *Acta Med Scand* 1981;**209**:393–396.

58. Yaniv, E., Preis, M., Hadar, T., Shvero, J. & Haddad, M. Antiestrogen therapy for hereditary hemorrhagic telangiectasia: a double-blind placebo-controlled clinical trial. *Laryngoscope* 2009;**119**:284–288.

59. Saba, H. I., Morelli, G. A. & Logrono, L. A. Brief report: treatment of bleeding in hereditary hemorrhagic telangiectasia with aminocaproic acid. *New Engl J Med* 1994;**330**:1789–1790.

60. Sabba, C., Pasculli, G., Cirulli, A., *et al.* Rendu-Osler-Weber disease: Experience with 56 patients. *Ann Ital Med Intern* 2002;**17**:173–179.

61. Lebrin, F., Srun, S., Raymond, K., *et al.* Thalidomide stimulates vessel maturation and reduces epistaxis in individuals with hereditary hemorrhagic telangiectasia. *Nat Med* 2010;**16**:420–428.

62. Simonds, J., Miller, F., Mandel, J. & Davidson, T. M. The effect of bevacizumab (avastin) treatment on epistaxis in hereditary hemorrhagic telangiectasia. *Laryngoscope* 2009;**119**:988–992.

63. Massoud, O. I., Youssef, W. I. & Mullen, K. D. Resolution of hereditary hemorrhagic telangiectasia and anemia with prolonged alpha-interferon therapy for chronic hepatitis C. *J Clin Gastroenterol* 2004;**38**:377–379.

64. Whitehead, K. J., Chan, A. C., Navankasattusas, S., *et al.* The cerebral cavernous malformation signaling pathway promotes vascular integrity via rho GTPases. *Nat Med* 2009;**15**:177–184.

65. Yin, L., Morishige, K., Takahashi, T., *et al.* Fasudil inhibits vascular endothelial growth factor-induced angiogenesis in vitro and in vivo. *Mol Cancer Ther* 2007;**6**:1517–1525.

66. Robinson, J. R., Jr, Awad, I. A., Magdinec, M. & Paranandi, L. Factors predisposing to clinical disability in patients with cavernous malformations of the brain. *Neurosurgery* 1993;**32**:730–735; discussion 735–736.

67. Safavi-Abbasi, S., Feiz-Erfan, I., Spetzler, R. F., *et al.* Hemorrhage of cavernous malformations during pregnancy and in the peripartum period: Causal or coincidence? Case report and review of the literature. *Neurosurg Focus* 2006;**21**:e12.

68. Bick, D. P. & Lau, E. C. Preimplantation genetic diagnosis. *Pediatr Clin N Am* 2006;**53**:559–577.

69. Pennell, P. B. Antiepileptic drugs during pregnancy: what is known and which AEDs seem to be safest? *Epilepsia* 2008;**49**(Suppl 9):43–55.

70. Marti, H. M. & Risau, W. Systemic hypocis changes the organ-specific distribution of vascular endothelial growth factor and its receptors. *Proc Natl Acad Sci USA* 1998;**95**:15809–15814.

Hemorrhage: new and recurrent

Colin B. Josephson and Rustam Al-Shahi Salman

Introduction

Preceding chapters have described the clinical and radiological features of cavernous malformations (CMs), but intracerebral hemorrhage (ICH) deserves special mention, partly because it is one of the more disabling problems caused by CMs, but also because ICH from CMs can be challenging to define, study, and quantify.

The supporting angioarchitecture in CMs is fragile and prone to hemorrhage [1]. Genetic studies of families in which CMs are inherited have identified three genes (CCM1 [encoding KRIT1], CCM2 [encoding OSM], and CCM3 [encoding PDCD10]) that appear to function as cytoskeletal scaffolding and adaptor proteins [2,3]. Immunohistochemical staining of human tissue has demonstrated that KRIT1 localizes to cerebral endothelium and the surrounding astrocytic foot processes and forms intracellular complexes with OSM and PDCD10 [3,4]. Disruption of this complex may result in failed lumen formation, disordered structure of the junctions between endothelial and neighboring cells, and impaired endothelial barrier function [5]. This compromises the blood–brain barrier and leads to chronic leakage of erythrocytes [6;7].

Although all CMs are characterized by surrounding hemosiderin deposition, their varied clinical manifestations – from being asymptomatic (estimated to affect 0.2–0.4% of the population [8;9]) to causing severe, disabling ICH – suggest that some CMs are intrinsically more likely to bleed than others.

The challenge of understanding hemorrhage from cavernous malformations

Reliable identification of an ICH is important for patients, clinicians, and researchers, but there are challenges. The main impediments to satisfactorily studying CMs, and thereby informing clinical practice, are their biological behavior, the diversity of their clinical manifestations, and the need for careful radiological investigation to detect both CMs following ICH as well as ICH following the diagnosis of a CM.

CMs are, by their nature, challenging to study

From an epidemiological point of view, the onset of disease, or inception point is unclear for CMs: they develop *de novo* over the course of an individual's lifetime, irrespective of whether they are inherited [10,11], appear to occur sporadically [12–19], or emerge following prior intracranial irradiation [20]. This makes the study of the risk of a first ICH difficult to establish, which seems to be the biggest question about CMs given the prevalence of asymptomatic CMs. Secondly, identifying the predictors of first ICH, and disentangling the predictors of recurrent ICH in the smaller population of people with symptomatic CMs, is complicated by the infrequency of symptomatic CMs, such that the overall statistical power of individual studies is limited by small sample sizes.

Research is inevitably biased by the vagaries of clinical practice

Some CMs presenting with an ICH will be obscured by the index bleed on computed tomography (CT) or magnetic resonance imaging (MRI) thus preventing the diagnosis of the underlying lesion unless delayed MRI is performed. The radiological investigation for a cause underlying ICH appears to be targeted at younger, normotensive patients in everyday European practice [21]. Older, hypertensive patients and patients

---

Cavernous Malformations of the Nervous System, ed. Daniele Rigamonti. Published by Cambridge University Press.
© Cambridge University Press 2011.

with more benign clinical courses may therefore be less likely to undergo the sometimes extensive investigation required to diagnose an underlying CM. Patients reporting non-focal clinical symptoms such as a headache or a generalized seizure, which might be due to ICH from a CM, do not always undergo brain imaging in everyday practice whether or not a CM diagnosis has already been established. In the absence of acute neurological deficits or coma, we have not delineated specific features, if any, of headaches and seizures that may be suggestive of an acute ICH. Investigation bias may lead to underestimation of the long-term risk of ICH because physicians may not further investigate episodes of minor or transient symptoms, such as a headache or focal sensory symptoms, if there is a known CM that is being conservatively managed. Reporting bias may also arise for patients who have opted for conservative treatment, who may refrain from presenting to medical attention for minor symptoms that may actually reflect a small but clinically symptomatic ICH.

The detection of CMs, and ICH due to them, is dependent on obtaining the right imaging modality at the right time

Unless new neurological symptoms are investigated swiftly with CT then the detection of ICH may be missed if MRI is not performed. This may have led to an underestimation of the risk of ICH in older studies, conducted when the availability and use of MRI was less widespread and before the development of hemosiderin-sensitive MRI sequences. Even when MRI is available, recognition of an old ICH on MRI can be difficult because the parenchyma surrounding a CM already contains blood products of different ages due to the chronic extravasation of erythrocytes. An ICH can partially or completely obscure a CM on MRI, and because ICH may take months to regress repeat scanning is often essential to reveal the underlying CM as a cause of the ICH [22]. Imaging may be difficult to interpret as evidence of a recent ICH, a change in CM size with no evidence of a recent hemorrhage, or a change in the signal characteristics [15] may all be seen on scans performed in response to a new or worsened focal neurological deficit (FND).

Furthermore, acute blood products in a CM may also be found incidentally on brain imaging [23], which seems to mandate a definition of ICH that requires both new clinical symptoms and new blood of the appropriate age on brain imaging.

The need for a definition of hemorrhage from a cavernous malformation

A systematic review of the literature identified 15 publications including at least 20 participants with follow-up data on ICH from familial or sporadic CMs [24]. There was variation in the detail and characteristics of the definitions of ICH, which ranged from unclear to explicit. One-quarter of the studies did not require clinical symptoms to accompany radiographic evidence of acute or subacute hemorrhage. Not all studies indicated the imaging modalities used to identify ICH and confirmation using relevant MRI sequences was not universally required. Examining both the consistency and variation between studies has helped identify clinical and radiological aspects of an ICH from a CM that require formal definition.

The Angioma Alliance definition of CM hemorrhage

A consensus statement on the clinical and imaging features of ICH from CMs was developed at a scientific workshop of the Angioma Alliance (Table 9.1). Clinical manifestations of ICH due to CMs include new focal neurological symptoms, or exacerbations of known deficits, that are anatomically referable to the site of the CM [24]. Conditions mimicking deficits attributed to the CM should be considered (Fig. 9.1): a detailed history is required to elicit features suggestive of a postictal Todd's paresis or migrainous aura. Describing the duration of symptoms as transient (<24 hours), persistent (>24 hours), or progressive can help categorize their severity and might help identify the mechanisms underlying them in future research studies [24].

The radiological evidence of new ICH that should accompany these symptoms is either new increased density on CT or met-hemoglobin or deoxyhemoglobin on MRI (Fig. 9.2) [25,26]. Ideally, a CT scan should be performed within a week of symptom onset [27], have a Hounsfield value consistent with acute blood, and demonstrate either interval change from a prior CT scan or resolution on a subsequent scan performed at least two weeks later [24]. An MRI performed within 2 weeks of the onset of symptoms may demonstrate the presence of met-hemoglobin or increasing signal dropout on gradient-recalled echo (GRE/T2*) sequences. The MRI signal abnormalities should be new when compared to prior scans and may evolve after 2 months.

Table 9.1 Angioma Alliance definition of a symptomatic hemorrhage in patients with a cavernous malformation of the brain [25]

1. A clinical event that satisfies the following criteria:
   a. Acute or subacute onset
   b. A new or worsened focal neurological deficit that can be anatomically referred to the site of the CM or symptoms indicative of an ICH (headache, seizure, impaired consciousness)

2. Objective evidence of a hemorrhage in the form of one of the following:
   a. Radiological evidence on MRI or CT
   b. Evidence of hemorrhage on surgical exposure
   c. Evidence of hemorrhage on pathological examination
   d. Evidence of hemorrhage on CSF examination (in very rare cases)

The presence of a hemosiderin halo or a change in the volume of a known CM is not sufficient in the absence of the above criteria.

MRI is advantageous because the imaging characteristics of the ICH last for longer than CT and change according to the stage of ICH evolution (Table 9.2). The physics behind this is complex and relies primarily on a combination of the ferromagnetic properties of iron and the integrity of the red cell membrane [28]. Initially, the erythrocyte membrane remains intact during the hyperacute stage of ICH. Oxygen remains bound to hemoglobin in a diamagnetic state and signal changes seen on T1 and T2 sequences are related to the increased spin density of the ICH compared to uninvolved brain tissue (Table 9.2). Within hours of the ICH, deoxyhemoglobin begins to form first at the periphery of the bleed and extends inwards towards the core. This appears as a thin rim of T2 hyperintensity that can be useful in distinguishing acute ICH from other pathological entities [29–31]. Deoxyhemoglobin is eventually converted into met-hemoglobin, causing a hyperintense signal on T1 and hypotense signal on T2 that is visualized in the early subacute period of the bleed. The red cell membranes eventually rupture and release met-hemoglobin into the surrounding interstitium during the late subacute phase resulting in a hyperintense appearance on both T1 and T2 [32]. Ferric iron is eventually liberated from met-hemoglobin following proteolysis and is engulfed by scavenging macrophages. It is then recycled into ferritin or concentrated within hemosiderin molecules causing T1 and T2 hypointensity [32]. The GRE sequence is an improvement on conventional parameters because it produces "signal drop-out" that is most pronounced in the hyperacute stage due to sequestering of iron within erythrocytes and during the chronic stages of ICH due to recycling and storage of iron within macrophages [33,34].

When brain imaging has not been performed, or is inconclusive, the Angioma Alliance definition allows acute ICH to be objectively confirmed on surgical exposure or pathological examination. Cerebrospinal fluid (CSF) can occasionally be of value if the CM is located close to or has bled towards the pial surface. In these circumstances, the CSF must be heavily and uniformly blood-stained or there should be evidence of either visible xanthochromia or, preferably, bilirubin on spectrophotometry [24].

Occasionally ancillary tests are not performed in response to focal neurological deficits (FND), or the modality and timing of these tests may conspire to leave uncertainty about whether ICH caused a patient's symptoms. In these circumstances, the episode should be labeled as an FND rather than a presumed ICH. An event is considered to be a non-hemorrhagic FND only if brain imaging has ruled out ICH.

The Angioma Alliance definition is designed to improve clinical practice and research design. The definition offers a clear algorithmic approach to the distinction of ICH, FND, and other symptoms (Figs. 9.1 and 9.2). This definition does not place any restrictions on the location of the new blood products on brain imaging, so long as they are present. CMs may change over time [15] and therefore a simple increase in CM size without concurrent evidence of new blood products on CT or MRI does not constitute radiological evidence of an acute ICH.

The definition encourages use of standard measures of impairment (the National Institutes of Health

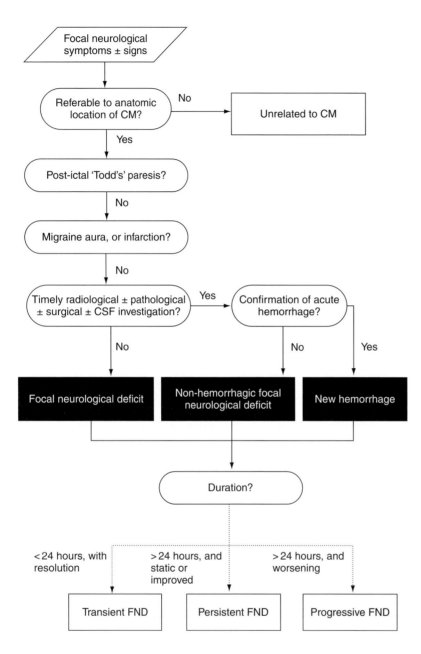

Figure 9.1. Algorithm for classifying focal neurological events (from Al-Shahi Salman et al., *Stroke* 2008 [24]).

Stroke Scale [36]), disability/handicap (the modified Rankin Scale [37]), and health-related quality of life (Short Form 12 or 36 or EQ–5D) at fixed time intervals following clinical presentation to give a measure of the effects on function; after all, a progressive FND causing a hemiparesis may have more impact on function than an ICH causing facial weakness. The pathophysiology of apparently non-hemorrhagic focal neurological deficits remains elusive, and their identification by the Angioma Alliance definition will facilitate their further study using higher magnet field strengths and different sequences such as susceptibility-weighted imaging and functional MRI [38–40]. Ultimately, more robust estimates of CM natural history and the prognosis for ICH will be facilitated by studies using consistent definitions.

Table 9.2 Characteristics of intracerebral hemorrhage on magnetic resonance imaging

	Hyperacute (<24 hrs)	Acute (1–3 days)	Early subacute (>3 days)	Late subacute (>7 days)	Chronic (>14 days)
T1W [33]	↔/↑	↔/↓	↑	↑	↔/↓
T2W [33]	↔/↑	↓	↓	↑	↓
Diffusion-weighted [36]	↑ & ↓	↓	↓	↑	↓

T1W = T1-weighted MRI; T2W = T2-weighted MRI; ↑ = hyperintense; ↔ = isointense; ↓ = hypointense.

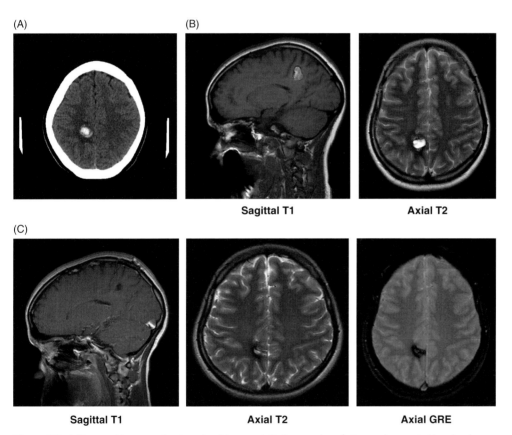

Sagittal T1   Axial T2

Sagittal T1   Axial T2   Axial GRE

Figure 9.2. A 21-year-old woman developed sudden-onset dizziness and confusion, and presented to a local emergency department where a same-day CT scan of the brain (A) revealed a right fronto-parietal intracerebral hemorrhage. A follow-up MRI scan 3 months later (B) revealed residual blood products. An MRI scan 12 months following presentation (C) revealed a cavernous malformation. T1 = T1 spin-echo sequence; T2 = T2 spin-echo sequence; GRE = gradient-recalled echo sequence.

Risk of hemorrhage from CMs

At the end of 2009 we systematically reviewed Ovid Medline (from 1966), Embase (from 1980), and the Cochrane Library for studies containing 20 or more adults with a diagnosis of a CM that used objective clinical outcomes to address the untreated clinical course of CMs (Table 9.3). We excluded any study that analyzed risk of ICH from the time of each patient's birth, because the assumption that CMs are congenital is potentially erroneous.

Table 9.3 Studies of the untreated clinical course of ≥20 participants with CMs (listed chronologically)

Study	Selection criteria	Patient source	Sample size	Mean duration of follow-up Years (range)	First hemorrhage rate % / year (95% CI)	Re-hemorrhage rate % / year (95% CI)
Robinson et al. [45]	–	1 hospital	66	2.2	0.7 (0.1 to 3.9)	
Zabramski et al. [10]	Familial	1 neurosurgery unit	21	2.2	6.5 (2.2 to 17.5)	
Fritschi et al. [43]	Brainstem	2 neurosurgery units + literature	41+98	2.5	–	21 (15.8 to 27.1)
Kondziolka et al. [46]	Conservative	1 neurosurgery unit	122	2.8	0.6	4.5
Aiba et al. [25]	–	1 neurosurgery unit	110	4.7	0.4 (0.1 to 2.2)	22.9
Kim et al. [64]	–	1 hospital	62	1.9	–	3.8
Porter et al. [41]	–	1 CM service	110	3.8	1.6 (0.8 to 3.3)	
Porter et al. [26]	Brainstem	1 neurosurgery unit	100	2	–	30.2 (25.2 to 35.9)
Moriarity et al. [44]	-	1 neurosurgery unit	68	5.2	3.1 (1.7 to 5.5)	
Labauge et al. [23]	Familial	Multicenter	33	2.1	4.3 (1.5 to 11.9)	–
Barker et al. [47]	Bled at presentation	1 neurosurgery unit	136	3.8	–	11.7 (9.3 to 14.7)
Kupersmith et al. [50]	Brainstem	1 clinic in neuro-ophthalmology	37	4.9	?	?
Hasegawa et al. [63]	Brainstem; bled at presentation	1 radiosurgery unit	83	4.3	–	33.9 (29.2 to 39.0)

Critical appraisal

Estimation of the risks of first or recurrent ICH due to CMs is limited by the short durations of follow-up and inconsistent definitions of ICH in the published studies [24]. All the published studies of outcome were based at large referral centers. Hospital-based studies can be limited by bias due to institution-specific rates of referral, investigation, and follow-up. Prospective population-based studies are ideal;

however, a precise evaluation of hemorrhagic events is difficult even in this setting because of the idiosyncrasies of local clinical practice. Furthermore, the period at risk in past studies has been variously calculated from the start of prospective follow-up or from first hemorrhage, which limits direct comparisons between certain studies. The findings may not be able to be generalized due to selection bias as the majority of participants were recruited from tertiary-care referral centers. No study attempted to assess clinical outcome blinded to prognostic features of interest. Some studies specified their working definition of a symptomatic hemorrhage [8,23,25,26,41–50]. Standard measures of outcome were rarely used and annualized hemorrhage rates were generally calculated using total (rather than first) events during the entire follow-up period. Comparing studies is difficult because hazard rates were not calculated at predetermined time points. Rates were sometimes calculated per CM rather than per patient, which complicates analysis because risks are relevant to patients rather than individual CMs (and multiple CMs in the same brain are not necessarily independent of each other).

Proportion of symptomatic CMs with ICH at first presentation

The first population-based study of the detection rate of CMs was conducted in the USA between 1965 and 1992 and involved retrospective review of the medical records of all adults with an intracranial vascular malformation in Olmsted County, Minnesota [51]. A prospective, population-based study of CMs in Scotland (The Scottish Intracranial Vascular Malformation Study; SIVMS), conducted during the years 1999–2010 (incident cases were enrolled in 1999–2003 and 2006–2010 but follow-up continued uninterrupted through all 10 years), found a higher detection rate of CMs in its first two years (0.56 per 100,000 adults per year; 95% confidence interval [CI] 0.41 to 0.75) than in the Olmsted county study (0.17 per 100,000 adults per year; 95% CI 0 to 0.34) [51,52], which is unsurprising because of the recent increase in the availability and uptake of MRI. In the Olmsted county study, neither of the two incident patients with a symptomatic CM presented with ICH, whereas in the Scottish population between 1999 and 2003, 17 (23%)

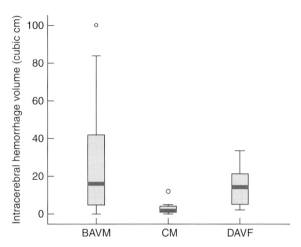

Figure 9.3. Box plot of volumes of hematomas among intracranial vascular malformations. Dark lines represent medians, boxes represent interquartile ranges, and outliers are indicated by open circles. BAVM, brain arteriovenous malformation; DAVF, dural arteriovenous fistula; CM, cavernous malformation. From Cordonnier et al., JNNP 2008 [53].

of 73 adults incident with a symptomatic CM had ICH at the time of first presentation [53].

ICHs related to CMs tend to be found in younger patients and are less debilitating (median Oxford Handicap Score [OHS] = 2, interquartile range [IQR] 2 to 3) than ICH related to arteriovenous malformations (AVMs; median OHS =3, IQR 2 to 5). Unlike AVMs, almost every bleed from a CM is purely intracerebral, and the volume of ICH due to CM is significantly smaller when compared to other IVMs, which probably explains the milder severity of ICH related to CMs (Fig. 9.3) [53].

Risk of first-ever ICH

The overall risk of developing a first-ever clinically significant ICH appears to be in the range of 0.4–0.6%/person-year over 3–5 years in patients with sporadic (solitary) CMs and no history of ICH at presentation [25,46] (Table 9.3). The rate of symptomatic ICH was slightly higher (1.4%/person-year) in a prospective cohort of 33 initially asymptomatic familial cases of CMs followed for a mean of 2.1 years [23].

Some studies have attempted to identify risk factors that increase the risk of ICH. Female sex appeared to confer a higher risk of first ever [25] and recurrent ICH [45] in retrospective studies, but not in a prospective cohort of familial CMs [10] or in cohorts that involved both retrospective and prospective follow-up [41,46]. Infratentorial lesions may confer a higher risk of future ICH (3.8%/year [95% CI 1.7 to 7.9] versus 0.4%/year [95% CI 0.1 to 2.1]) [41], but this was not reproduced in another study [44]. The number and size of CMs do not appear to increase the risk of ICH [44,45].

The risk of re-bleeding following a first hemorrhage

The risk of recurrent ICH after a first ICH in cohorts of patients with CMs in any location varied between 3.8 and 33.9% per year (Table 9.3). However, the risk of recurrent ICH appears to be much higher from brainstem CMs, ranging from 21 to 33.9% per year (Table 9.3). Other studies found that re-bleeding appears to be more common in young patients (<40 years of age) [25,47], especially in females [25].

Temporal clustering of ICHs may be a characteristic feature of CMs and may be a particularly prominent feature over the first 2 years following first-ever ICH [47,54]. If confirmed in other studies, clustering would have a major impact on how we interpret studies of therapeutic efficacy. However, as already mentioned, reporting bias may explain the apparent temporal clustering and decline in frequency of recurrent ICH over time.

Discussion

Standards for future studies

There is a clear need for further carefully designed studies of the risk of ICH from CMs (Table 9.4) [24]. Cohorts should be enrolled at a clearly defined inception point within the disease process (such as at the point of diagnosis, first ICH, second ICH or first treatment) that is consistent across all patients. Prospective population-based data collection is ideal, but if a retrospective design is unavoidable then the period of risk should not be assumed to encompass the patient's entire lifespan because the evidence that CMs are congenital is lacking and there is clear evidence of *de novo* cavernoma occurrence [10,15,23,49,55]. Comparison of studies would be easier if outcomes include objective, pre-defined clinical events (such as

Table 9.4 Ideal characteristics for studies of hemorrhage risk and outcome in patients with cavernous malformations of the brain [25]

1. Radiological or pathological certainty of the diagnosis at baseline

2. Prospective follow-up from a clearly defined point in the disease process
   a. If retrospective, the "lifetime period of risk" must not be assumed

3. Population-based

4. A sample size > 20

5. Objective, pre-defined clinical outcomes
   a. Clinical events (hemorrhage or focal neurological deficits defined according to the Angioma Alliance definition)
   b. Case fatality
   c. Clinical outcomes according to validated measures of disability

6. Outcome assessments assessed:
   a. Blinded to prognostic features of interest
   b. Stratified by treatment
   c. Quantified at specified intervals from the time of diagnosis or treatment

7. Completeness of follow-up > 90%

8. Duration of follow-up > 1 year

ICH, FND, standardized measures of disability, and death). Risk factors that are of particular interest to clinicians and patients include the characteristics of the ICH (e.g. first versus recurrent), patient age and sex, and CM anatomical location and number (i.e. single or multiple lesions). Outcome assessors should be blinded to prognostic features of interest and stratify outcome by treatment. To generate meaningful data, duration and completeness of follow-up should be ≥1 year and ≥90% respectively.

Future directions

In conjunction with current and future knowledge about the epidemiology of sporadic and familial CMs, studies of patients with familial CM may help unravel the biological mechanisms leading to CM formation and rupture. Familial CMs display a tendency to develop *de novo* over the course of a patient's lifespan [10,15,55,56] and may have a higher propensity for ICH than sporadic cases [10,23]. It is hoped that the molecular mechanisms involved in promoting CM development and rupture might help identify reliable biomarkers of risk of future hemorrhage, as well as targets for rational drug design and directed therapeutic manipulation.

A better understanding of pathophysiology may also lead to clarification of the mechanisms behind apparent non-hemorrhagic focal neurological deficits. It may be that the term is erroneous and that microscopic bleeds undetectable by current imaging techniques may be accountable for the symptoms. Conversely, metabolic aberrations, cortical spreading depression, or ischemic events may be alternative explanations.

The external validity (generalizability) of studies could be enhanced by a consistent definition of ICH due to CM. A universal definition could facilitate comparison and combination of studies by using sensitivity analysis (for example, by combining hemorrhagic and potentially hemorrhagic focal neurological deficits in studies with delayed or incomplete brain imaging). This approach could also improve statistical power by combining non-hemorrhagic FND, potentially hemorrhagic FND, and definite ICH to increase the number of outcome events.

Single studies conducted on rare diseases, such as CMs, often lack the power to detect small but clinically meaningful results [57]. Type II errors (false-negative results) are surprisingly common in clinical research and are generally due to under-powering of studies [57,58]. This problem can be circumvented through the use of meta-analytic techniques. Data from several small but comparable studies can be quantitatively amalgamated to achieve precise estimates of outcome measures or uncover effects that may have otherwise gone undetected.

A variation on this approach is the individual patient data (IPD) meta-analysis. It offers several advantages over conventional methods [59–61]. Publication bias and study-specific variations in time-point analysis, lengths of follow-up, and methods of statistical analysis and reporting can constrain classical meta-analyses. An IPD approach circumvents these limitations through central processing of individual patient data from both published and unpublished datasets. This allows researchers to use consistent analysis for all patients across studies, to use up-to-date data, to avoid biases related to aggregate data in meta-

regression, and to investigate subgroups of interest [62]. This technique would offer an ideal approach to the analysis of event rates and prognosis in CMs.

Cavernous malformations of the brain are rare and symptomatic ICHs are uncommon. To organize and design a study of large enough power to reliably describe the natural history and treatment efficacy can be cumbersome from both an organizational and an economic perspective. However, we aim to undertake this IPD meta-analysis of CM prognosis, and the many CM databases that exist [10,23,41,44,46,52,63] could help define the risks and many potential predictors of first and recurrent hemorrhage from CMs.

References

1. Wong, J. H., Awad, I. A. & Kim, J. H. Ultrastructural pathological features of cerebrovascular malformations: a preliminary report. *Neurosurgery* 2000;**46**:1454–1459.

2. Leblanc, G. G., Golanov, E., Awad, I. A. & Young, W. L. Biology of vascular malformations of the brain. *Stroke* 2009;**40**:e694–e702.

3. Hilder, T. L., Malone, M. H., Bencharit, S., *et al.* Proteomic identification of the cerebral cavernous malformation signaling complex. *J Proteome Res* 2007;**6**:4343–4355.

4. Guzeloglu-Kayisli, O., Amankulor, N. M., Voorhees, J., *et al.* KRIT1/cerebral cavernous malformation 1 protein localizes to vascular endothelium, astrocytes, and pyramidal cells of the adult human cerebral cortex. *Neurosurgery* 2004;**54**:943–949.

5. Whitehead, K. J., Chan, A. C., Navankasattusas, S., *et al.* The cerebral cavernous malformation signaling pathway promotes vascular integrity via Rho GTPases. *Nat Med* 2009;**15**:177–184.

6. Clatterbuck, R. E., Eberhart, C. G., Crain, B. J. & Rigamonti, D. Ultrastructural and immunocytochemical evidence that an incompetent blood-brain barrier is related to the pathophysiology of cavernous malformations. *J Neurol Neurosurg Psychiatry* 2001;**71**:188–192.

7. Tu, J., Stoodley, M. A., Morgan, M. K. & Storer, K. P. Ultrastructural characteristics of hemorrhagic, nonhemorrhagic, and recurrent cavernous malformations. *J Neurosurg* 2005;**103**:903–909.

8. Del Curling, O., Jr., Kelly, D. L., Jr., Elster, A. D. & Craven, T. E. An analysis of the natural history of cavernous angiomas. *J Neurosurg* 1991;**75**:702–708.

9. Morris, Z., Whiteley, W. N. & Longstreth, W. T., Jr., *et al.* Incidental findings on brain magnetic resonance imaging: systematic review and meta-

analysis. *BMJ* 2009;**339**:b3016. doi: 10.1136/bmj. b3016.:b3016.

10. Zabramski, J. M., Wascher, T. M., Spetzler, R. F., *et al.* The natural history of familial cavernous malformations: results of an ongoing study. *J Neurosurg* 1994;**80**:422–432.

11. Brunereau, L., Levy, C., Laberge, S., Houtteville, J. & Labauge, P. De novo lesions in familial form of cerebral cavernous malformations: clinical and MR features in 29 non-Hispanic families. *Surg Neurol* 2000;**53**:475–482.

12. Agazzi, S., Maeder, P., Villemure, J. G. & Regli, L. De novo formation and growth of a sporadic cerebral cavernous malformation: implications for management in an asymptomatic patient. *Cerebrovasc Dis* 2003;**16**:432–435.

13. Cakirer, S. De novo formation of a cavernous malformation of the brain in the presence of a developmental venous anomaly. *Clin Radiol* 2003;**58**:251–256.

14. Campeau, N. G. & Lane, J. I. De novo development of a lesion with the appearance of a cavernous malformation adjacent to an existing developmental venous anomaly. *AJNR Am J Neuroradiol* 2005;**26**:156–159.

15. Clatterbuck, R. E., Moriarity, J. L., Elmaci, I., *et al.* Dynamic nature of cavernous malformations: a prospective magnetic resonance imaging study with volumetric analysis. *J Neurosurg* 2000;**93**:981–986.

16. Detwiler, P. W., Porter, R. W., Zabramski, J. M. & Spetzler, R. F. De novo formation of a central nervous system cavernous malformation: implications for predicting risk of hemorrhage. Case report and review of the literature. *J Neurosurg* 1997;**87**:629–632.

17. Fender, L. J., Lenthall, R. K. & Jaspan, T. De novo development of presumed cavernomas following resolution of *E. coli* subdural empyemas. *Neuroradiology* 2000;**42**:778–780.

18. Labauge, P., Brunereau, L., Coubes, P., *et al.* Appearance of new lesions in two nonfamilial cerebral cavernoma patients. *Eur Neurol* 2001;**45**:83–88.

19. Massa-Micon, B., Luparello, V., Bergui, M. & Pagni, C. A. De novo cavernoma case report and review of literature. *Surg Neurol* 2000;**53**:484–487.

20. Nimjee, S. M., Powers, C. J. & Bulsara, K. R. Review of the literature on de novo formation of cavernous malformations of the central nervous system after radiation therapy. *Neurosurg Focus* 2006 Jul 15; **21**:e4.

21. Cordonnier, C., Klijn, C. J., van Beijnum, J. & Al-Shahi Salman, R. Radiological investigation of spontaneous intracerebral hemorrhage: systematic review and trinational survey. *Stroke* 2010;**41**:685–690.

22. Wardlaw, J. M., Keir, S. L., Seymour, J., *et al.* What is the best imaging strategy for acute stroke? *Health Technol Assess* 2004;**8**: iii, ix–iii, 180.

23. Labauge, P., Brunereau, L., Laberge, S. & Houtteville, J. P. Prospective follow-up of 33 asymptomatic patients with familial cerebral cavernous malformations. *Neurology* 2001;**57**:1825–1828.

24. Al-Shahi Salman, R., Berg, M. J., Morrison, L. & Awad, I. A. Hemorrhage from cavernous malformations of the brain: definition and reporting standards. Angioma Alliance Scientific Advisory Board. *Stroke* 2008;**39**:3222–3230.

25. Aiba, T., Tanaka, R., Koike, T., *et al.* Natural history of intracranial cavernous malformations. *J Neurosurg* 1995;**83**:56–59.

26. Porter, R. W., Detwiler, P. W., Spetzler, R. F., *et al.* Cavernous malformations of the brainstem: experience with 100 patients. *J Neurosurg* 1999;**90**:50–58.

27. Dennis, M. S., Bamford, J. M., Molyneux, A. J., Warlow, C. P. Rapid resolution of signs of primary intracerebral haemorrhage in computed tomograms of the brain. *Br Med J (Clin Res Ed)* 1987;**295**:379–381.

28. Gomori, J. M., Grossman, R. I., Goldberg, H. I., Zimmerman, R. A. & Bilaniuk, L. T. Intracranial hematomas: imaging by high-field MR. *Radiology* 1985;**157**:87–93.

29. Linfante, I., Llinas, R. H., Caplan, L. R. & Warach, S. MRI features of intracerebral hemorrhage within 2 hours from symptom onset. *Stroke* 1999;**30**:2263–2267.

30. Patel, M. R., Edelman, R. R. & Warach, S. Detection of hyperacute primary intraparenchymal hemorrhage by magnetic resonance imaging. *Stroke* 1996;**27**:2321–2324.

31. Wiesmann, M., Mayer, T. E., Yousry, I., Hamann, G. F. & Bruckmann, H. Detection of hyperacute parenchymal hemorrhage of the brain using echo-planar T2*-weighted and diffusion-weighted MRI. *Eur Radiol* 2001;**11**:849–853.

32. Smith, E. E., Rosand, J. & Greenberg, S. M. Imaging of hemorrhagic stroke. *Magn Reson Imaging Clin N Am* 2006;**14**:127–40, v.

33. Bradley, W. G., Jr. MR appearance of hemorrhage in the brain. *Radiology* 1993;**189**:15–26.

34. Liang, L., Korogi, Y., Sugahara, T., *et al.* Detection of intracranial hemorrhage with susceptibility-weighted MR sequences. *AJNR Am J Neuroradiol* 1999;**20**:1527–1534.

35. Kang, B. K., Na, D. G., Ryoo, J. W., *et al.* Diffusion-weighted MR imaging of intracerebral hemorrhage. *Korean J Radiol* 2001;**2**:183–191.

36. Brott, T., Adams, H. P., Jr., Olinger, C. P., et al. Measurements of acute cerebral infarction: a clinical examination scale. *Stroke* 1989;**20**:864–870.

37. Banks, J. L. & Marotta, C. A. Outcomes validity and reliability of the modified Rankin scale: implications for stroke clinical trials: a literature review and synthesis. *Stroke* 2007;**38**:1091–1096.

38. Pinker, K., Stavrou, I., Szomolanyi, P., et al. Improved preoperative evaluation of cerebral cavernomas by high-field, high-resolution susceptibility-weighted magnetic resonance imaging at 3 Tesla: comparison with standard (1.5 T) magnetic resonance imaging and correlation with histopathological findings – preliminary results. *Invest Radiol* 2007;**42**:346–351.

39. de Souza, J. M., Domingues, R. C., Cruz, L. C., Jr., et al. Susceptibility-weighted imaging for the evaluation of patients with familial cerebral cavernous malformations: a comparison with t2-weighted fast spin-echo and gradient-echo sequences. *AJNR Am J Neuroradiol* 2008;**29**:154–158.

40. Thickbroom, G. W., Byrnes, M. L., Morris, I. T., et al.. Functional MRI near vascular anomalies: comparison of cavernoma and arteriovenous malformation. *J Clin Neurosci* 2004;**11**:845–848.

41. Porter, P. J., Willinsky, R. A., Harper, W. & Wallace, M. C. Cerebral cavernous malformations: natural history and prognosis after clinical deterioration with or without hemorrhage. *J Neurosurg* 1997;**87**:190–197.

42. Cantu, C., Murillo-Bonilla, L., Arauz, A., et al. Predictive factors for intracerebral hemorrhage in patients with cavernous angiomas. *Neurol Res* 2005;**27**:314–318.

43. Fritschi, J. A., Reulen, H. J., Spetzler, R. F. & Zabramski, J. M. Cavernous malformations of the brain stem. A review of 139 cases. *Acta Neurochir (Wien)* 1994;**130**(1–4):35–46.

44. Moriarity, J. L., Wetzel, M., Clatterbuck, R. E., et al. The natural history of cavernous malformations: a prospective study of 68 patients. *Neurosurgery* 1999;**44**:1166–1171.

45. Robinson, J. R., Awad, I. A. & Little, J. R. Natural history of the cavernous angioma. *J Neurosurg* 1991;**75**:709–714.

46. Kondziolka, D., Lunsford, L. D. & Kestle, J. R. The natural history of cerebral cavernous malformations. *J Neurosurg* 1995;**83**:820–824.

47. Barker, F. G., min-Hanjani, S., Butler, W. E., et al. Temporal clustering of hemorrhages from untreated cavernous malformations of the central nervous system. *Neurosurgery* 2001;**49**:15–24.

48. Abdulrauf, S. I., Kaynar, M. Y. & Awad, I. A. A comparison of the clinical profile of cavernous malformations with and without associated venous malformations. *Neurosurgery* 1999;**44**:41–46.

49. Labauge, P., Brunereau, L., Levy, C., Laberge, S. & Houtteville, J. P. The natural history of familial cerebral cavernomas: a retrospective MRI study of 40 patients. *Neuroradiology* 2000;**42**:327–332.

50. Kupersmith, M. J., Kalish, H., Epstein, F., et al. Natural history of brainstem cavernous malformations. *Neurosurgery* 2001;**48**:47–53.

51. Brown, R. D., Jr., Wiebers, D. O., Torner, J. C. & O'Fallon, W. M. Incidence and prevalence of intracranial vascular malformations in Olmsted County, Minnesota, 1965 to 1992. *Neurology* 1996;**46**:949–952.

52. Al-Shahi, R., Bhattacharya, J. J., Currie, D. G., et al. Prospective, population-based detection of intracranial vascular malformations in adults: the Scottish Intracranial Vascular Malformation Study (SIVMS). *Stroke* 2003;**34**:1163–1169.

53. Cordonnier, C., Al-Shahi Salman, R., Bhattacharya, J. J., et al. Differences between intracranial vascular malformation types in the characteristics of their presenting haemorrhages: prospective, population-based study. *J Neurol Neurosurg Psychiatry* 2008;**79**:47–51.

54. Tung, H., Giannotta, S. L., Chandrasoma, P. T. & Zee, C. S. Recurrent intraparenchymal hemorrhages from angiographically occult vascular malformations. *J Neurosurg* 1990;**73**:174–180.

55. Kattapong, V. J., Hart, B. L. & Davis, L. E. Familial cerebral cavernous angiomas: clinical and radiologic studies. *Neurology* 1995;**45**:492–497.

56. Labauge, P., Laberge, S., Brunereau, L., Levy, C. & Tournier-Lasserve, E. Hereditary cerebral cavernous angiomas: clinical and genetic features in 57 French families. Societe Francaise de Neurochirurgie. *Lancet* 1998;**352**:1892–1897.

57. Egger, M. & Smith, G. D. Meta-analysis. Potentials and promise. *BMJ* 1997;**315**:1371–1374.

58. Collins, R., Keech, A., Peto, R., Sleight, P., et al. Cholesterol and total mortality: need for larger trials. *BMJ* 1992;**304**:1689.

59. Stewart, L. A. & Tierney, J. F. To IPD or not to IPD? Advantages and disadvantages of systematic reviews using individual patient data. *Eval Health Prof* 2002;**25**:76–97.

60. Stewart, L. A. & Clarke, M. J. Practical methodology of meta-analyses (overviews) using updated individual patient data. Cochrane Working Group. *Stat Med* 1995;**14**:2057–2079.

61. Stewart, L. A. & Parmar, M. K. Meta-analysis of the literature or of individual patient data: is there a difference? *Lancet* 1993;**341**:418–422.

62. Simmonds, M. C., Higgins, J. P., Stewart, L. A., *et al.* Meta-analysis of individual patient data from randomized trials: a review

of methods used in practice. *Clin Trials* 2005;**2**:209–217.

63. Hasegawa, T., McInerney, J., Kondziolka, D., *et al.* Long-term results after stereotactic radiosurgery for patients with cavernous malformations. *Neurosurgery* 2002;**50**:1190–1197.

64. Kim, D. S., Park, Y. G., Choi, J. U., Chung, S. S. & Lee, K. C. An analysis of the natural history of cavernous malformations. *Surg Neurol* 1997;**48**:9–17.

Cavernous malformations and epilepsy: medical management of seizures and the presurgical evaluation of medically intractable epilepsy

Gregory K. Bergey

Introduction

Cavernous malformations are common vascular malformations. Cavernomas are estimated to occur in about 0.5–0.7% of the population, although postmortem studies suggest the incidence may be even higher [1], and make up about 10–20% of intracranial vascular malformations [2]. Seizures are probably the most common presenting symptom [2,3]. Although the majority of cavernomas may be clinically occult or detected as incidental findings, the frequent occurrence of these lesions means that they are a common cause of symptomatic epilepsy. It is difficult to accurately know the percentage of patients with cavernomas who have seizures because many patients may have asymptomatic cavernomas and do not seek medical attention. Treatment of seizures due to cavernomas is an important part of the management of patients with these lesions.

Although cavernomas are congential (whether genetic or not) rather than acquired lesions, they are dynamic, both pathologically and with regard to hemorrhage and epileptogenesis [4]. This is evidenced by the fact that most seizures due to cavernomas do not begin until after a number of years. Since seizures originate from cerebral cortex or mesial temporal regions, cavernomas located in the cortical, immediate subcortical regions, or adjacent to the amygdala or hippocampus are more likely to be epileptogenic. Cavernomas in the brainstem, cerebellum, or deep white matter will not produce seizures, but can, of course, hemorrhage. Patients with multiple cavernomas are statistically more likely to have seizures than are those with solitary lesions, but (see below) seizures may originate from only one of the multiple lesions. The natural history of cavernomas, even those that do not have overt hemorrhages, is to have evolution of the surrounding hemosiderin ring. The development of this hemosiderin ring probably is associated with increased epileptogenicity. Animal models have demonstrated that iron injected into the cortex can produce focal seizures [5,6]. Overt hemorrhage associated with a cavernoma, even though typically self-limited, may produce seizures if the hemorrhage involves adjacent cortical regions or mesial temporal structures (e.g. hippocampus, amygdala). It is known that hemorrhagic strokes, such as those associated with emboli, typically involve the cortex and are more epileptogenic than bland infarcts or strokes involving deep structures [7]. Patients may present with seizures at the time of an acute overt hemorrhage (Fig. 10.1). After the hemorrhage is resorbed over the following months, the cavernoma may be less epileptogenic than before, but some increased propensity toward seizures remains. Once a cavernoma becomes epileptogenic it will probably remain so unless removed surgically. Therefore patients with symptomatic cavernomas who are begun on antiepileptic therapy will require life-long therapy unless the cavernoma is removed.

This chapter will focus on the medical management of these patients with cavernomas and seizures and, where indicated, the presurgical evaluation. The indications for cavernoma resection are different for epilepsy and hemorrhage. While some patients may have readily controlled seizures and not require surgery, many (probably 40–50%) will develop medically

Cavernous Malformations of the Nervous System, ed. Daniele Rigamonti. Published by Cambridge University Press.
© Cambridge University Press 2011.

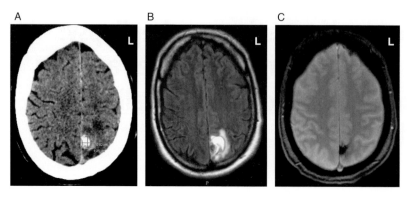

Figure 10.1. Panel A is a non-contrast CT done at the time of presentation when the patient had a partial seizure with secondary generalization. A left parieto-occipital hemorrhage is seen. MRI at the time of presentation (panel B) revealed only the hemorrhage and could not define any underlying lesion. A full angiogram 3 months later was unremarkable. Panel C: T2 gradient-echo sequences 6 months after presentation reveals the hemosiderin deposition and underlying cavernous malformation. The patient has been seizure-free on antiepileptic medications for over 18 months.

intractable epilepsy. The cavernomas that produce seizures are often favorably located, many occurring in the frontal and temporal lobes [8], and resection produces seizure freedom in a large percentage of patients. Therefore seizure surgery should be routinely considered early in patients who continue to have disabling seizures despite medical therapy.

Medical management of patients with seizures and cavernous malformations

Seizures due to cavernomas often present in young adults (e.g. 20–40 years of age) although certainly earlier or later presentations occur. Because cavernomas are focal lesions, the seizures associated with these malformations are partial seizures, either simple partial (without alteration of consciousness) or complex partial (with alteration of consciousness) with or without secondary generalization. This is true even if the history is only one of generalized tonic-clonic seizures; generalized tonic-clonic seizures due to cavernomas will always have a partial onset. This partial onset, although often recognized in the clinical history, may not be apparent when seizures originate from silent brain regions (e.g. orbitofrontal) or propagate rapidly (e.g. neocortical) and do not produce focal symptomatology prior to secondary generalization. Simple partial seizures are seizures without alteration of consciousness. In these instances the ictal manifestations will reflect the affected region of the brain (e.g. sensory, occipital, motor). For instance, a patient with simple partial seizures originating from the occipital cortex may only have transient (typically < 60 seconds, sometimes much shorter) visual phenomena. While, in theory, simple partial seizures, since they do not by definition produce alteration of

consciousness, might be thought not to require antiepileptic therapy, treatment with antiepileptic drug therapy (AED) is recommended in patients with symptomatic cavernomas because of the potential for future propagation producing complex partial or generalized symptoms. If an individual already on AED therapy, however, is only experiencing simple partial seizures and there are no alterations of consciousness, it is not necessary to increase or add medication unless the simple partial events are particularly frequent or distressing to the patient.

All available antiepileptic drugs (AEDs), with the exception of ethosuximide, are effective against partial seizures with or without secondary generalization. Patients not having surgical resections, and even some who do (see below), will need life-long therapy. AEDs should therefore be selected with this understanding and the considerations of the individual patient. For instance, in female patients of child-bearing age, AEDs that have increased risk during pregnancy (e.g. valproate, phenobarbital) should be avoided [9]. Other powerful enzyme-inducing AEDs (e.g. phenytoin, carbamazepine) have the potential for drug interactions and may also potentiate bone mineral density loss in older patients [10]. If tolerated, levetiracetam and lamotrigine can be effective for partial seizures and have favorable side-effect profiles. Lacosamide, pregabalin, and oxcarbazepine are also alternatives, recognizing that oxcarbazepine, while having much less hepatic induction than does carbamazepine, has an increased potential to produce significant hyponatremia (via an SIADH-like mechanism), particularly in older patients. Other AEDs may be considered for individual patients, again recognizing that the selection is for long-term therapy. If there is a need for rapid introduction, levetiracetam, phenytoin, or valproate can be used. In most patients, however, rapid loading is not required and AED selection can be individualized.

In the United States, most newer AEDs are approved as adjunctive therapy for complex partial seizures with or without secondary generalization because the FDA until just recently required difficult, and probably unethical, trial designs that included placebo or low-dose active control arms [11,12]. In addition to the older AEDs (e.g. phenytoin, carbamazepine, valproate, phenobarbital), topiramate and oxcarbazepine have FDA indications for initial monotherapy and lamotrigine has FDA approval for conversion to monotherapy. However, it is generally felt that all AEDs effective as adjunctive therapy are effective as monotherapy and this would be demonstrated by non-inferiority or equivalency trials, which are accepted by regulatory bodies elsewhere and by the FDA in other disease states (e.g. oncology, infectious disease). Indeed levetiracetam and lamotrigine have approval for initial monotherapy in the European Union and zonisamide is approved for initial monotherapy in Japan. AED selection should therefore be based on the appropriateness for the given patient; AED use as initial monotherapy, even if not FDA approved, does not deviate from the standards of medical care.

There is no indication for prophylactic antiepileptic drug therapy in patients with cavernomas that have not yet produced seizures. Although controlled trials addressing this question have not been performed, it is known that in patients with brain tumors, AED prophylaxis does not prevent seizures [13–15] and it is unlikely that the situation would be different with cavernomas. Late-postraumatic epilepsy is not prevented by AED prophylaxis (for review, see Temkin [16]). Since many patients with late-posttraumatic epilepsy have high risk head injuries (e.g. hemorrhagic contusion, subdural hematoma) with associated hemorrhage and later hemosiderin deposition, these patients have some similarities to patients with cavernomas.

After the patient with a cavernoma has experienced a seizure, the patient should be placed on AED therapy with appropriate restrictions to activity until it is established that disabling seizures have been controlled. While the classic definition of epilepsy is recurrent seizures, the definition of epilepsy has recently been appropriately revised to be at least one seizure with an enduring predisposition to have seizures [17]. Therefore if a patient has a seizure thought due to a cavernous malformation, treatment after a single seizure, whether partial or secondarily generalized, is appropriate since the cavernous malformation represents this "enduring predisposition".

Patients with a cavernoma may undergo resective surgery for other indications without ever having had seizures. Although there are no formal guidelines for AED prophylaxis prior to craniotomy, there are good data supporting this practice [18]. In patients with cavernomas who have not had seizures, AED prophylaxis prior to resection is warranted. Levetiracetam offers the ability to be introduced rapidly, being non-sedating, having few allergic reactions, no hepatic induction or drug interactions, and being available as a parenteral formulation. Introducing levetiracetam at 500 mg bid will provide a steady state concentration in less than 2 days (~35 hours because of the levetiracetam $t \frac{1}{2}$ of 7 h). If necessary levetiracetam can be orally loaded [19] with 1500 mg given as a single dose followed by maintenance dosing; peak levels are reached in 45 minutes after a single oral dose [20]. In recent unblinded comparative trials of seizure control after craniotomy for brain tumors, levetiracetam offered equal efficacy and fewer side effects than phenytoin [21,22]. Occasional irritability, behavioral side effects, and sedation have been reported with acute levetiracetam loading (two of 78 patients in Zachenhofer *et al.* [23]); none of the 37 patients orally loaded [19] had behavioral side effects. Serious behavioral changes (e.g. psychosis) are no more common with levetiracetam than any other AED. Phenytoin and valproate can also be loaded rapidly and are alternatives to levetiracetam. Levetiracetam, phenytoin (the prodrug fosphenytoin is preferred), and valproate are all available as parenteral formulations. A newly approved AED lacosamide is also available in oral and parenteral formulations, but reports of its use in acute situations are limited to date [24,25]. After recovery from resective surgery, patients who have no previous history of seizures are candidates for early withdrawal of AEDs.

Presurgical evaluation of patients with medically intractable epilepsy

This discussion will focus on when surgery is appropriate for seizure control in patients with cavernous malformations. Other chapters in this volume will address the indications for surgery for recurrent hemorrhage or progressive neurological deficits. Since the hemorrhages from cavernomas are often self-limited compared with arteriovenous malformations, intractable epilepsy is the most common

Table 10.1 Treatment of cavernous malformations and seizures. This presents a diagrammatic treatment plan; details of the presurgical evaluation are in the text.

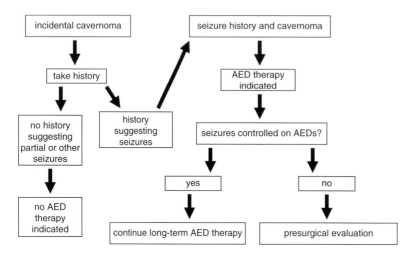

Treatment of Cavernous Malformations and Seizures

indication for resection of cavernomas. As mentioned, the incidence of medically refractory seizures in patients with seizures due to cavernomas is significant, not surprising in light of the symptomatic structural etiology for the seizures. A landmark study [26] examined the response to AED therapy and the identification of refractory epilepsy. In this group of 525 patients with new-onset epilepsy, which included idiopathic, cryptogenic, and symptomatic epilepsy, only 13% had their seizures controlled with a second AED after a first drug failed, and if seizures failed to be controlled with adequate trials of two AEDs (i.e. good doses or levels and not failure due to side effects) then they reported only 1% of this group had their seizures controlled with a third AED. Medical intractability therefore can be defined as failing adequate trials of two or three AEDs. Consideration should then be given to the assessment of surgical candidacy for these patients. In patients with lesional symptomatic partial epilepsy these data support considering resective surgery in patients who are excellent surgical candidates (e.g. mesial temporal sclerosis, cavernous angioma) after the patient has failed to have disabling seizures (i.e. seizures with associated alteration of consciousness) controlled with trials of two medications. This is particularly true of cavernomas that are in favorable locations (e.g. anterior frontal or temporal), remote from eloquent areas. There is certainly no justification for trials of many AEDs in these patients since the chance for seizure control after surgery is > 70% compared to < 5% with additional medication trials. As in all considerations for seizure surgery, major comorbidities may influence surgical candidacy, but many patients with cavernomas are young, otherwise healthy individuals, whose seizures represent the major impact on their quality of life.

Important questions in the presurgical evaluation of patients with medically intractable epilepsy and cavernous malformations are listed in Table 10.1 and discussed below. As is the case with any consideration for epilepsy surgery, establishing the lesion as the symptomatic cause of the seizures, and considering the relative risks of resective surgery are important. Cavernomas commonly involve the temporal lobe [8]; fortunately the more surgically challenging locations (e.g. deep brain, brainstem) are not regions producing seizures.

Imaging

The imaging of cavernomas with MRI and other techniques is discussed in detail in other chapters, but is an important part of the presurgical evaluation for intractable epilepsy and so will be considered in this context. The evaluation when a patient first presents with history of a seizure or seizures often is the first determination of the presence of a cavernous malformation. As is the case with all new-onset partial seizures, MRI is the imaging technique of choice because CT, although quite good at detecting acute hemorrhage, may miss many less obvious lesions, particularly in the mesial temporal lobe regions. At times an acute hemorrhage may make determination of the underlying cavernoma difficult, but by the time seizures are determined to be medically intractable there will have been resolution of these acute changes.

Any consideration of seizure surgery requires the determination that the cavernoma is the cause of the intractable epilepsy. In some instances this may be easier than in others. As mentioned above, lesions in deep white matter, brainstem, etc. are unlikely to be epileptogenic whereas those in cortical or mesial temporal regions are much more likely to be symptomatic causes. While the presence of multiple cavernomas does not preclude surgical consideration, it is critical that one be certain that solitary malformations are indeed single lesions. MRI is very sensitive at detecting cavernous lesions, and these lesions produce a characteristic MRI picture of a heterogeneous signal on T1 and T2 imaging with the surrounding hemosiderin ring producing a hypointense signal [27,28]. Gradient-echo sequences (Fig. 10.3) are even more sensitive in detecting cavernomas than the routine MRI sequences and should be done on patients prior to consideration for epilepsy surgery in order to identify all cavernomas [29]. Small lesions can still be missed due to MRI slice thickness, but this can be addressed later if ictal EEG recordings are discordant with the identified lesions.

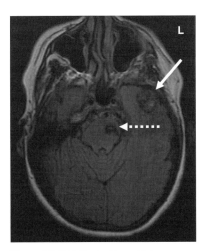

Figure 10.2. Patient with multiple cavernous malformations, two shown on T2 FLAIR MRI imaging. The left temporal cavernoma (solid arrow) is the cause of the patient's seizures. The pontine cavernoma (dotted arrow) is not epileptogenic nor are cavernomas (not illustrated) in the white matter of the left occipital lobe, and both left and right parietal white matter.

While resection of the cavernoma itself may be sufficient to eliminate the risk of subsequent hemorrhage, it is felt that optimal seizure control and the opportunity for AED reduction occurs with resection of not only the cavernoma but the surrounding hemosiderin ring [30–33], although no controlled studies have been done. Assessment of the extent of hemosiderin deposition is particularly important when the cavernoma is in or near eloquent cortex since this may limit the ability to do a broad resection.

Multiple cavernomas

About 80% of patients have solitary cavernomas, but 20% have multiple cavernomas. These patients with multiple cavernomas often have a familial history with a pattern of autosomal dominant inheritance [34,35]. This is discussed in detail elsewhere in this volume. In the past such multifocal lesions in patients with cavernomas or other disorders such as tuberous sclerosis were thought to make such patients suboptimal surgical candidates; however, it is now appreciated that even if multiple cavernomas are epileptogenic, often only one of the cavernomas is the cause of the medically refractory seizures [36] and resection of that cavernoma will offer a high chance of seizure freedom [37]. Therefore these patients with multiple lesions, if they have medically refractory disabling seizures, are appropriate candidates for resective seizure surgery. It is of critical importance to determine which cavernoma is producing the medically refractory seizures. When surgery is done for recurrent hemorrhages, the offending cavernoma can be easily identified. When surgery is contemplated due to intractable epilepsy the assessment can be more complicated in patients with multiple cavernomas. While lesion location and the history of previous hemorrhage may be suggestive, it is important to have more definitive evidence. In the epilepsy monitoring unit AEDs are typically reduced or discontinued during the monitoring period in order to record a number of seizures within a reasonable period of time. Careful correlation with the clinical features of the refractory seizures is important since AED reduction could unmask interictal activity or other seizures that were previously controlled with medications. This information, if not assessed properly, can confound the presurgical evaluation.

EEG monitoring

In patients with solitary cavernomas and medically intractable epilepsy, it is still recommended that inpatient continuous video-EEG monitoring be performed

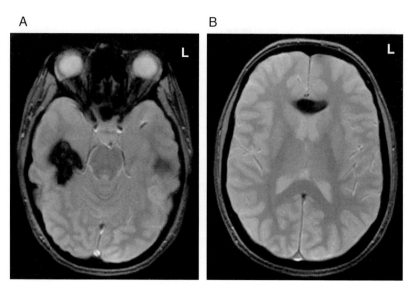

Figure 10.3. Another patient with medically intractable complex partial seizures with multiple cavernous malformations, one large cavernoma in the right temporal lobe, and another in the anterior corpus callosal region as shown on T2 gradient-echo sequences. Continuous video-EEG monitoring revealed seizures to be originating from the right temporal lobe, but independent anterior right frontal spikes were also prominent in the interictal period. The patient had resection of the temporal cavernoma and is now seizure-free (on AED monotherapy), indicating that the temporal cavernoma was the cause of the medically refractory partial seizures, but that the anterior cavernoma has some epileptogenic potential that is suppressed by medications.

to confirm that the cavernoma is the source of the patient's medically intractable partial seizures. On occasion dual pathology may be present (e.g. dysplasia or mesial temporal abnormalities). During the inpatient video monitoring, AEDs are often reduced to capture several seizures; the hope is that seizure onset will be concordant with the known cavernoma. If there is a prominent interictal spike focus consistent with the cavernous malformation, fewer ictal events are necessary for the presurgical planning.

Continuous video-EEG monitoring is even more critical in patients with cavernomas located in regions (e.g. deep white matter) thought not to be epileptogenic or when multiple cavernomas are present (Fig. 10.3). At times, if the multiple cavernomas are spaced far apart, scalp monitoring may be sufficient to indicate which cavernoma is producing the seizures, but in these instances multiple seizures should be recorded to confirm this, particularly if interictal activity suggests potential multifocality. In other instances if the multiple candidate cavernomas are located in close proximity, intracranial monitoring may be necessary to determine which cavernoma is the epileptogenic focus. The possibility that AED withdrawal may unmask a secondary focus that was previously controlled with medication exists, but this has not been systematically studied. The patient should confirm that the seizures occurring during the monitoring period are clinically similar to those occurring on medication at home.

Magnetoencephalography (MEG) may provide confirmative information. MEG maps interictal spikes so is most useful when there are prominent and frequent interictal spikes [38]. MEG mapping in these instances can be helpful when there are multiple cavernomas. MEG does not eliminate the need for ictal-EEG monitoring or subdural grid mapping when indicated.

Mapping of eloquent cortex

Many cavernomas producing seizures are located in the frontal and temporal lobes. If the lesion of interest is near language or motor areas, fMRI may be sufficient to determine hemispheric dominance and the location of motor areas since there is good concordance with language lateralization found with the intracarotid amobarbital procedure (IAP) or Wada test [39]. It is important to recognize, however, that cavernomas near eloquent areas of interest may affect the lateralization index of the fMRI and produce discordant (compared to IAP) language lateralization due to effects on BOLD generation or disturbance of brain normalization [40]. Magnetoencephalography (MEG) can also supplement the fMRI in the mapping of language or motor areas [41]. If, however, consideration is being given to resection of mesial temporal structures, particularly in the dominant temporal lobe, then the IAP remains an important determination of localization of memory since neither fMRI or MEG are non-invasive tests with equivalent reliability. Resection of mesial temporal structures (e.g. hippocampus) that are important in verbal memory can produce significant verbal memory deficits, in contrast

A B

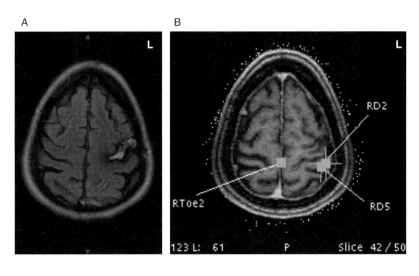

Figure 10.4. Patient with intractable focal motor seizures (right hand) originating from left frontal cavernoma with previous history of acute hemorrhage several years ago. Panel A illustrates cavernoma on MRI T2 FLAIR imaging. Panel B illustrates magnetic source imaging (MSI) for localization of somatosensory cortex for right toe, and the second and fifth digits of right hand (green boxes), indicating that the cavernoma involved the primary motor cortex. Interictal spikes were not sufficient for reliable source localization on MEG (not shown) but suggested a region near the cavernoma. The patient was operated upon awake with successful removal of the cavernoma and no increased post-operative motor deficit. MSI done by R. Knowlton of the University of Alabama.

to the resection of dysfunctional mesial temporal structures (e.g. mesial temporal lobe sclerosis).

Knowledge about the proximity of eloquent areas (e.g. motor, language, memory) is important because optimal outcomes regarding seizure freedom appear to be related to resection of not only the cavernoma (which would eliminate any future risk of hemorrhage) but also the surrounding hemosiderin ring [30–33]. Location of the cavernoma in or near eloquent areas may limit the ability to make a broad resection of the hemosiderin staining. In instances where the cavernoma is in motor or speech areas, consideration should be given to performing awake craniotomy to guide the resection and minimize postoperative deficits.

Dual pathology

Surgical candidacy of patients with cavernous malformations who are refractory to medical therapy needs to assess not only whether the cavernoma is single or multiple, but whether dual pathology exists. Cortical venous malformations are the most common coexistent pathology and are more common in patients with sporadic and solitary cavernomas [42,43]. Fortunately developmental venous anomalies are usually benign and asymptomatic; recognition of the possible association is important in any presurgical planning. Very rarely cortical dysplasias may coexist with cavernomas; in these instances consideration that the dysplasia may be the epileptogenic cause needs careful consideration [44–46].

Another concern is the potential coexistence of mesial temporal epileptogenicity, even if overt mesial temporal sclerosis is not present. Whether years of uncontrolled seizures can kindle the adjacent mesial temporal structures in humans is not resolved. If the mesial temporal region is abnormal on imaging and is not needed to support verbal memory (i.e. nondominant temporal lobe or dysfunction dominant temporal lobe determined by Wada testing) then adjacent mesial temporal areas can be resected. If, however, there is concern about resecting functional hippocampus, the resection should be confined to the lesion to minimize post-operative deficits.

Role of intracranial monitoring in the presurgical evaluation

Chronic intracranial monitoring with subdural grid and strip arrays may be useful, if there are multiple proximal candidate cavernomas that could be epileptogenic. In addition subdural arrays can provide functional mapping of language and motor areas if the cavernoma is near these important regions. A recent publication [8] reports 173 patients, 102 presenting with epilepsy, 61 with cavernomas in the temporal lobe who had intraoperative electrocorticography with resection of areas with active spiking. The authors claimed that using electrocorticography in these temporal lobe patients resulted in more extensive resections and improved seizure-free outcomes early, but at 2 years there was no significant difference between the seizure-free groups (79% seizure-free without electro-corticography, 83% seizure-free with electrocorticography). Whether any trend toward benefit merely reflected more extensive resection of the surrounding hemosiderin or more extensive resection of mesial temporal structures is not clear. The cautions about removing functional hippocampal structures have been addressed above.

Resective vs. stereotactic surgery for intractable epilepsy

While stereotactic radiosurgery has been reported to reduce the risk of subsequent recurrent hemorrhage [47,48], its use in the treatment of cavernous angiomas is much less established than in arteriovenous malformations; this is also discussed in accompanying chapters. Regardless of the utility of radiosurgery for treatment of recurrent hemorrhages, this treatment modality is less effective than resection in the control of intractable epilepsy. Although one small series reports 64% seizure freedom (nine of 14 patients) in the group treated with radiosurgery, this group had 87% (13 of 15 patients) free of disabling seizures after resective surgery [49]. This difference did not reach statistical significance because the study was underpowered with too few patients. In a large series of 125 patients [50], 28 with seizures, 53% were considered to have a "good" outcome but this study grouped Engel grade II (occasional disabling seizures) with the Engel grade I (no disabling seizures). Other articles [51–53] report good outcomes of between 25 and 60% but again these studies group Engel grade I and II.

The goal of seizure surgery is to render patients free of disabling seizures. While the use of radiosurgery to treat cavernomas in the deep brain regions or brainstem may be appropriate, these locations do not produce seizures. Examining the outcomes of temporal lobe surgery (not limited to cavernomas), Engel grade I outcomes of 48–84% of patients are seizure-free [54]. This is a heterogeneous group of patients; positive predictive features include those patients with MRI evidence of mesial temporal sclerosis or a circumscribed lesion (e.g. cavernoma, ganglioglioma) and a presurgical evaluation showing concordant epileptiform abnormalities. Long-term seizure control, freedom from disabling seizures (Engel grade I), is high after surgical resection of the cavernomas, with rates of 70–85% reported [32,55,56].

Typically it may take 1 year or more for the full benefits of radiosurgery treatment, whether for ablation of the vascular malformation to reduce the risk of hemorrhage or for seizure control. The first year after radiosurgery can be accompanied by significant local tissue reaction, at times with worsening seizures, and requiring corticosteroid therapy [57]. It is not surprising that radiosurgery would be less successful than resective surgery for seizure control since the lesion still remains. Therefore for the treatment of intractable epilepsy due to cavernomas, resective surgery is the preferred surgical treatment in most patients. Fortunately, most cavernomas that are epileptogenic are in brain regions that are readily surgically accessible.

Reduction or discontinuation of antiepileptic medications

While this chapter focuses on the presurgical evaluation of patients with cavernous malformations and medically intractable epilepsy, a brief comment regarding management of patients after surgical resection is warranted. Patients with symptomatic cavernomas producing partial seizures are not good candidates for withdrawal from AED therapy if the cavernoma remains even if they have been seizure-free for several years and the routine EEG is normal. While it is conceivable that in some patients seizures were triggered by an acute hemorrhage and that with resorption of the acute bleed epileptogenicity has diminished, the lesion and the remaining hemosiderin remain and the risk of seizure recurrence off medications is probably significant; therefore AED withdrawal is not recommended. Intractable epilepsy is the most common indication for surgical resection of cavernomas. Reasonable expectations for the patient undergoing such a resection are freedom from disabling seizures (complex partial or secondarily generalized) and a reduction in antiepileptic medication. The chance of becoming seizure-free is > 70% and it is reasonable to reduce AEDs to monotherapy by the first year after surgery if the patient is seizure-free (or only has occasional auras or simple partial seizures). Whether the patient can come off all AEDs is a complicated and unresolved question that has not been addressed with good evidence-based trials. We know that patients who are seizure-free for 1 year after temporal lobectomy for all reasons (e.g. mesial temporal sclerosis, etc.) have a 15–20% risk of seizure recurrence over the next 10 years [54]. This recurrence typically occurs with attempts at withdrawal of AEDs. The general trend at major epilepsy centers is to leave patients on small amounts of a single AED for prolonged periods of time. The availability of new second-generation AEDs that have excellent side-effect profiles (e.g. lamotrigine, levetiracetam) facilitates this decision. Patients with solitary cavernomas that have been resected, where the resection includes the surrounding hemosiderin ring, and where secondary epileptogenesis (e.g. adjacent mesial structures) is not a concern, may be candidates for AED withdrawal, but only after a prolonged period of seizure freedom (~ 4 years) and with restriction of activities during the period of withdrawal.

Summary

Cavernous malformations are a common cause of symptomatic partial seizures. While many patients with symptomatic cavernomas can have their seizures controlled with medications, almost half develop medically intractable epilepsy. In these patients, resective seizure surgery offers an excellent chance for seizure control. When the lesion is favorably located in temporal or frontal lobe regions and not involving eloquent cortex, consideration for seizure surgery is appropriate early, after the patient has failed to have disabling seizures controlled by two AEDs. In other patients with multiple cavernomas, or cavernomas near or in eloquent areas, some delay may be warranted, but these patients also can have excellent outcomes following surgery although more extensive evaluations may be required.

References

1. McCormick, W. F., Hardman, J. M. & Boulter, T. R. Vascular malformations ("angiomas") of the brain, with special reference to those occurring in the posterior fossa. *J Neurosurg* 1968;**28**:241–251.

2. Aiba, T., Tanaka, R., Koike, T., *et al.* Natural history of intracranial cavernous malformations. *J Neurosurg* 1995;**83**:56–59.

3. Porter, P. J., Willinsky, R. A., Harper, W. & Wallace, M. C. Cerebral cavernous malformations: natural history and prognosis after clinical deterioration with or without hemorrhage. *J Neurosurg* 1997;**87**:190–197.

4. Clatterbuck, R. E., Moriarity, J. L., Elmaci, I., *et al.* Dynamic nature of cavernous malformations: a prospective magnetic resonance imaging study with volumetric analysis. *J Neurosurg* 2000;**93**:981–986.

5. Willmore, L. J., Sypert, G. W., Munson, J. V. & Hurd, R. W. Chronic focal epileptiform discharges induced by injection of iron into rat and cat cortex. *Science* 1978;**200**:1501–1503.

6. Sharma, V., Babu, P. P., Singh, A., Singh, S. & Singh, R. Iron-induced experimental cortical seizures: electroencephalographic mapping of seizure spread in the subcortical brain areas. *Seizure* 2007;**16**:680–690.

7. Leone, M. A., Tonini, M. C., Bogliun, G., *et al.*, ARES (Alcohol Related Seizures) Study Group. Risk factors for a first epileptic seizure after stroke: a case control study. *J Neurol Sci* 2009;**277**:138–142.

8. Van Gompel, J. J., Rubio, J., Cascino, G. D., Worrell, G. A. & Meyer, F. B. Electrocorticography-guided resection of temporal cavernoma: is electrocorticography warranted and does it alter the surgical approach? *J Neurosurg* 2009;**110**:1179–1185.

9. Harden, C. L., Meador, K. J., Pennell, P. B., *et al.* American Academy of Neurology; American Epilepsy Society. Management issues for women with epilepsy – Focus on pregnancy (an evidence-based review): II. Teratogenesis and perinatal outcomes: Report of the Quality Standards Subcommittee and Therapeutics and Technology Subcommittee of the American Academy of Neurology and the American Epilepsy Society. *Epilepsia* 2009;**50**:1237–1246.

10. Bergey, G. K. Initial treatment of epilepsy: special issues in treating the elderly. *Neurology* 2004;**63**(10 Suppl 4): S40–8.

11. French, J. A. & Schachter, S. A workshop on antiepileptic drug monotherapy indications. *Epilepsia* 2002;**43**(Suppl 10):3–27.

12. French, J. A., Wang, S., Warnock, B. & Temkin, N. Historical control monotherapy design in the treatment of epilepsy. *Epilepsia* 2010;**51**:1936–1943.

13. Glantz, M. J., Cole, B. F., Forsyth, P. A., *et al.* Practice parameter: anticonvulsant prophylaxis in patients with newly diagnosed brain tumors. Report of the Quality Standards Subcommittee of the American Academy of Neurology. *Neurology* 2000;**54**:1886–1893.

14. Sirven, J. I., Wingerchuk, D. M., Drazkowski, J. F., Lyons, M. K. & Zimmerman, R. S. Seizure prophylaxis in patients with brain tumors: a meta-analysis. *Mayo Clin Proc* 2004;**79**:1489–1494.

15. Mikkelsen, T., Paleologos, N. A., Robinson, P. D., *et al.* The role of prophylactic anticonvulsants in the management of brain metastases: a systematic review and evidence-based clinical practice guideline. *J Neurooncol* 2010;**96**:97–102.

16. Temkin, N. R. Preventing and treating posttraumatic seizures: the human experience. *Epilepsia* 2009;**50** (Suppl 2):10–13.

17. Fisher, R. S. & Leppik, I. Debate: when does a seizure imply epilepsy? *Epilepsia* 2008;**49**(Suppl 9):7–12.

18. Temkin, N. R. Prophylactic anticonvulsants after neurosurgery. *Epilepsy Curr* 2002;**2**:105–107.

19. Koubeissi, M. Z., Amina, S., Pita, I., Bergey, G. K. & Werz, M. A. Tolerability and efficacy of oral loading of levetiracetam. *Neurology* 2008;**70**:2166–2170.

20. Ramael, S., Daoust, A., Otoul, C., *et al.* Levetiracetam intravenous infusion: a randomized, placebo-controlled safety and pharmacokinetic study. *Epilepsia* 2006;**47**:1128–1135.

21. Milligan, T. A., Hurwitz, S. & Bromfield, E. B. Efficacy and tolerability of levetiracetam versus phenytoin after supratentorial neurosurgery. *Neurology* 2008;**71**:665–669.

22. Lim, D. A., Tarapore, P., Chang, E., *et al.* Safety and feasibility of switching from phenytoin to levetiracetam monotherapy for glioma-related seizure control following craniotomy: a randomized phase II pilot study. *J Neurooncol* 2009;**93**:349–354.

23. Zachenhofer, I., Donat, M., Oberndorfer, S. & Roessler, K. Perioperative levetiracetam for prevention of seizures in supratentorial brain tumor surgery. *J Neurooncol* 2011;**101**:101–106.

24. Chung, S., Sperling, M. R., Biton, V., *et al.*, SP754 Study Group. Lacosamide as adjunctive therapy for partial-onset seizures: a randomized controlled trial. *Epilepsia* 2010;**51**:958–967.

25. Krauss, G., Ben-Menachem, E., Mameniskiene, R., *et al.*, SP757 Study Group. Intravenous lacosamide as short-term replacement for oral lacosamide in partial-onset seizures. *Epilepsia* 2010;**51**:951–957.

26. Kwan, P. & Brodie, M. J. Early identification of refractory epilepsy. *New Engl J Med* 2000;**342**: 314–319.

27. Rigamonti, D., Drayer, B. P., Johnson, P. C., *et al.* The MRI appearance of cavernous malformations (angiomas). *J Neurosurg* 1987;**67**:518–524.

28. Rivera, P. P., Willinsky, R. A. & Porter, P. J. Intracranial cavernous malformations. *Neuroimaging Clin N Am* 2003;**13**:27–40.

29. Campbell, P. G., Jabbour, P., Yadla, S. & Awad, I. A. Emerging clinical imaging techniques for cerebral cavernous malformations: a systematic review. *Neurosurg Focus* 2010;**29**:E6.

30. Baumann, C. R., Schuknecht, B., Lo Russo, G., *et al.* Seizure outcome after resection of cavernous malformations is better when surrounding hemosiderin-stained brain also is removed. *Epilepsia* 2006;**47**:563–566.

31. Hammen, T., Romstöck, J., Dörfler, A., *et al.* Prediction of postoperative outcome with special respect to removal of hemosiderin fringe: a study in patients with cavernous haemangiomas associated with symptomatic epilepsy. *Seizure* 2007;**16**:248–253.

32. Stavrou, I., Baumgartner, C., Frischer, J. M., Trattnig, S. & Knosp, E. Long-term seizure control after resection of supratentorial cavernomas: a retrospective single-center study in 53 patients. *Neurosurgery* 2008;**63**:888–896.

33. Bernotas, G., Rastenyte, D., Deltuva, V., *et al.* Cavernous angiomas: an uncontrolled clinical study of 87 surgically treated patients. *Medicina (Kaunas)* 2009;**45**:21–28.

34. Rigamonti, D., Hadley, M. N., Drayer, B. P., *et al.* Cerebral cavernous malformations. Incidence and familial occurrence. *New Engl J Med* 1988;**319**:343–347.

35. Riant, F., Bergametti, F., Ayrignac, X., Boulday, G. & Tournier-Lasserve, E. Recent insights into cerebral cavernous malformations: the molecular genetics of CCM. *FEBS J* 2010;**277**:1070–1075.

36. Kivelev, J., Niemelä, M., Kivisaari, R., *et al.* Long-term outcome of patients with multiple cerebral cavernous malformations. *Neurosurgery* 2009;**65**:450–455.

37. Rocamora, R., Mader, I., Zentner, J. & Schulze-Bonhage, A. Epilepsy surgery in patients with multiple cerebral cavernous malformations. *Seizure* 2009;**18**:241–245.

38. Stefan, H., Scheler, G., Hummel, C., *et al.* Magnetoencephalography (MEG) predicts focal epileptogenicity in cavernomas. *J Neurol Neurosurg Psychiatry* 2004;**75**:1309–1313.

39. Arora, J., Pugh, K., Westerveld, M., *et al.* Language lateralization in epilepsy patients: fMRI validated with the Wada procedure. *Epilepsia* 2009;**50**:2225–2241.

40. Wellmer, J., Weber, B., Urbach, H., *et al.* Cerebral lesions can impair fMRI-based language lateralization. *Epilepsia* 2009;**50**:2213–2224.

41. Kamada, K., Sawamura, Y., Takeuchi, F., *et al.* Expressive and receptive language areas determined by a non-invasive reliable method using functional magnetic resonance imaging and magnetoencephalography. *Neurosurgery* 2007;**60**:296–305.

42. Petersen, T. A., Morrison, L. A., Schrader, R. M. & Hart, B. L. Familial versus sporadic cavernous malformations: differences in developmental venous anomaly association and lesion phenotype. *AJNR Am J Neuroradiol* 2010;**31**:377–382.

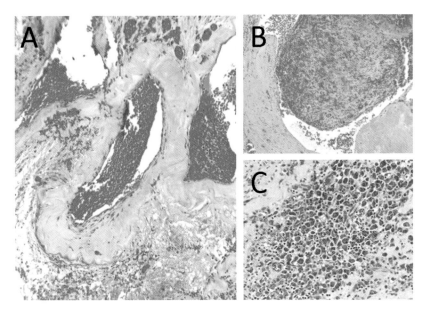

Figure 1.1 (A) The back-to-back blood vessels of cavernous malformations have thick, amorphous walls. (B) The blood vessel shown here contains a recent thrombus. (C) Densely packed hemosiderin-laden macrophages are often found within or around the rim of a cavernous angioma.

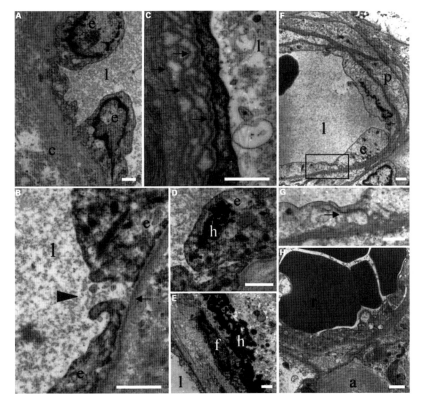

Figure 1.2 Electron micrographs of cavernous malformations (A-E) and microvessels in adjacent normal brain (F-H). (A) Ultrastructurally, these lesions consist of endothelial cells (e) lining vascular sinusoid lumens (l) and surrounded by a dense collagenous matrix (c). No perivascular cells were seen and the endothelial basal lamina was in direct contact with the collagenous matrix. (B) Gaps (arrowhead) between adjacent endothelial cells were seen in cavernous malformations where the lumen (l) was exposed directly to the basal lamina (arrow). (C) In focal areas, the basal lamina (arrows) demonstrated multiple abnormal layers. (D,E) Haemosiderin (h) could be seen within endothelial cells (D) and within microns of the lumens of the vascular sinusoids (E). A rare fibroblast profile (f) is seen in (E) in the connective tissue matrix. (F) A cerebral microvessel from brain tissue adjacent to a lesion demonstrates typical encircling pericytes (p) separating the endothelial cell basal lamina from the neuropil. A red blood cell (r) is noted in the lumen. (G) Magnification of the boxed area in F demonstrates a tight junction (arrow) between adjacent endothelial processes. (H) Another microvessel from the surrounding brain is being contacted by an astrocyte foot process (a) containing abundant intermediate filaments. Scale bar shown in all images represents 1 μm. Reproduced from [49] with permission from BMJ Publishing Group.

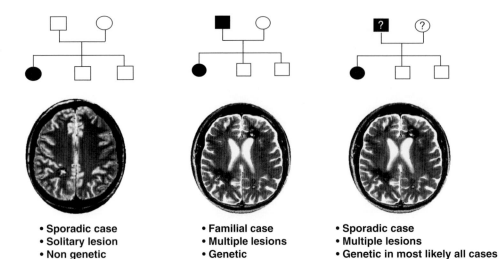

- Sporadic case
- Solitary lesion
- Non genetic

- Familial case
- Multiple lesions
- Genetic

- Sporadic case
- Multiple lesions
- Genetic in most likely all cases

Figure 4.1 Multiplicity of CCM lesions is a hallmark of the familial form of the disease. Left panel: a sporadic, non-genetic case with a unique lesion on cerebral MRI. Middle panel: a familial case with multiple lesions. Right panel: a sporadic case with multiple lesions which is most likely a genetic case due to either an incomplete clinical penetrance or a *de novo* mutation.

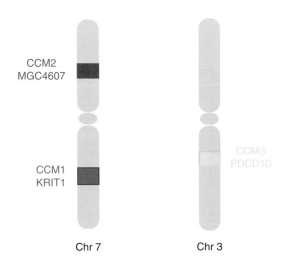

Figure 4.2 CCM genetic loci and genes. Three CCM genes have been mapped on chromosomes 7 (CCM1 and CCM2) and 3 (CCM3). The vast majority of CCM gene mutations are loss of function mutations.

CCM1/Krit1

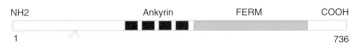

NH2   Ankyrin   FERM   COOH

1   736

Figure 4.3 The three CCM genes encode for three unrelated proteins, krit1 (CCM1) which contains several ankyrin domains and a FERM domain, mgc4607, also called malcavernin, which contains a PTB (phosphotyrosine binding) domain, and pdcd10, a protein involved in apoptosis.

CCM2/Malcavernin

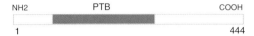

NH2   PTB   COOH

1   444

CCM3/pdcd10

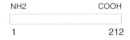

NH2   COOH

1   212

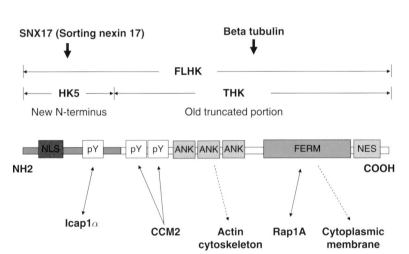

Figure 5.2 The domains and their functions of the CCM1 gene. The schematic diagram summarizes the domains and functions of full-length krit1 based on our current knowledge. Solid arrow lines indicate the confirmed interactions with a specific domain. Dashed arrow lines indicate proposed interactions based on the domain's well-known functions. Arrowheads indicate the confirmed interactions with an undefined binding site.

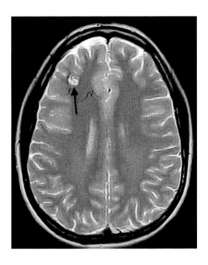

Figure 12.1 Axial T2-weighted MR image of a patient presenting with new-onset generalized seizure at age 33, in the absence of alcohol or drug intake or trauma. Seizure semiology, pre-ictal and post-ictal symptoms and interictal electroencephalogram (EEG) were not helpful in localizing the seizure focus, and seizures did not recur on anticonvulsant medications. Gradient-echo images did not reveal other lesions and contrast-enhanced imaging did not reveal an associated overt venous developmental anomaly. Because of the patient's occupation as a driver, and his young age, he elected to undergo microsurgical excision of the solitary right frontal CCM (arrow), along with the surrounding hemosiderin-stained brain parenchyma ("lesionectomy-plus"). The patient remained seizure-free postoperatively, was tapered off anticonvulsants after 1 year, and has resumed driving and normal life without seizure restrictions. Continued medical therapy with anticonvulsants would also have been appropriate. If his seizures were intractable or longstanding, or if seizures persisted after lesionectomy, more extensive brain mapping with interictal and ictal-onset recording would be performed, allowing resection of epileptogenic brain tissue adjacent to the lesion.

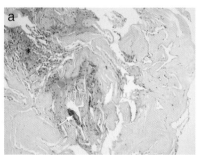
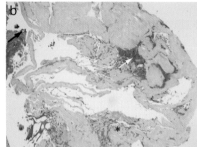

Figure 13.1 Low power (40×
magnification) hematoxylin and eosin
(H&E) stained sections of a spinal CM (A)
and a cerebral CM (B) show that the
histopathological features of the two
lesions are identical. The sections show
thin-walled sinusoids of endothelial cells
associated with thrombosis (white arrow;
pink stain), calcification (black arrow; dark
blue stain), and hemosiderin deposits
(brownish pigment within the cytoplasm
of macrophages (*)). Used with permission
from Barrow Neurological Institute.

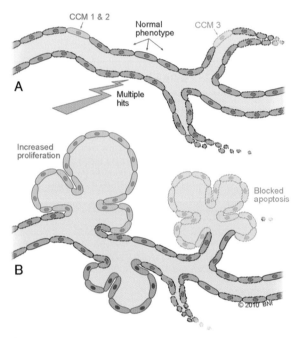

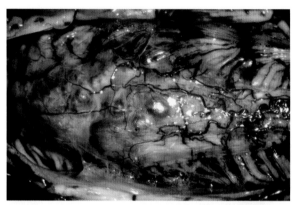

Figure 13.4 Intraoperative photograph of a spinal CM identified by
its distinct bluish discoloration. Although these lesions may be readily
identified using microscopic magnification, intraoperative
ultrasonography may be needed to identify lesions without an
exophytic component. Used with permission from Barrow
Neurological Institute.

Figure 13.2 Although the origin of cavernous malformations is
unknown, several mutations in important regulators of proliferation,
differentiation, and the apoptotic machinery have been identified.
Mutations regulating the decision of an endothelial cell to proliferate
or differentiate (CCM1 and CCM2) cause unregulated growth of
vasculature, while those involved in the apoptotic machinery (CCM3)
interrupt the finely orchestrated pruning mechanism, further
exacerbating the unregulated growth phenotype of this lesion. CM
may form after exposure to radiation. Radiation may stimulate or
block pathways similar to those in mutations identified in the familial
cases, resulting in unregulated growth of endothelial cells and
formation of CMs. Used with permission from Barrow Neurological
Institute.

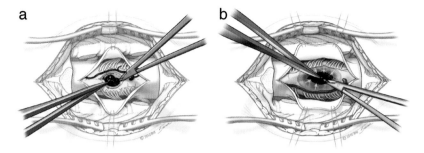

a

b

Figure 13.5 Schematic representation of the surgical technique used to resect spinal CMs, which are typically small, low-flow lesions with a mulberry-like appearance. The surgical technique used to remove these lesions is similar to that used to resect benign intramedullary spinal cord tumors. Using MRI guidance, the location of the lesion is identified. The dura is opened sharply over the lesion. The lesion is identified by its bluish discoloration. Care is taken to dissect sharply within the gliotic plane surrounding the lesion to avoid injury to normal spinal tissue. The use of electrocoagulation should be minimized, and hemosiderin-stained tissue should be preserved as much as possible. Although (A) smaller lesions are amenable to en bloc resection, (B) larger lesions should be decompressed internally and then dissected circumferentially to minimize trauma to the spinal cord. The lesion bed should be inspected carefully before closure to prevent leaving remnant spinal CM, which could give rise to recurrent disease. Used with permission from Barrow Neurological Institute.

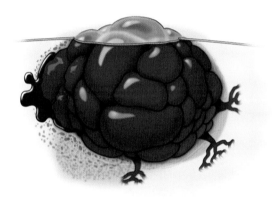

Figure 13.6 CMs are frequently associated with other vascular anomalies. During the resection of intramedullary spinal CMs, it is essential to identify and preserve any cryptic venous malformations. These cryptic malformations often serve as the primary blood supply for watershed regions adjacent to CMs, and their removal may result in ischemic damage to critical spinal tracts, resulting in permanent neurological devastation. Used with permission from Barrow Neurological Institute.

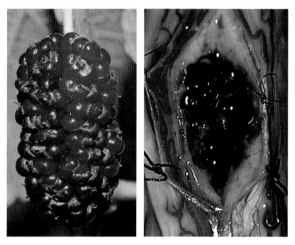

Figure 14.1 Comparison between a cavernous malformation (same case as depicted in MRI studies of spinal cord lesion in Fig. 14.3) and a mulberry. Note multiple lobules and variegated appearance of the lesion.

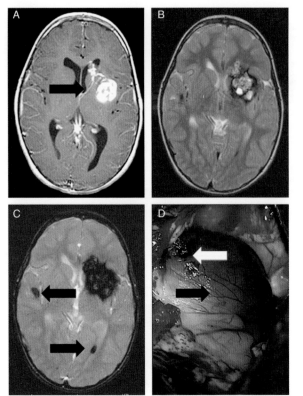

Figure 14.2 MRI appearance of cavernous malformations. (A) T1 post-contrast axial study of left frontal lesion; note irregular enhancement and presence of associated developmental venous malformation (arrow). (B) T2 images demonstrating "popcorn" appearance of lesion with multiple small cysts and darker rim of hemosiderin on periphery. (C) Susceptibility images reveal "bloom" of previous hemorrhages and highlight other lesions within this patient (arrows). (D) Operative correlation of radiographic studies with greenish, hemosiderin-stained surrounding tissue (black arrow) and darker, "mulberry"-like malformation (white arrow).

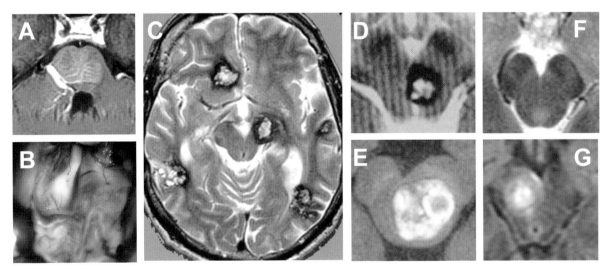

Figure 15.1 (A) T1-W contrast-enhanced axial MRI showing a large pontine venous malformation found in a 54-year-old female. (B) Intraoperative view of the surface of the rhomboid fossa in a 30-year-old male showing a large superficial venous malformation (CVM). The patient underwent surgery for removal of a cavernous malformation (not seen in this image) that was located more superiorly and had no direct contact to this CVM. (C) T2-W axial MRI showing multiple intracerebral cavernous malformations including a lesion within the left midbrain tegmentum. (D) T2-W axial MRI taken in a 55-year-old female furnishes evidence of a small cavernous malformation within the left part of the midbrain tectum. (E) More than 2 years later this lesion clearly increased in size, mostly due to intrinsic proliferative activity. (F) T2-W axial MRI taken at the level of the midbrain in a 31-year-old female who suffered from hereditary disease. Multiple cerebral cavernous malformations were found in this patient but none was initially located within the brainstem. (G) Two years later the patient presented with a left-sided hemiparesis caused by a hemorrhagic *de novo* cavernous malformation within the right midbrain tegmentum.

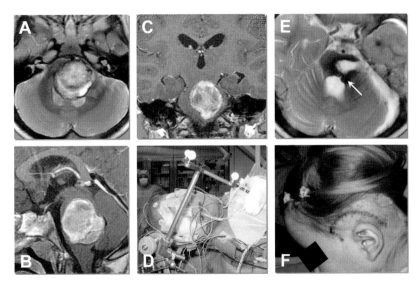

Figure 15.3 T2-W axial (A) and T1-W contrast-enhanced MRI in sagittal (B) and coronal plane (C), taken in a 3.5-year-old girl who presented with right-sided hemiparesis, unable to walk alone. The images demonstrate a large intrapontine cavernous malformation with an extensive intralesional hematoma. Surgery was performed in the acute stage, and the lesion was accessed from laterally via a left-sided subtemporal transtentorial approach with the patient in the supine position (D). Total removal of the cavernoma is demonstrated on postoperative MRI, and the parenchymal tissue dorsal to the resection cavity (arrow) has remained intact (E). The postoperative photograph of this girl shows the skin incision in the left temporal region (F).

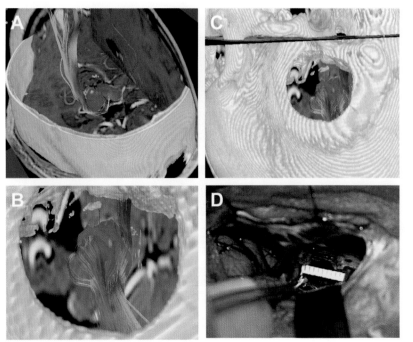

Figure 15.4 Visualization of the corticospinal tract, medial lemniscus and cavernoma within the right midbrain and upper pons in a 38-year-old male (same patient as shown in Fig. 15.6). (A) View from superiorly, anteriorly and laterally showing the tracts located lateral to the cavernoma. The multi-modality 3D data set consists of a tri-planar MRI; the cavernoma was segmented from the MRI, the skull from CT scans, and the fiber tracts derived from DTI. (B, C) Surgical perspective through a simulated temporal craniotomy. Note the corticospinal tract along the anterior margin of the cavernoma and the sensory fibers along its dorsal portion. The surgical corridor was chosen between both tracts. (D) Intraoperative photograph showing the subtemporal approach and cavernoma exposure through a small vertical brainstem opening in the planned position. The vein of Labbé and tributaries at the base of the temporal lobe have been dissected free and spared throughout the procedure.

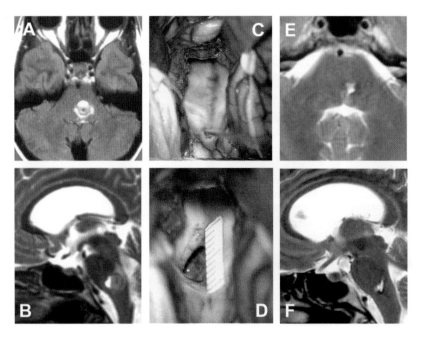

Figure 15.5 Preoperative T1-W axial (A) and T2-W sagittal MRI (B) of a 36-year-old female who presented with internuclear ophthalmoplegia. Surgery was performed via the floor of the fourth ventricle with the patient placed in the sitting position. The rhomboid fossa showed a slight yellowish discoloration and excavation in the midline (C). The lesion was exposed through a midline incision below the facial colliculus (D). Total removal of the lesion is demonstrated on postoperative T2-W MRI in axial (E) and sagittal plane (F).

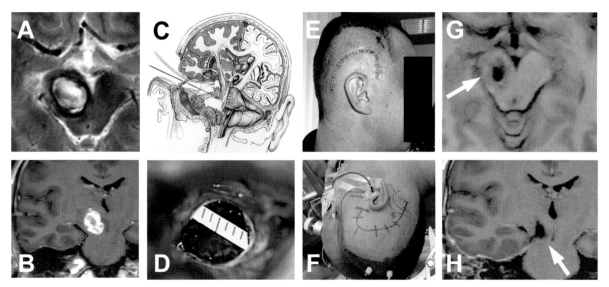

Figure 15.6 This 38-year-old male presented with a left-sided hemiparesis and diplopia. A large and hemorrhagic cavernous malformation is seen in the depth of the right midbrain tegmentum on T2-W axial (A) and T1-W coronal MRI (B). The lesion was exposed via a right-sided subtemporal route, as illustrated by Peter Roth (C). The opening on the surface of the brainstem (approximately 7 mm) remained smaller than the initial diameter of the lesion (D). The skin incision on the right temporal region can be seen both on the postoperative photograph of the patient (E) and marked on the skin in the operating room (F). Total removal of the lesion without damage of the temporal lobe or the brainstem is demonstrated on postoperative MRI in axial (G) and coronal plane (H). The arrows point to the resection cavity. No additional neurological deficits occurred postoperatively.

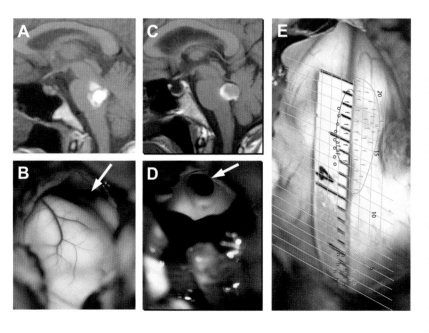

Figure 15.7. (A) Sagittal T1-W non-enhanced MRI showing a large intraaxial cavernous malformation with fresh intralesional hematoma. The lesion is bulging subependymally into the fourth ventricle and has been approached via the rhomboid fossa using the telovelar exposure. (B) The intraoperative photograph taken in this patient shows the left side of the upper rhomboid fossa below the aqueduct (arrow) bulging into the fourth ventricle. (C) Sagittal T1-W MRI showing a similar lesion in another patient. More than half of the cavernous malformation is bulging exophytically into the fourth ventricle. This lesion was also exposed via the telovelar midline approach. (D) The intraoperative photograph demonstrates that the lesion broke into the fourth ventricle through the ependyma of the rhomboid fossa. Superiorly, the aqueduct is visible (arrow). (E) Mapping the rhomboid fossa using a millimeter scale placed in longitudinal direction. The measurement in the caudal-cranial direction commenced at the obex. The area of facial nerve response is marked with "f" and is encircled on both sides. Obviously, this area clearly differs between the left and right side.

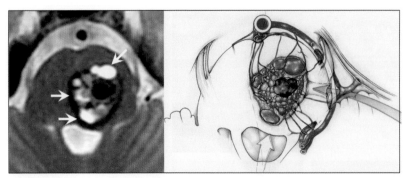

Figure 15.8 Left: axial non-enhanced T1-W MRI of a male showing a large pontine cavernoma at the level of the trigeminal root. The lesion contains several areas of fresh hematoma cavities (arrows). Right: the artistic illustration by Peter Roth highlights the various parts of which the lesion is composed: multiple caverns, several hematoma cavities and the vascular supply. Although access via the rhomboid fossa would have yielded the shortest distance to the lesion (white arrow), the malformation was approached and totally removed from laterally (green arrow).

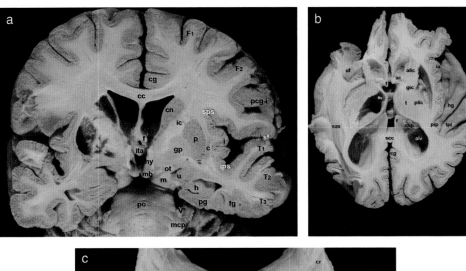

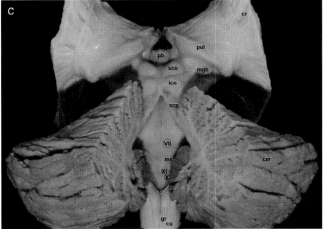

Figure 16.1 In order to demonstrate some of the eloquent locations in which cavernous malformations may be located, cadaver brains are shown. The anatomical locations of the cavernous malformations from the cases presented in this chapter can be seen in these images. (a) Coronal section of a cadaver brain through the foramen of Monro, anterior view. The putamen, globus pallidus and caudate nucleus of the right hemisphere are removed using the fiber dissection technique to reveal the internal capsule. Various eloquent locations of the brain are demonstrated. Note the close relationship of the superior periinsular sulcus with the internal capsule. (b) Axial section of a cadaver brain through the foramen of Monro, superior view. Right-sided the putamen, globus pallidus, and caudate nucleus are dissected away to demonstrate the anterior limb of the internal capsule and the lateral extension of the anterior commissure. Together with the left-sided putamen, globus pallidus, caudate nucleus and thalamus, the left frontal, temporal, and insular cortex are removed in order to demonstrate the lateral extension of the anterior commissure joining to the sagittal stratum. The anterior and posterior limbs of the internal capsule are also illustrated. Asterisk denotes the mammillothalamic tract of Vicq d'Azyr. (c) Posterior view of the brain stem and thalamus with neighboring corona radiata of cadaver specimen is shown. Vermis of the cerebellum dissected away, therefore the floor of the fourth ventricle is exposed. Bilateral cerebral hemispheres are also removed but part of the corona radiata near the thalamus is preserved. Abbreviations: ac, anterior commissure; alic, anterior limb of internal capsule; alv, atrial portion of lateral ventricle; aps, anterior periinsular sulcus; c, claustrum; cc, corpus callosum; cer, cerebellum; cg, cingulate gyrus; chp, choroid plexus; cis, central insular sulcus; cn, caudate nucleus; cr, corona radiata; cu, cuneate fasciculus; f, fornix; F1, superior frontal gyrus; F2, middle frontal gyrus; fg, fusiform gyrus; gic, genu of internal capsule; gp, globus pallidus; gr, gracile fasciculus; h, hippocampus; hg, Heschl gyrus; hy, hypothalamus; i, insula; ia, insular apex; ic, internal capsule; ico, inferior colliculus; ips, inferior periinsular sulcus; ita, interthalamic adhesion; m, midbrain; mb, mamillary body; mcp, middle cerebellar peduncle; mgb, medial geniculate body; ms, medullary striae of fourth ventricle; o, obex; ot, optic tract; p, putamen; pb, pineal body; pcg-i, inferior portion of precentral gyrus; pg, parahippocampal gyrus; pip, posterior insular point; plic, posterior limb of internal capsule; po, pons; pul, pulvinar of thalamus; sas, sagittal stratum; scc, splenium of corpus callosum; sco, superior colliculus; scp, superior cerebellar peduncle; sf, sylvian fissure; sps, superior peri-insular sulcus; t, thalamus; T1, superior temporal gyrus; T2, middle temporal gyrus; T3, inferior temporal gyrus; tpl, temporal planum; u, uncus; uf, uncinate fasciculus. Roman numbers in circles indicate the nuclei of the corresponding cranial nerves.

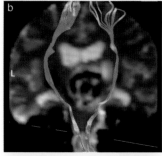

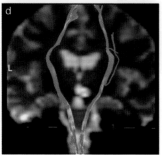

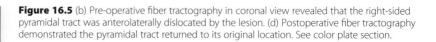

Figure 16.5 (b) Pre-operative fiber tractography in coronal view revealed that the right-sided pyramidal tract was anterolaterally dislocated by the lesion. (d) Postoperative fiber tractography demonstrated the pyramidal tract returned to its original location. See color plate section.

43. Rigamonti, D. & Spetzler, R. F. The association of venous and cavernous malformations. Report of four cases and discussion of the pathophysiological, diagnostic, and therapeutic implications. *Acta Neurochir (Wien)* 1988;**92**:100–105.

44. Maciunas, J. A., Syed, T. U., Cohen, M. L., *et al.* Triple pathology in epilepsy: coexistence of cavernous angiomas and cortical dysplasias with other lesions. *Epilepsy Res* 2010;**91**:106–110.

45. Takebayashi, S., Hashizume, K., Uchida, K. & Tanaka, T. [A case of coexistence with cavernous angioma and focal cortical dysplasia]. *No To Shinkei* 2006;**58**:245–249 (in Japanese).

46. Giulioni, M., Zucchelli, M., Riguzzi, P., *et al.* Co-existence of cavernoma and cortical dysplasia in temporal lobe epilepsy. *J Clin Neurosci* 2007;**14**:1122–1124.

47. Kondziolka, D., Lunsford, L. D., Flickinger, J. C. & Kestle, J. R. Reduction of hemorrhage risk after stereotactic radiosurgery for cavernous malformations. *J Neurosurg* 1995;**83**:825–831.

48. Monaco, E. A., Khan, A. A., Niranjan, A., *et al.* Stereotactic radiosurgery for the treatment of symptomatic brainstem cavernous malformations. *Neurosurg Focus* 2010;**29**:E11.

49. Hsu, P. W., Chang, C. N., Tseng, C. K., *et al.* Treatment of epileptogenic cavernomas: surgery versus radiosurgery. *Cerebrovasc Dis* 2007;**24**:116–120.

50. Liu, K. D., Chung, W. Y., Wu, H. M., *et al.* Gamma knife surgery for cavernous hemangiomas: an analysis of 125 patients. *J Neurosurg* 2005;**102**(Suppl):81–86.

51. Hasegawa, T., McInerney, J., Kondziolka, D., *et al.* Long-term results after stereotactic radiosurgery for patients with cavernous malformations. *Neurosurgery* 2002;**50**:1190–1197.

52. Lunsford, L. D., Khan, A. A., Niranjan, A., *et al.* Stereotactic radiosurgery for symptomatic solitary cerebral cavernous malformations considered high risk for resection. *J Neurosurg* 2010;**113**:23–29.

53. Shih, Y. H. & Pan, D. H. Management of supratentorial cavernous malformations: craniotomy versus gammaknife radiosurgery. *Clin Neurol Neurosurg* 2005;**107**:108–112.

54. Spencer, S. & Huh, L. Outcomes of epilepsy surgery in adults and children. *Lancet Neurol* 2008;**7**:525–537.

55. Baumann, C. R., Acciarri, N., Bertalanffy, H., *et al.* Seizure outcome after resection of supratentorial cavernous malformations: a study of 168 patients. *Epilepsia* 2007;**48**:559–563.

56. Chang, E. F., Gabriel, R. A., Potts, M. B., *et al.* Seizure characteristics and control after microsurgical resection of supratentorial cerebral cavernous malformations. *Neurosurgery* 2009;**65**:31–37.

57. Bartolomei, F., Hayashi, M., Tamura, M., *et al.* Long-term efficacy of gamma knife radiosurgery in mesial temporal lobe epilepsy. *Neurology* 2008;**70**:1658–1663.

The pros and cons of conservative and surgical treatment of cavernous malformations

Pablo F. Recinos, Sheng-Fu Larry Lo and Daniele Rigamonti

Introduction

Cavernous malformations (CMs) of the nervous system were once poorly understood entities. With the advent and use of computed tomography (CT) and magnetic resonance imaging (MRI), our ability to diagnose and understand their behavior has advanced. As our knowledge of their natural history has increased, it has become clear that certain CMs require treatment while others do not. However, the ability to predict the behavior of individual CMs remains beyond our current limitations. Currently, management of CMs is based on the clinical presentation, the anatomical location of the lesion, and our knowledge of behavior patterns based on these two factors.

Traditionally, CMs have been managed either conservatively or with surgery. More recently, radiosurgery has evolved as a possible treatment option. We present a systematic review of the management of CMs based on presentation and anatomical location. We also present algorithms based on current knowledge to guide the management of CMs.

Management considerations based on seizure history

Seizure activity presents in 23–50% of patients harboring cavernous malformations (Fig. 11.1) [1]. Supratentorial lesions are more prone to be epileptogenic than infratentorial lesions. However, no association has been found between the presence of a CM in a particular cerebral lobe and an increased risk of seizure development [2]. When a patient presents with a first-time seizure and is found to have a mass lesion on imaging, the first objective is to determine whether the lesion is the etiology of the seizure or whether it is an incidental finding. If a CM is diagnosed and if seizure symptoms correspond to the location of the lesion, then a causative relationship is established and treatment is initiated. In cases where the CM is found to be in a non-epileptogenic location (e.g. infratentorial, in the brainstem, or in the deep white matter) or other possible seizure etiologies are present (e.g. alcohol, drugs, or trauma), the management of the CM and seizures are considered individually [3].

Epilepsy produced by CMs can be treated medically or surgically. The first-line option for seizures produced by CMs is medical. After a patient has a first-time seizure, the likelihood of seizure recurrence must be weighed against the risks of placing the patient on chronic anticonvulsant therapy [3]. Although newer anticonvulsants tend to have a reduced side-effect profile compared to older drugs, they are not always appropriate or indicated (e.g. pregnancy). When medical therapy is initiated, anticonvulsants are prescribed according to seizure characteristics.

There is a paucity of studies available that have studied medical therapy alone for the treatment of seizures caused by a CM. Churchyard *et al.* reported a series of 16 patients in which 13 patients had supratentorial CMs and presented with seizures. Out of those 13 patients, only one patient required surgical excision due to intractable epilepsy, while the rest had seizures controlled by anticonvulsants. Their study was limited by short follow-up time in four patients. Notably, none of the 13 patients who presented with seizures had a subsequent hemorrhage. This study demonstrated that a select group of patients suffering seizures from a CM could be successfully managed with medical therapy alone [4].

There have been numerous studies that have examined surgery as a treatment for epilepsy caused by CMs.

Cavernous Malformations of the Nervous System, ed. Daniele Rigamonti. Published by Cambridge University Press.
© Cambridge University Press 2011.

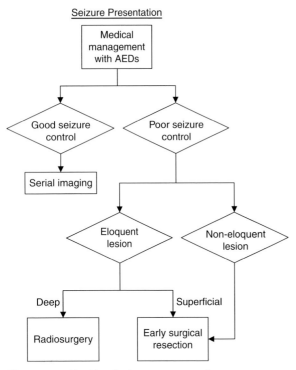

Seizure Presentation

Figure 11.1. Algorithm for the management of cavernous malformations presenting with seizures.

In 1999, Moran *et al.* published a review of 268 reported cases of supratentorial CMs that had seizures. Out of those patients, 228 (84%) were reported to be seizure-free, 21 (8%) had improved seizure control, 16 (6%) had no change in epilepsy, and 5 (2%) had worse control of their seizures [2]. Effectively, 92% of patients had results that were improved from their baseline after surgical excision of the CM. Similar results have been reflected in subsequent series [5–7].

The timing of surgery to remove a CM that causes seizures has also been shown to affect patient outcomes. Ferroli *et al.* reported a series of 163 patients with CM-related seizures who had pure lesionectomy. Post-resection, 98.4% (63/64) of patients having experienced a single seizure or sporadic convulsions were seizure-free. In contrast, 68.7% (68/99) were seizure-free and 10.1% (10/99) had decreased seizure frequency in the subset of patients who presented with a long clinical history of seizures [5]. Cohen and colleagues performed a retrospective analysis of 51 patients who underwent pure lesionectomy for the resection of a CM. They observed that in patients with only one preoperative seizure and those with a seizure history of less than

2 months, 100% of patients were seizure-free. In the group experiencing 2–5 preoperative seizures and those with a 2–12 month seizure history 75–80% of patients were seizure-free, while in the group having experienced greater than five preoperative seizures and those with greater than a 12-month seizure history only 50–55% of patients were seizure-free [8]. In both the study by Ferroli *et al.* and that by Cohen and co-workers, a pure lesionectomy was performed without resection of surrounding cortex [5,8]. Given that patients with a longer seizure history had a lower rate of seizure-free outcomes, the brain tissue surrounding the lesions may have undergone changes and become epileptogenic.

Some authors have argued that as a CM builds a surrounding hemosiderin ring, through either hemorrhage or chronic seizures, the surrounding brain parenchyma undergoes changes that can make it epileptogenic. Therefore, the effect of surgical resection of a CM plus its surrounding hemosiderin ring versus resection of only the CM was examined. Baumann and co-workers performed a retrospective study of 31 patients with chronic epilepsy caused by a CM who underwent surgical resection. In all cases, there was a hemosiderin ring surrounding the CM. Out of the 31 patients, 14 were treated by total lesionectomy with complete resection of the surrounding hemosiderin ring while 17 were treated with total lesionectomy with partial or no resection of the surrounding hemosiderin ring. In the first 2 years after surgery, both groups had a comparable rate of being seizure-free (Engel class I). However, 3 years post-operatively, the group with complete hemosiderin ring excision had a higher seizure-free rate compared to the group with partial or no hemisiderin ring excision (59% vs. 46% respectively) [9]. Similarly, Stavrou *et al.* performed a retrospective study of 53 patients with supratentorial CMs treated with microsurgery. In the subgroup of patients with a seizure history of less than 2 years, those having a lesionectomy with excision of the hemosiderin ring had a significantly higher seizure-free outcome compared to those treated by lesionectomy without excision of the hemosiderin ring. However, excision of the hemosiderin ring did not affect outcome in patients with a preoperative seizure history of greater than 2 years [10].

Another aspect that has been investigated in patients with a long history of epilepsy secondary to a CM was the effect of a tailored surgical resection of the lesion and associated seizure focus (as determined by preoperative studies). Paolini and colleagues reported on a series of eight patients with intractable temporal lobe epilepsy (mean 2 years, range 1–43 years) secondary to a CM. Preoperative clinical and electrical monitoring with EEG or video-EEG were obtained and a focused resection was subsequently performed. Two underwent lesionectomy with excision of surrounding hemosiderin and gliosis, four underwent lesionectomy with antero-mesial temporal lobectomy, and two underwent lesion-ectomy with extended temporal lobectomy. Six out of the seven patients available at one year were completely seizure-free (Engel IA), while the other patient was classified as Engel IB [11]. Although these results are certainly promising, larger studies need to be performed to further validate these findings.

Management considerations based on anatomical location

Non-eloquent, lobar

See Fig. 11.2.

The anatomical location of a CM is a critical factor that directly affects the risks and benefits of both con-servative and surgical management. The management of hemispheric, non-eloquent CMs is straightforward and the least controversial. Asymptomatic lobar CMs that are found incidentally in non-eloquent areas should always be managed with observation. In this clinical scenario, the main risks are future hemorrhage

and seizure development. Given that massive hemor-rhage is not characteristic of CMs, any hemorrhagic event in a non-eloquent, lobar location is unlikely to produce significant morbidity. Lobar, non-eloquent lesions that present with progressive neurological deficit, recurrently hemorrhage, or are associated with intractable seizures should be surgically resected [3,7,12,13]. Microsurgical resection of these lesions is generally safe and curative [14].

Eloquent cortex and deep supratentorial

See Fig. 11.3.

Management of CMs that are located in eloquent cortex or in deep supratentorial regions requires a case-by-case evaluation. The main complications from lesions in these locations are also seizure development, hemorrhagic events, and focal neurological deficits related to hemorrhage. In a recent meta-analysis, the annual risk of hemorrhage in the basal ganglia and thalamus was found to be between 2.8% and 4.1% [15]. However, a single hemorrhagic event can have devastating neurological consequences given that a large number of critical pathways are packed into a focused space. When a hemorrhage does occur as a result of a deep CM, the risk of significant, long-term morbidity ranged from 15 to 33% [16,17]. Although this risk is higher than the risk observed in other loca-tions, it is possible that hemorrhages in the basal ganglia and thalamus are much more likely to present clinically

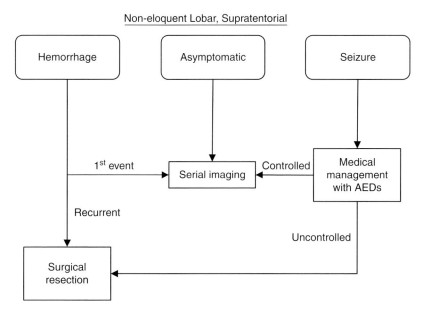

Non-eloquent Lobar, Supratentorial

Figure 11.2. Algorithm for the management of cavernous malformations located in non-eloquent, supratentorial cortex.

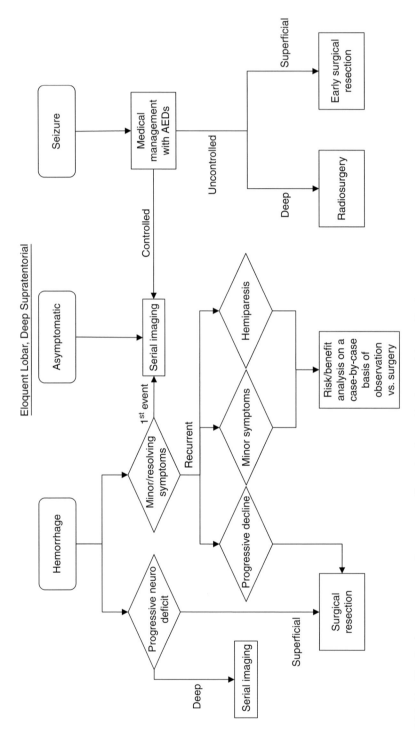

Figure 11.3. Algorithm for the management of cavernous malformations located in eloquent lobar and/or deep cortex.

than hemorrhages in non-eloquent areas. Conversely, an invasive, surgical approach to the basal ganglia and thalamus also carries a risk of devastating complications. Gross *et al.* performed a meta-analysis of patients with CMs of the basal ganglia and thalamus that were reported in surgical series. Out of 103 patients, 71 (89%) had complete lesion resection, 10 (10%) suffered permanent, long-term morbidity as a result of surgery, and two (1.9%) died from surgery [15]. The position of the lesion within the eloquent structures (e.g. if it reaches a pial or ependymal surface or it is embedded deep within a critical structure) may also affect the relative risk of surgery. The use of electrophysiological monitoring, frameless stereotactic guidance systems, and integration of functional MRI with intraoperative navigation has allowed such high-risk lesions to be resected in a more precise and safe manner [18,19]. Overall, it is not surprising that both the natural history and surgical outcomes of basal ganglia and thalamic CMs are associated with a higher morbidity and mortality compared to CMs in non-eloquent locations. Therefore, patients with incidentally found CMs in eloquent cortex or deep structures should be managed with observation and serial MRIs on a yearly or bi-yearly basis. If seizures occur as a result of the CMs, they should be managed with anticonvulsants. After a first hemorrhage, the patient's clinical status will influence management. If symptoms and/or a focal deficit are present but are minor and improve, continued observation is indicated. Surgical intervention can be considered if there is both a significant, non-resolving neurological deficit and if the lesion reaches an ependymal or pial surface [15]. After a second hemorrhage, the patient is at increased risk for temporal clustering of hemorrhagic events and surgery should be strongly considered to eliminate future risk of hemorrhage or worsening neurological deficit [15,20]. Since surgery is not typically performed in the acute phase of the hemorrhage, the patient's clinical status nonetheless influences management. If the patient makes a swift improvement in clinical status, continued conservative management may again be indicated since mortality from a CM hemorrhage is rare. Conversely, if the patient presents profoundly hemiparetic, it is unknown how much benefit is afforded to the patient with surgical resection despite the surgical risks being much lower. Therefore, surgery should be performed only if it is determined there is a favorable risk/benefit ratio.

Brainstem

See Fig. 11.4.

The management paradigm of brainstem CMs is similar to that of CMs in eloquent cortex and deep locations. The main complication of brainstem CMs is hemorrhage and neurological deficit as a result of hemorrhage. The hemorrhage rate of brainstem CMs in natural history studies was found to be 2.33–4.1%, while in surgical studies it ranged from 2.68 to 6.8% per patient-year prior to intervention [21]. The rebleed rates have also been examined and have been found to be between 5 and 21.5% in natural history studies and ranged from 17.7% per patient-year to 1.9 hemorrhages per patient-year prior to intervention in surgical series [22–26]. Temporal clustering of recurrent hemorrhage has also been shown to occur in brainstem CMs [27,28].

A hemorrhage in the brainstem can resemble brainstem stroke syndromes and be neurologically devastating. Conservative management carries the risk of future hemorrhages, which can result in permanent neurological deficits. Abe *et al.* reported a cohort of 30 patients with brainstem CMs that were managed by observation. Twenty-one percent of patients suffered severe neurological symptoms after having initially suffered minor symptoms as a result of a hemorrhage. They also reported that 6.8% of patients experienced persistent neurological deficit after 1 month with no signs of improvement [29].

Likewise, surgery carries significant risks. Gross *et al.* performed a comprehensive review of 78 studies that covered the natural history, surgical outcomes, and radiosurgical outcomes of brainstem CMs. In the surgical series, complete resection was achieved in 684 out of 745 cases (92%). Initial postoperative morbidity ranged from 29% to 67% in larger series, but was often temporary. Out of 683 patients, 85% had improvement of clinical symptoms, 14% had worsening of symptoms, and 1.9% died from complications related to surgery [21]. Thus, the morbidity and mortality of conservative management versus surgical management must be considered when counseling the patient.

After an initial hemorrhage, observation is recommended due to the fact that some CMs have a more benign course than others. Brainstem CMs producing two or more hemorrhagic events are likely to follow a more aggressive course. If the lesion comes to a pial or ependymal surface on preoperative MRI, surgery

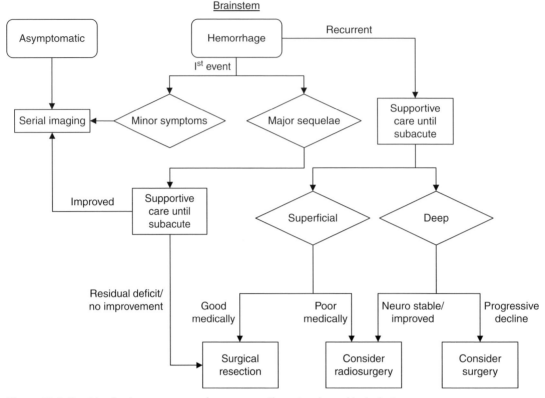

Figure 11.4. Algorithm for the management of cavernous malformations located in the brainstem.

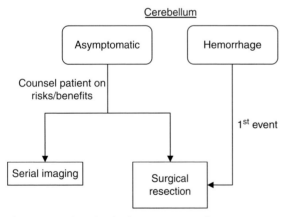

Figure 11.5. Algorithm for the management of cavernous malformations located in the cerebellum.

should be strongly considered [13,21,27,28]. Although some surgical series have reported good results in resecting deep-seated brainstem lesions, other series have reported significant worsening in clinical status when a lesion is deep-seated compared to one that comes to the surface (9% versus 29% respectively) [13,24,30,31]. Therefore, a more conservative approach is advocated for deep-seated brainstem CMs, unless there is clear, progressive neurological deterioration.

Cerebellum

See Fig. 11.5.

Cerebellar CMs are unique in that they can reach large sizes, cause massive hemorrhages, and can have potentially fatal consequences [32,33]. The natural history of CMs located in the cerebellum is not well understood given most of the data available are limited to select case reports. A retrospective series by de Oliveira *et al.* reported on the surgical outcomes of 10 patients with cerebellar CMs. All patients presented in the acute phase of hemorrhage and had an average lesion size of 4.6 cm. They were treated as an emergency given the risk of further mass effect from hemorrhage. Two patients had concomitant hydrocephalus and had a shunt placed. All of the patients had a good or excellent outcome, with only two patients having residual sequellae from the event (ataxia in one and nystagmus in the other) [34]. Therefore, microsurgical resection is a reasonable option for cerebellar CM presenting after a single hemorrhage, especially if there is risk for further hemorrhagic expansion within the posterior fossa [12,14].

Spinal intramedullary

See Fig. 11.6.

Spinal intramedullary (IM) CMs are rare entities that account for 5% of all IM lesions in adults and 1% of IM lesions in children [35,36]. The main complications of IMCMs result from hemorrhage and the associated mass effect within the spinal cord. In a comprehensive review of 107 reported cases, Zevgaridis estimated the hemorrhage rate of IMCMs to be 1.4% per lesion per year [37]. It has been well documented that IMCMs can behave aggressively, exhibiting a high propensity to hemorrhage and producing devastating neurological deficits [36,38,39]. However, it is also known that IMSCMs can have a prolonged, benign course. Kharkar *et al.* reported a series of 14 patients, ten of whom were managed conservatively and four of whom were managed with surgery. Of the 10 patients who were managed conservatively, all but one patient was the same or improved compared to presentation over a mean follow-up time of 6.7 years. The status of the patient who worsened neurologically was confounded

by concomitant amyotrophic lateral sclerosis [40]. Although this study was clearly limited by a selection bias, it clearly highlighted that not all IMCMs have a course that results in progressive worsening. Overall, the natural history of IMCMs is poorly understood because most of our current understanding stems from data from surgical series.

Most reported IMCM cases in the literature have been managed surgically. Jallo *et al.* reported a series of 26 patients and reviewed 186 patients in the literature who had an IMCM treated with microsurgical resection. In the short term, up to 50% of patients were transiently worse than they were preoperatively. Long-term outcomes, however, were favorable with 102 (61%) demonstrating improvement, 53 (31%) remaining clinically unchanged, and 13 (8%) with a worse outcome compared to preoperative status [41]. Surgery is certainly a definitive option for patients with symptomatic IMCMs in eliminating the risk of future hemorrhage. For patients who rapidly deteriorate in the acute phase and for whom conservative management is felt to be too risky, surgery is indicated. However, if a patient can be supportively managed to the subacute phase, a reassessment of the patient's clinical status is warranted. For patients who have improved neurologically, conservative management should be highly considered. For patients who are unchanged neurologically or who have progressively

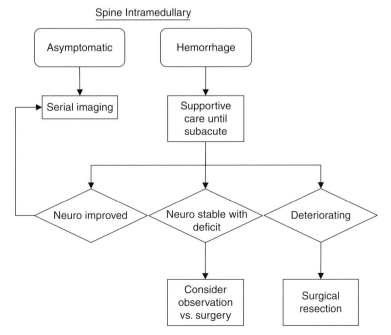

Figure 11.6. Algorithm for the management of intramedullary spinal cord cavernous malformations.

deteriorated in the subacute phase, microsurgical resection should be strongly considered in order to avoid further progression of symptoms and sequelae from hemorrhagic events.

Radiosurgical treatment of cavernous malformations

The most recent treatment modality for CMs is stereotactic radiotherapy. Currently, its use is usually reserved for CMs that are poorly accessible by microsurgical approaches, such as deep lesions in the brainstem. Some authors have also advocated its use in patients who are not good surgical candidates and have CMs that exhibit highly aggressive behavior. Despite the emerging body of evidence supporting its use as an alternative to microsurgical resection for certain lesions, a prospective randomized controlled trial to confirm its efficacy is unavailable at this time. Here, we will review the clinical outcome studies of radiosurgery for CM treatment and discuss its limitations.

Defining efficacy in radiosurgical treatment of CMs is challenging. Unlike high-flow arteriovenous malformations (AVMs) where clear neuroimaging criteria exist based on size to gauge the success of treatment, a reduction in size is an unreliable method to determine treatment efficacy of CMs. Clatterbuck et al. and Kim et al. both concluded that CMs are dynamic lesions that may spontaneously regress as part of their natural course [42,43]. Therefore, clinical reduction in hemorrhage rate is often used as a measure of the therapeutic efficacy of radiosurgery. A recent comprehensive review of the literature pertaining to the radiosurgical treatment of CMs by Pham et al. reported pre-treatment hemorrhage rates ranging from 13% to 36% per person-year when calculated from the first hemorrhage event, or 2% to 6.4% if the lesion was presumed to be present from birth. After treatment with radiosurgery, annual hemorrhage rates ranged from 1.6% to 8% per person-year. Their review included gamma knife (GK), linear accelerator (LA), proton beam (PB), and helium ion Bragg peak (HB) as types of radiation used, with the majority of the studies using gamma knife [44].

Some studies have suggested that the significant decrease in postradiation hemorrhage rates greater than 2 years following radiosurgical treatment of CMs may reflect an intrinisic lesion change as seen in AVMs treated with radiosurgery [44,45]. Hemorrhage rates after 1 year ranged from 7.3% to 22.4%, which decreased to 0.8% to 5.2% following a 2-year latency period [1]. The change in hemorrhage rate may represent a gradual luminal narrowing following radiosurgery over a 2 to 3 year period similar to that observed with AVMs treated with radiosurgery. Conversely, this could simply reflect the temporal clustering phenomenon described by Barker et al., who demonstrated that for the first 2.5 years following an initial hemorrhagic event of an untreated CM, the monthly hemorrhage rate was 2%. The hemorrhage rate decreased to less than 1% per month following this initial period of increased hemorrhage risk [20]. Therefore, the observations made following radiosurgery may simply reflect the natural history of CMs and not a benefit conferred by the treatment.

Seizure control is another clinical parameter that has been used to study the efficacy of radiosurgery, though it has been examined to a lesser extent compared to hemorrhage rates. Of the 291 patients reviewed by Pham et al. treated with GK, LA, PB, and HB, 89 patients (31%) were reported to be seizure-free following radiosurgery with or without anticonvulsants [44]. In the same population, 102 patients (35%) had a reduction in the number of seizures experienced. Only 11 patients (3.7%) had an increase in seizure frequency following radiosurgery, with two cases (18%) attributed to transient radiation-induced edema. The mechanism of increased seizure frequency in the other nine patients was not well defined. In a study by Régis et al. using GK to treat cerebral CMs in 49 patients, the location of the CM was found to be an important predictor of post-treatment seizure control rate. Only two out of 14 patients (14%) with CMs in the mesotemporal region became seizure-free whereas six out of seven patients and four out of four patients became seizure-free with CMs located in the laterotemporal (86%) and central regions (100%), respectively [46]. Seizure type was also prognostic in the same study. Ten out of 13 patients (77%) who presented with simple-partial seizures became seizure-free compared to five out of 18 patients (28%) who presented with complex-partial seizures. Gender, age, and duration of epilepsy did not appear to have any prognostic value in this study [46].

Despite the fact that radiosurgery is less invasive than open surgery, the complications from radiosurgery cannot be trivialized. Across all studies reviewed using GK, LA, PB, and HB, the morbidity rates ranged from 2.5% to 59% and the mortality ranged from 0% to 8.3% [44]. The permanent morbidity and mortality rates appear to be dependent on the location of the lesion, with lobar lesions having the most favorable rates of 0% to 13% compared to 0% to 54% for lesions located in the basal ganglia, thalamus, and brainstem. Furthermore, most studies suggest that brainstem lesions have higher complication rates from radiosurgery compared to deep lesions of the basal ganglia and thalamus, with rates ranging from 8% to 25% for brainstem lesions compared to 0% to 22% for basal ganglia and thalamic lesions [47,48]. The mean tumor margin dose in the studies reviewed ranged from 12.1 Gy to 25 Gy. As expected, complications were more prevalent in the studies with higher radiation doses, highlighted by the morbidity rates of 2.5% and 59% occurring at 12.1 Gy and 18 Gy, respectively [47,48].

Radiosurgery is a minimally invasive treatment modality with a negligible recovery time. Radiosurgery is also able to treat deep lesions that are inaccessible by microsurgical techniques. However, the long-term outcomes and the optimal radiation dose need to be further investigated to clearly define the role radiosurgery will play in the treatment of CMs. The efficacy of radiosurgery in preventing recurrent hemorrhages is controversial based on the current evidence available. The pretreatment hemorrhage rates in radiosurgical studies ranged from 2% to 6.4% per person-year while the post-treatment hemorrhage rates ranged from 1.6% to 8%. Although hemorrhage rates decreased 2 years following radiosurgery to 0.8% to 5.2% per person-year, this may simply reflect the natural history of CMs rather than a meaningful effect of radiosurgery.

Radiosurgery appears to be a reasonable alternative to surgery for CMs that produce seizures and are located in a surgically inaccessible area, with a 31% seizure-free rate, 35% seizure-reduction rate, and with only 3.7% of patients reporting an increase in seizure frequency post treatment. This is especially true of lesions that are extratemporal that present with simple partial seizures. For lesions that are anatomically accessible, surgery is the preferred treatment modality as seizure-free rates reported in the literature range from 70% to 97% [8,49–51]. This is highlighted by a study where Shih *et al.* offered both surgical and radiosurgical treatment options for their cohort of 30 patients who presented with seizures. Higher seizure-free rates were achieved by surgical resection (79%) compared to radiosurgery (25%), although prospective, randomized trials comparing these treatment modalities are still needed [51].

Summary

The management of CMs of the nervous system consists of three basic strategies: conservative/medical, surgery, and radiosurgery. It is clear that some CMs tend to have a benign course and others behave more aggressively although the factors that influence the behavior of a CM remain a mystery. A basic knowledge of the natural history of CMs and of the outcomes of surgery and radiosurgery are necessary in order to appropriately counsel patients with a newly diagnosed CM. Management strategies are based on the presentation and the anatomical location of the CM. Incidentally found CMs in the nervous system are always treated conservatively with serial imaging. Patients who present with seizures attributable to a CM should always be treated medically. If medical therapy fails, surgical resection should be recommended if feasible. For epileptogenic lesions that are surgically inaccessible, treatment with radiosurgery may be considered. The management of CMs presenting with hemorrhage depends on the anatomical location of the lesion. The risks and benefits of both conservative and surgical management need to be carefully considered as they are dramatically different based on the location of the CM and its relationship to the surrounding anatomical structures. Currently, there is no clear role for radiosurgery in the treatment of CMs that present with hemorrhage.

References

1. Batra, S., Lin, D., Recinos, P. F., Zhang, J. & Rigamonti, D. Cavernous malformations: natural history, diagnosis and treatment. *Nat Rev Neurol* 2009;**5**:659–670.

2. Moran, N. F., Fish, D. R., Kitchen, N., *et al.* Supratentorial cavernous haemangiomas and epilepsy: a review of the literature and case series. *J Neurol Neurosurg Psychiatry* 1999;**66**:561–568.

3. Awad, I. & Jabbour, P. Cerebral cavernous malformations and epilepsy. *Neurosurg Focus* 2006;**21**:e7.

4. Churchyard, A., Khangure, M. & Grainger, K. Cerebral cavernous angioma: a potentially benign condition? Successful treatment in 16 cases. *J Neurol Neurosurg Psychiatry* 1992;**55**:1040–1045.

5. Ferroli, P., Casazza, M., Marras, C., *et al.* Cerebral cavernomas and seizures: a retrospective study on 163 patients who underwent pure lesionectomy. *Neurol Sci.* 2006;**26**:390–394.

6. Yeon, J. Y., Kim, J. S., Choi, S. J., *et al.* Supratentorial cavernous angiomas presenting with seizures: surgical

outcomes in 60 consecutive patients. *Seizure* 2009;**18**:14–20.

7. Baumann, C. R., Acciarri, N., Bertalanffy, H., *et al.* Seizure outcome after resection of supratentorial cavernous malformations: a study of 168 patients. *Epilepsia* 2007;**48**:559–563.

8. Cohen, D. S., Zubay, G. P. & Goodman, R. R. Seizure outcome after lesionectomy for cavernous malformations. *J Neurosurg* 1995;**83**:237–242.

9. Baumann, C. R., Schuknecht, B., Lo Russo, G., *et al.* Seizure outcome after resection of cavernous malformations is better when surrounding hemosiderin-stained brain also is removed. *Epilepsia* 2006;**47**:563–566.

10. Stavrou, I., Baumgartner, C., Frischer, J. M., Trattnig, S. & Knosp, E. Long-term seizure control after resection of supratentorial cavernomas: a retrospective single-center study in 53 patients. *Neurosurgery* 2008;**63**:888–896; discussion 97.

11. Paolini, S., Morace, R., Di Gennaro, G., *et al.* Drug-resistant temporal lobe epilepsy due to cavernous malformations. *Neurosurg Focus* 2006;**21**(1):e8.

12. Amin-Hanjani, S., Ojemann, R. G. & Ogilvy, C. S. Surgical management of cavernous malformations of the nervous system. In H. H. Schmidek and D. W. Roberts, eds., *Schmidek & Sweet Operative Neurosurgical Techniques: Indications, Methods, and Results*, 5th ed. (Philadelphia: Saunders Elsevier, 2006), pp. 1307–1324.

13. Bertalanffy, H., Benes, L., Miyazawa, T., *et al.* Cerebral cavernomas in the adult. Review of the literature and analysis of 72 surgically treated patients. *Neurosurg Rev* 2002;**25**:1–53; discussion 4–5.

14. D'Angelo, V. A., De Bonis, C., Amoroso, R., *et al.* Supratentorial cerebral cavernous malformations: clinical, surgical, and genetic involvement. *Neurosurg Focus* 2006;**21**:e9.

15. Gross, B. A., Batjer, H. H., Awad, I. A. & Bendok, B. R. Cavernous malformations of the basal ganglia and thalamus. *Neurosurgery* 2009;**65**:7–18; discussion 19.

16. Porter, P. J., Willinsky, R. A., Harper, W. & Wallace, M. C. Cerebral cavernous malformations: natural history and prognosis after clinical deterioration with or without hemorrhage. *J Neurosurg* 1997;**87**:190–197.

17. Pozzati, E. Thalamic cavernous malformations. *Surg Neurol* 2000;**53**:30–9; discussion 9–40.

18. Zhao, J., Wang, Y., Kang, S., *et al.* The benefit of neuronavigation for the treatment of patients with intracerebral cavernous malformations. *Neurosurg Rev* 2007;**30**:313–318; discussion 9.

19. Conrad, M., Schonauer, C., Morel, C., Pelissou-Guyotat, I. & Deruty, R. Computer-assisted resection of supra-tentorial cavernous malformation. *Minim Invasive Neurosurg* 2002;**45**:87–90.

20. Barker, F. G., Amin-Hanjani, S., Butler, W. E., *et al.* Temporal clustering of hemorrhages from untreated cavernous malformations of the central nervous system. *Neurosurgery* 2001;**49**:15–24; discussion 25.

21. Gross, B. A., Batjer, H. H., Awad, I. A. & Bendok, B. R. Brainstem cavernous malformations. *Neurosurgery* 2009;**64**:E805–818; discussion E18.

22. Aiba, T., Tanaka, R., Koike, T., *et al.* Natural history of intracranial cavernous malformations. *J Neurosurg* 1995;**83**:56–59.

23. Kondziolka, D., Lunsford, L. D. & Kestle, J. R. The natural history of cerebral cavernous malformations. *J Neurosurg* 1995;**83**:820–824.

24. Bruneau, M., Bijlenga, P., Reverdin, A., *et al.* Early surgery for brainstem cavernomas. *Acta Neurochir (Wien)* 2006;**148**:405–414.

25. Sandalcioglu, I. E., Wiedemayer, H., Secer, S., Asgari, S. & Stolke, D. Surgical removal of brain stem cavernous malformations: surgical indications, technical considerations, and results. *J Neurol Neurosurg Psychiatry* 2002;**72**:351–355.

26. Kupersmith, M. J., Kalish, H., Epstein, F., *et al.* Natural history of brainstem cavernous malformations. *Neurosurgery* 2001;**48**:47–53; discussion 54.

27. Pozzati, E., Acciarri, N., Tognetti, F., Marliani, F. & Giangaspero, F. Growth, subsequent bleeding, and de novo appearance of cerebral cavernous angiomas. *Neurosurgery* 1996;**38**:662–669; discussion 669–670.

28. Tung, H., Giannotta, S. L., Chandrasoma, P. T. & Zee, C. S. Recurrent intraparenchymal hemorrhages from angiographically occult vascular malformations. *J Neurosurg* 1990;**73**:174–180.

29. Abe, M., Kjellberg, R. N. & Adams, R. D. Clinical presentations of vascular malformations of the brain stem: comparison of angiographically positive and negative types. *J Neurol Neurosurg Psychiatry* 1989;**52**:167–175.

30. Bouillot, P., Dufour, H., Roche, P. H., *et al.* [Angiographically occult vascular malformations of the brain stem. Apropos of 25 cases]. *Neurochirurgie* 1996;**42**:189–200; discussion 201.

31. Ferroli, P., Sinisi, M., Franzini, A., *et al.* Brainstem cavernomas: long-term results of microsurgical resection in 52 patients. *Neurosurgery* 2005;**56**:1203–1212; discussion 1212–1214.

32. Hayashi, T., Fukui, M., Shyojima, K., Utsunomiya, H. & Kawasaki, K. Giant cerebellar hemangioma in an infant. *Childs Nerv Syst* 1985;**1**:230–233.

33. de Tribolet, N., Kaech, D. & Perentes, E. Cerebellar haematoma due to a cavernous angioma in a child. *Acta Neurochir (Wien)* 1982;**60**:37–43.

34. de Oliveira, J. G., Rassi-Neto, A., Ferraz, F. A. & Braga, F. M. Neurosurgical management of cerebellar cavernous malformations. *Neurosurg Focus* 2006;**21**:e11.

35. Spetzger, U., Gilsbach, J. M. & Bertalanffy, H. Cavernous angiomas of the spinal cord clinical presentation, surgical strategy, and postoperative results. *Acta Neurochir (Wien)* 1995;**134**:200–206.

36. Deutsch, H., Jallo, G. I., Faktorovich, A. & Epstein, F. Spinal intramedullary cavernoma: clinical presentation and surgical outcome. *J Neurosurg* 2000;**93**(1 Suppl):65–70.

37. Zevgaridis, D., Medele, R. J., Hamburger, C., Steiger, H. J. & Reulen, H. J. Cavernous haemangiomas of the spinal cord. A review of 117 cases. *Acta Neurochir (Wien)* 1999;**141**:237–245.

38. Sandalcioglu, I. E., Wiedemayer, H., Gasser, T., *et al.* Intramedullary spinal cord cavernous malformations: clinical features and risk of hemorrhage. *Neurosurg Rev* 2003;**26**:253–256.

39. McCormick, P. C., Michelsen, W. J., Post, K. D., Carmel, P. W. & Stein, B. M. Cavernous malformations of the spinal cord. *Neurosurgery* 1988;**23**:459–463.

40. Kharkar, S., Shuck, J., Conway, J. & Rigamonti, D. The natural history of conservatively managed symptomatic intramedullary spinal cord cavernomas. *Neurosurgery* 2007;**60**:865–872; discussion 872.

41. Jallo, G. I., Freed, D., Zareck, M., Epstein, F. & Kothbauer, K. F. Clinical presentation and optimal management for intramedullary cavernous malformations. *Neurosurg Focus* 2006;**21**:e10.

42. Clatterbuck, R. E., Moriarity, J. L., Elmaci, I., *et al.* Dynamic nature of cavernous malformations: a prospective magnetic resonance imaging study with volumetric analysis. *J Neurosurg* 2000;**93**:981–986.

43. Kim, D. S., Park, Y. G., Choi, J. U., Chung, S. S. & Lee, K. C. An analysis of the natural history of cavernous malformations. *Surg Neurol* 1997;**48**:9–17; discussion 18.

44. Pham, M., Gross, B. A., Bendok, B. R., Awad, I. A. & Batjer, H. H. Radiosurgery for angiographically occult vascular malformations. *Neurosurg Focus* 2009;**26**:E16.

45. Chang, S. D., Levy, R. P., Adler, J. R., Jr., *et al.* Stereotactic radiosurgery of angiographically occult vascular malformations: 14-year experience. *Neurosurgery* 1998;**43**:213–220; discussion 220–221.

46. Regis, J., Bartolomei, F., Kida, Y., *et al.* Radiosurgery for epilepsy associated with cavernous malformation: retrospective study in 49 patients. *Neurosurgery* 2000;**47**:1091–1097.

47. Liu, K. D., Chung, W. Y., Wu, H. M., *et al.* Gamma knife surgery for cavernous hemangiomas: an analysis of 125 patients. *J Neurosurg* 2005;**102**(Suppl):81–86.

48. Pollock, B. E., Garces, Y. I., Stafford, S. L., *et al.* Stereotactic radiosurgery for cavernous malformations. *J Neurosurg* 2000;**93**:987–991.

49. Amin-Hanjani, S., Ogilvy, C. S., Candia, G. J., Lyons, S. & Chapman, P. H. Stereotactic radiosurgery for cavernous malformations: Kjellberg's experience with proton beam therapy in 98 cases at the Harvard Cyclotron. *Neurosurgery* 1998;**42**:1229–1236; discussion 1236–1238.

50. Cappabianca, P., Alfieri, A., Maiuri, F., *et al.* Supratentorial cavernous malformations and epilepsy: seizure outcome after lesionectomy on a series of 35 patients. *Clin Neurol Neurosurg* 1997;**99**:179–183.

51. Shih, Y. H. & Pan, D. H. Management of supratentorial cavernous malformations: craniotomy versus gammaknife radiosurgery. *Clin Neurol Neurosurg* 2005;**107**:108–112.

Surgical treatment of cavernous malformations associated with epilepsy

Mahua Dey and Issam Awad

Introduction and lesion definition

Cerebral cavernous malformations (CCM) are a common vascular anomaly affecting more than 0.5% of the population [1]. The lesions, which may affect any brain region, consist of clusters of dilated vascular sinusoids of varying size, filled with blood or thrombus at different stages of organization. The gross lesion appearance has been likened to that of a mulberry. The so-called "caverns" comprising the lesion are lined with endothelium, but otherwise lack mature vessel angioarchitecture [2,3]. They grow by a process of vascular cavern proliferation in the setting of repetitive intralesional hemorrhages [4]. Lesions typically exhibit hallmarks of previous perilesional hemorrhage, including gliosis and hemosiderin deposit [4]. Patients harboring CCMs are predisposed to a lifetime risk of epilepsy or focal neurological deficits related to hemorrhage or lesion proliferation [5]. Hemorrhage from CCM lesion is less likely apoplectic than with higher-flow arteriovenous anomalies [1,6,7].

Because of their often isodense appearance related to subacute hemorrhage or microcalcifications, CCMs are commonly missed or misdiagnosed on computed tomographic scans of the brain. These lesions are angiographically occult, with very sluggish blood flow, or stasis and thrombus at different stages of organization within the caverns. The CCMs are best detected on magnetic resonance (MR) images, where they are characterized by a mixed signal within the lesion itself on T1- and T2-weighted sequences, surrounded by a ring of T2 hypointensity from hemosiderin, reflecting blood leakage (Figs. 12.1 and 12.2). Smaller CCM lesions may only be revealed by gradient-echo MR images, in which they can be identified because of the lesions' hemorrhagic signal (Fig. 12.3). The MR appearance of CCMs is highly sensitive and specific [8].

Sporadic versus familial CCM disease

In 60 to 80% of cases CCMs are unassociated with family history, and these typically reflect solitary lesions, or less likely focal clusters of lesions near a developmental venous anomaly or in a previously irradiated brain region (Fig. 12.4). The remaining cases manifest an autosomal dominant inheritance pattern with variable clinical expression, and typically involve multifocal lesions scattered throughout the brain in a volume distribution [1] some of which may only be revealed by gradient-echo MR (Fig. 12.3), or other specialized imaging techniques. Three distinct gene foci on chromosomes 7q, 7p, and 3q have each been linked to familial CCM [9]. The identified proteins encoded by CCM genes interact with the endothelial cytoskeleton during angiogenesis, and are expressed in neural tissue, thus explaining the occurrence of these lesions in the central nervous system [9,10]. The familial form is most prevalent in Hispanic Americans of Mexican descent, who manifest a "common founder mutation" [11].

Capillary malformations and CCMs

Capillary vascular malformations, also known as capillary telangiectases, are vascular malformations that consist of a collection of dilated capillaries with normal intervening brain parenchyma [12]. Most commonly located in the pons, they are typically an incidental finding at autopsy, although in some cases symptomatic capillary malformations have been revealed on MR images as indistinct patches of punctuate contrast enhancement [13–15]. Capillary malformations may also be found in association with more clinically overt lesions, such as CCMs or venous malformations. Microscopically, the vessel walls of capillary malformations appear similar to those of normal capillaries, lined with a single layer of vascular endothelium. While both

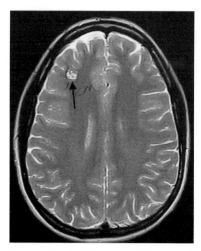

Figure 12.1. Axial T2-weighted MR image of a patient presenting with new-onset generalized seizure at age 33, in the absence of alcohol or drug intake or trauma. Seizure semiology, pre-ictal and post-ictal symptoms and interictal electroencephalogram (EEG) were not helpful in localizing the seizure focus, and seizures did not recur on anticonvulsant medications. Gradient-echo images did not reveal other lesions and contrast-enhanced imaging did not reveal an associated overt venous developmental anomaly. Because of the patient's occupation as a driver, and his young age, he elected to undergo microsurgical excision of the solitary right frontal CCM (arrow), along with the surrounding hemosiderin-stained brain parenchyma ("lesionectomy-plus"). The patient remained seizure-free postoperatively, was tapered off anticonvulsants after 1 year, and has resumed driving and normal life without seizure restrictions. Continued medical therapy with anticonvulsants would also have been appropriate. If his seizures were intractable or longstanding, or if seizures persisted after lesionectomy, more extensive brain mapping with interictal and ictal-onset recording would be performed, allowing resection of epileptogenic brain tissue adjacent to the lesion. See color plate section.

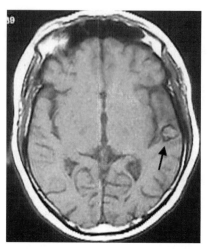

Figure 12.2. Axial T1-weighted MR image of a patient presenting with recurrent partial complex seizures, including prolonged post-ictal dysphasia, despite optimal anticonvulsant medications. The patient was otherwise highly functional, except for subtle difficulties in verbal domain on speech and neuropsychological testing. Gradient-echo images did not reveal other lesions and contrast-enhanced imaging did not reveal an associated overt venous developmental anomaly. The interictal EEG revealed left temporal epileptogenic activity. Because of eloquent lesion location, in or adjacent to temporal lobe speech areas, a CCM lesionectomy was performed. The patient remained seizure-free after surgery, except for brief auras of speech arrest without partial complex semiology or generalization. He has remained on anticonvulsant medications. If seizures recur and become intractable again, he would be evaluated with subdural electrodes (lateral and mesiobasal) to map the location and extent of epileptogenic brain, and guide a tailored temporal lobe resection at subsequent procedure.

capillary telangiectases and CCMs represent dilated capillaries, the presence of hemorrhage (identifiable on MR imaging or histopathological examination) is a cardinal difference that clearly distinguishes CCMs from capillary malformations. The association of CCMs and capillary malformations in the same patient has been recognized for many years, but the exact prevalence of this association remains uncertain, in view of diagnostic insensitivity of current imaging modalities for non-hemorrhagic capillary ectasia. Any causation or evolution between the two lesion types remains speculative, but raises the question about a more diffuse cerebrovascular anomaly in patients with apparently solitary CCM lesions.

"Capillary telangiectasiae" (capillary malformations) should not be confused with micro-arteriovenous malformations of hereditary hemorrhagic telangiectasia (Osler-Weber-Rendu disease), the latter affecting brain, skin, mucosa and lungs in association with gene loci

unrelated to CCM disease and lesions of different histology than CCM [16].

Cerebral venous malformations and CCMs

The most common cerebrovascular malformation is the venous malformation, also known as venous angioma or developmental venous anomaly (DVA). This lesion rarely bleeds, except in association with a CCM [17,18]. The DVA is composed of abnormally enlarged venous channels separated by normal neural parenchyma. The anomaly reflects regional venous dysmorphism arranged in a radial pattern extending from a dilated central venous trunk, and there is paucity of other normal venous drainage in the region of the anomaly [19]. Sporadic non-familial CCMs are often associated with a DVA, detected on contrast-enhanced T1-weighted MR sequences, while multifocal CCMs associated with autosomal dominant inheritance and the three gene loci of CCM disease are rarely associated with DVA [17,20].

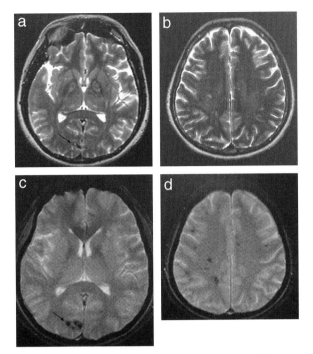

Figure 12.3. Axial T2-weighted MR images in a patient with longstanding generalized seizures, and family history of multiple first-degree bleed relatives with seizures or stroke at young age. A right occipital pole anomaly was noted consistent with subtle CCM (A), without clear relationship to the patient's seizures, and EEG revealed bifrontal and Rolandic spike-wave activity. No other lesions were noted in the brain on conventional MRI sequences (B). Gradient-echo images were performed and better delineated the occipital CCM (C), and revealed numerous other CCM lesions elsewhere in the brain (D), consistent with familial CCM disease. Seizures have been treated medically, and it is unclear whether resection of any single CCM would affect his epilepsy syndrome, unless seizures become more clearly localizable by clinical semiology or EEG.

Mixed lesions and the spectrum of angiographically occult vascular malformations

Despite the apparently distinct clinical, imaging, and pathological profiles of the various cerebral vascular malformations, some CCM lesions exhibit mixed or transitional features, implying related pathobiological mechanisms [15,21–24]. Portions of CCMs may, like arteriovenous or venous malformations, exhibit partial or complete mature vessel wall elements, and many CCMs appear to arise in close proximity to DVAs or capillary malformations as noted above. Various cerebrovascular malformations may be associated with skin lesions in rare syndromic settings, as with hereditary hemorrhagic telangiectasia (Osler-Weber-Rendu disease noted above) and encephalofacial angioma (Sturge-Weber disease). The skin lesions that occur infrequently in association with familial CCMs have been characterized as hyperkeratotic angioma [25], but their precise prevalence and clinical significance have not been well studied.

Mechanisms of epilepsy

The evolution of modern neuroimaging has greatly enhanced the diagnosis and treatment of localization-related epilepsy. Many types of seizures previously classified as cryptogenic have been reclassified as lesional epilepsies. Lesional epilepsy is thought to be a direct consequence of a focal brain lesion of neoplastic,

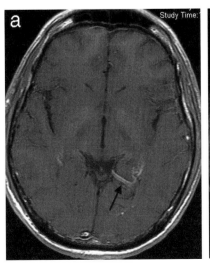
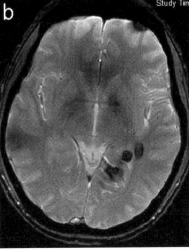

Figure 12.4. Axial T1-weighted MRI with contrast in a patient with new-onset symptoms of vague visual auras that have cleared after starting anticonvulsant medications. He had undergone previous neuraxis irradiation in childhood after resection of a cerebellar medulloblastoma. The scan reveals a left mesiotemporal developmental venous anomaly (A). The gradient-echo images (B) reveal multiple associated hemorrhagic lesions consistent with CCMs (B). The patient is highly functional, including excellent memory and speech function, and the lesions have remained stable during several years of ongoing surveillance. Because of the sprawling nature of the lesions in highly eloquent brain, a curative lesionectomy surgery cannot be performed safely.

vascular, dysgenetic, traumatic, or ischemic origin that may be amenable to surgical treatment, with resection offering the potential for cure or significant reduction in seizure frequency. Localization-related epilepsy is also likely to be affected by individual predisposition, as lesions of identical type, size, and location may cause varying manifestations (including seizure disorders of varying degrees of severity) in different patients. Predisposition may also play a role in seizure intractability, propensity for pharmacological seizure control, and surgical outcome – the likelihood of cure or recurrence of epilepsy after lesion excision.

The CCMs in supratentorial locations adjacent to cortical structures are most likely associated with epilepsy (Figs. 12.1 and 12.2). Seizure semiology and pre-ictal and post-ictal symptoms often, but not always, reflect lesion laterality or locale. Lesions adjacent to mesiotemporal or limbic structures frequently result in partial complex seizures, with or without secondary generalization (Fig. 12.5).

Epileptogenesis in adjacent brain tissue

Epileptic seizures are the most common clinical presentation of supratentorial CCMs. The malformed blood vessels do not typically include functioning neural tissue and are not intrinsically epileptogenic. However, they can induce seizures through their effect on the surrounding brain tissue due to recurrent microhemorrhage leading to gliosis, deposits of blood breakdown products, and cellular and humoral inflammatory responses [10]. Overt hemorrhage from CCMs may create encephalomalacia and cortical scars that may be independently epileptogenic. These sequelae are often observed on MR imaging and may be associated with focal neurological deficits.

These alterations in adjacent brain tissue may induce epileptic activity that depends on the presence of the hemorrhagic vascular malformation and may not support epileptic activity in the absence of that primary lesion. Other changes in adjacent brain tissue may represent permanent (independent) epileptogenic foci. In these cases, selective resection of the lesion revealed on MR studies may not be sufficient to abolish all the seizures. There is thought to be a spectrum of maturation of epileptogenicity, and the duration of epileptogenicity is thought to be important in the establishment of independent seizure foci. Thus, lesion-related epilepsy is postulated to be more likely permanent or independent of the instigating pathology after a longer

duration of seizures. CCM-related epilepsy has been shown to induce different firing patterns in adjacent hippocampal tissue slices than epilepsy associated with neoplasia [26].

Epileptogenesis in remote brain regions

Lesions may induce changes in brain tissue located at a significant distance from the primary epileptogenic focus, and this may contribute to an epilepsy syndrome, and even to independent distant foci of epileptogenicity. The limbic structures, and to a lesser extent the neocortex, may "learn" to generate seizures independently and may become secondarily epileptogenic after repeated exposure to the seizures caused by an epileptogenic lesion. Over time, network relationships may be altered in such a way that leads to secondary epileptogenesis in these remote regions [27]. This process has been most frequently demonstrated with structural lesions adjacent to mesiotemporal and other limbic structures (parahippocampal, cingulate, frontobasal), and is less likely to occur in other neocortical locations. The demonstration of dual epileptogenic activity in association with a single CCM does not necessarily imply that the second focus, the one that is more remote from the lesion, will remain active after lesion excision. In fact, this seems to be uncommon in the setting of seizure disorders associated with a solitary vascular malformation (Fig. 12.5). For this reason, a staged approach is often best in such cases: the lesion and surrounding epileptogenic brain tissue are excised during an initial operation, and more extensive investigations of the remaining epileptogenicity and possible further treatment for it are performed only in those uncommon cases in which seizures persist after lesionectomy. The more frequent, recalcitrant and long-standing the seizures, the more likely a secondary focus will remain as an independent source of seizures after primary lesion excision. This observation has led to the recommendation of early surgical intervention when medical therapy fails to control seizures [28].

Multiple lesions

Dual and multifocal lesions are important to the understanding of the pathogenesis of epilepsy, and such cases require more careful surgical planning. When patients are known to harbor multiple structural lesions, more extensive preoperative investigations and tailoring of interventions are required for seizure control [29–31].

Cerebral cavernous malformations are frequently associated with multifocal vascular lesions, any one of which may contribute to epileptogenesis. While larger lesions or those most recently associated with bleeding or other clinical manifestations are more likely to be the source of seizures than smaller lesions or those with less apparent clinical importance, this cannot be taken for granted (Fig. 12.3). Resection of the wrong lesion will not only fail to control seizures, but it may also result in catastrophic functional sequelae when the remaining epileptogenic lesion is located in the contralateral temporal or frontal lobe. In the setting of cerebral vascular malformations, it is important to use the most sensitive imaging studies to identify or exclude multifocal structural pathological conditions that may be contributing to epileptogenicity. Gradient-echo or susceptibility-weighted MR images must be performed to identify or exclude multiple foci of occult hemorrhage (Figs. 12.3 and 12.4).

Medical therapies

The first-line treatment for seizures associated with vascular malformation is always medical. Different anticonvulsant agents are associated with varying degrees of effectiveness for different seizure types; several newer drugs are associated with fewer side effects and may be more safely prescribed even for pregnant women. After a patient's first seizure, a decision is typically made about whether to prescribe anticonvulsant medication. This decision is based on the risk of seizure recurrence and on the potential risks associated with chronic antiepileptic therapy. Whenever a structural lesion is identified on imaging studies, a decision must also be made about its probable relationship to the seizure disorder. In the setting of solitary cortical CCM, and certainly when seizure symptoms clearly correspond to the lesion location, this relationship is easy to establish. In other cases, such as those involving infratentorial or subcortical vascular anomalies or seizures precipitated by alcohol, drugs, or trauma, the possibility of an incidental lesion should be considered, especially when seizure symptoms do not suggest appropriate localization. Venous malformations are extremely common in the general population and often occur together with various neurological symptoms, including seizures, without any causal relationship. Electrophysiological studies may be helpful in this regard, especially when they yield positive results with appropriate lateralization or the identification of an epileptogenic focus; negative results on electroencephalography do not rule out epileptogenicity for a lesion. When seizures are thought to be caused by CCMs, long-term anticonvulsant therapy is indicated, as the seizures will probably recur and may progress to intractability. A drug should be chosen on the basis of the seizure and the individual patient's tolerance for the potential side effects of different anticonvulsant medications. The selected drug is almost always initially prescribed as monotherapy. Only when seizures recur despite verified compliance and therapeutic doses of this agent is a second agent added. Patients with CCMs in cortical locations are subject to a prospective lifetime risk of new seizures. This risk is greatest with CCMs situated in temporal, frontal, and perilimbic locations, and may affect occupational clearance (for example, in professional drivers, crane operators or airplane pilots). Clinical history is important in managing such cases, and care should be taken to elicit information about auras or other symptoms that may represent seizure activity. Nevertheless, prophylactic treatment is rarely indicated for these patients unless epileptic activity has been established.

Lesion excision

Resection of vascular malformations may be undertaken to prevent future hemorrhage and/or for seizure control. Lesionectomy is associated with excellent postoperative seizure control in many patients. The likelihood of postoperative seizure control following simple lesion excision is greater in patients with less intractable preoperative epilepsy and also in patients with extratemporal lesions [32,33]. Unlike temporal lobectomy, there are no anatomically standard operations for performing a simple lesionectomy, although resection of adjacent hemosiderin-stained brain tissue is often advocated in less-eloquent brain locations (Fig. 12.1).

In patients with temporal lobe lesions and intractable epilepsy, lesionectomy without resection of mesiotemporal lobe structures has documented relatively low seizure control rates, ranging from 20 to 45% [32,34,35]. Still, the cognitive consequences of up-front resection of mesiotemporal structures must be carefully considered and highly individualized, especially in patients with shorter-duration and less recalcitrant seizures, and in patients with good neuropsychological function (preserved material-specific memory), or when lesions involve speech areas (Fig. 12.2). Often lesionectomy is performed as a first procedure, and only those patients with persistent uncontrolled seizures are subjected to epilepsy surgery evaluation and a second resective procedure.

In cases of extratemporal lesional resection, more favorable seizure control rates are reported, varying from 65 to 95% [32,33]. Most patients in whom seizures are fully controlled postoperatively will still require long-term anticonvulsant therapy, although often with fewer agents and at lower dosages than they required preoperatively. When the decision is made to reduce or discontinue anticonvulsant therapy, it is important to taper the dosage cautiously to avoid precipitating new or recurrent seizures. Of patients who harbor a single CCM, undergo lesionectomy for treatment of recent-onset, localization-related seizures, and are seizure-free postoperatively, up to half may be successfully tapered off all anticonvulsant medications [36–39]. This promising outcome, and its associated positive impact on quality of life, may play a role in the decision to excise a solitary accessible cortical CCM, even when seizures are not truly intractable to medical therapy.

Lesionectomy and corticectomy

Resection of structural lesions may be limited to resection of the lesion alone or may entail resection of the lesion and the epileptogenic cortex. A tailored resection may be performed to avoid the eloquent cortex. Many studies [33,34,40,41] have compared lesionectomy with the combination of lesionectomy and corticectomy, but the results have been controversial. A meta-analysis evaluating seizure outcome following either lesionectomy or the combination of lesionectomy and corticectomy concluded that at 2-year follow up, the prevalence of persistent seizures following lesionectomy ranged from 1.4 to 4 times the prevalence following the more extensive resective procedures. Low-grade gliomas, gangliogliomas, and vascular malformations were most successfully treated with lesionectomy and corticectomy [42]. In contrast, patients with fewer seizures before presentation, shorter preoperative seizure histories, or seizures that responded to antiepileptic medications were more likely to be seizure-free following lesionectomy alone [43–49]. Several studies have shown that complete lesion excision is necessary for seizure control in the majority of patients who harbor a CCM that has been shown to be responsible for their seizures [33]. It also

is well documented that lesion excision alone may not always suffice for seizure control, especially in patients with truly intractable epilepsy. Many patients who have had persistent intractable seizures following lesion excision have had lesions in the temporal lobe [32]. Some of these patients became seizure-free after additional resection of epileptogenic brain tissue in the same region.

When epileptogenic brain tissue is resected in addition to the lesion during a first operation, it may provide the patient with seizure control and spare him or her a second surgical intervention. But the potential functional impact of resection of additional brain tissue must be considered, especially when contemplating resection of mesial structures in the presence of high or normal material-specific memory function, or resection involving other eloquent areas (such as the dominant temporal neocortex). Intraoperative electrocorticography is sometimes performed to further delineate the extent of the cortical epileptogenic zone. This technique may provide prognostic information by indicating the areas of residual electric discharges after the resection of the vascular malformation or what was thought to be the seizure focus [50,51]. It is important to remember, however, that residual spikes in adjacent brain areas do not reliably predict residual epileptogenicity, nor does their absence guarantee postoperative seizure control [50,51].

Disconnection surgery

Multiple subpial transections are mainly used to treat patients with partial epilepsies associated with epileptic foci within eloquent cortical regions [52]. The technique, which involves interrupting the gray matter columns, can inhibit synchronization and spread of seizure activity with less drastic effects on eloquent function [53–56]. Most patients who have undergone multiple subpial transections in eloquent brain tissue have had subtle and transient postoperative deficits that correspond to the transected areas and are most pronounced in the first week after surgery [57–60]. Corpus callosotomy is another palliative treatment that may be beneficial for patients with multiple or poorly lateralized epileptogenic foci, secondarily generalized tonic-clonic seizures, and injurious drop attacks (those that result in falls and injury) due to tonic or atonic seizures [61–63]. Elimination or a more than 80% reduction in seizures has been reported in 70% of patients who underwent this treatment

[61,62,64]. Complications specific to this procedure consist of acute disconnection syndromes; these are more common after total callosotomy [65].

Neuroaugmentative surgery

Vagus nerve stimulation is a palliative treatment for intractable seizures. Published data document seizure reduction rates varying from 35 to 75% in the setting of various seizure types, with most patients remaining on anticonvulsants postoperatively. Related side effects can include voice alteration, hoarseness, throat or neck pain, headache, cough, dyspnea, vocal cord paralysis, and aspiration [66–69]. The procedure is technically relatively simple, but it is very important to talk with patients before surgery about their expectations regarding outcome. To our knowledge, no results have been reported for vagus nerve stimulation applied specifically to the treatment of seizures associated with cerebrovascular malformations. Deep brain stimulation has been attempted for the modulation of seizure activity, with electrode stimulation targets in the cerebellum; in the anterior, centromedian, and ventralis intermedius thalamic nuclei; and in the caudate nucleus [70,71]. Stimulation of the hippocampus has recently been used in an attempt to block temporal lobe seizures [72]. Stimulation of the subthalamic nucleus has been shown to reduce daytime seizures by 80% [70].

Management strategies

First seizure

Surgery is rarely considered for seizure control in patients presenting with a first seizure associated with a known or newly diagnosed vascular malformation. Lesion excision may be performed for the purpose of preventing future hemorrhage, and in rare cases, especially those involving solitary and accessible CCMs, to provide patients with a chance to discontinue anticonvulsant medications. Medical treatment is typically initiated to try to determine whether a patient's seizures may be classified as intractable. Cerebral cavernous malformations are known to be more epileptogenic than other cerebrovascular anomalies, as they are more frequently associated with seizures in general and with intractable seizures in particular. The exact mechanisms by which CCMs cause seizures are unknown, although a number of electrophysiological and pathophysiological theories

have been proposed. These include changes in neurotransmitter levels (γ-aminobutyric acid and somatostatin), free radical formation, and altered second messenger function [73]. Morphological changes have also been identified, including alterations in vascular supply, neuronal cell loss, glial proliferation, and subtle subcortical disconnections [37]. It is commonly believed that the breakdown products caused by repeated microhemorrhages deposit ferric ions, which are known to be highly epileptogenic, into the cortex around the lesion. In animals, the injection of ferric ions into the cortex and subcortical regions creates a potent and reproducible model of recurrent and intractable seizures [78]. These different pathophysiological mechanisms may present opportunities for developing more specific targeted anticonvulsant strategies. Cerebral cavernous malformations in the rolandic or perirolandic cortex, as well as near limbic areas (temporal lobe and cingulate gyrus lesions), are typically the most epileptogenic. Lesion size may represent an additional factor in epileptogenicity. A final issue that must be considered is the possibility that the CCM identified on imaging may represent an incidental finding and may not play any role in seizure onset. This may be the situation in up to 6% of cases of patients with CCMs and epilepsy [74]. In some cases, CCMs may represent structural lesions coexistent with mesial temporal sclerosis. Although there is only minimal risk of hemorrhage in capillary telangiectasia, there are reports in the literature describing the association of capillary malformation with seizures and hemorrhage [75,76]. Seizures can occur as a direct result of hemorrhage caused by the capillary malformation, and such a hemorrhage is likely to convert the lesion into a CCM. Venous angiomas are rarely associated with seizures. Moreover these lesions are usually difficult to relate causally and topographically to an epileptogenic zone [77–79]. These lesions are typically observed as incidental findings during diagnostic evaluations. Venous angiomas are often associated with CCMs, and seizures in this setting are probably due to the CCM rather than the venous angioma [77–80]. Rarely, brain dysmorphisms (gyral or lobar developmental anomalies) may be associated with regional venous dysmorphism. In those instances, the venous anomaly is an index for associated dysmorphic brain tissue that may be epileptogenic. Careful electrophysiological studies as well as interictal and ictal functional imaging are indicated in these cases to explore whether the lesion is associated with an epileptogenic zone.

Controlled seizures

Surgical intervention is not typically warranted in CCMs with well-controlled epilepsy unless there is another indication carefully articulated. Lesion excision may be contemplated to prevent hemorrhage without any expectation of improving seizure control. Resection of a vascular malformation might be undertaken for seizure control in patients who are not compliant with their antiepileptic medication regimen. Similarly, patients who do not want to continue to take antiepileptic medications because of concerns about adverse effects or other issues may also benefit from resection of associated solitary CCM. In these cases, it is very important to take into account the location of the malformation and the feasibility of the procedure, weighing the risks and potential benefits, and to remember that enhanced seizure control or discontinuation of medication cannot be guaranteed. Patients with CCMs have a lower risk of apoplectic hemorrhage than those harboring AVMs, but lesions with prior overt hemorrhage or demonstrated growth are often considered for excision to prevent further neurological sequelae.

Prognosis and outcome of intractable seizures

Patients who have solitary CCMs associated with uncontrolled epilepsy and symptoms related to lesion location are candidates for surgical excision of the CCM with the goal of improving seizure control. Overall analysis of the published outcome data demonstrates symptom improvement in the majority of such patients [1,7,81]. Among patients treated with surgical resection of the offending lesion, 50 to 90% were seizure-free postoperatively with or without anticonvulsant therapy [1,7,81]. Persistent seizures have been reported in conjunction with incomplete lesion resection. In order to maximize the likelihood of seizure control, excision of the CCM should be accompanied, whenever feasible (that is, in non-eloquent brain regions), by resection of the gliotic hemosiderin-stained brain parenchyma surrounding the lesion [7,38,77]. There is no evidence that extensive preoperative mapping or additional brain tissue excision at initial surgery will improve seizure outcome beyond what can be obtained with lesionectomy and resection of perilesional gliotic brain tissue in cases of solitary CCMs and intractable epilepsy. In the rare cases in which patients suffer residual or recurrent seizures after lesionectomy, a second operation may be considered for resection of residual lesion and/or adjacent or remote epileptogenic brain tissue. As in other cases of localization-related epilepsy, such repeated operations require comprehensive preoperative and intraoperative mapping as well as functional studies. When there is any question whatsoever about the relationship of a CCM to an intractable seizure disorder, patients should not undergo empiric lesion resection in the remote hope that intractable epilepsy might resolve. Instead, detailed preoperative mapping and recording should be performed. This is particularly true in cases involving multiple CCMs, in which a single epileptogenic lesion is not always easy to isolate. In these cases, careful preoperative mapping and other diagnostic studies must be performed before resection of a specific lesion is proposed for seizure control.

Conclusions

The direct relationship between CCMs and seizures is not always clear. Prolonged preoperative mapping and careful recording are mandatory for clarifying cases in which the lesion may not be the primary epileptogenic source, may simply be incidental or unrelated to the seizure disorder, or in cases involving multifocal lesions. In patients harboring a solitary CCM that is believed to be epileptogenic, optimum seizure control is achieved through complete resection of the lesion, along with surrounding hemosiderin-stained brain tissue, if the lesion is in a non-eloquent location.

The threshold for considering lesion excision depends on the projected natural history of the lesion as well as its surgical accessibility. In the different scenarios, patients and their family members should be advised of all expectations related to the various treatment options under consideration.

References

1. Robinson, J. R., Awad, I. A. & Little, J. R. Natural history of the cavernous angioma. *J Neurosurg* 1991;**75**:709–714.

2. Robinson, J. R., Jr., Awad, I. A., Masaryk, T. J. & Estes, M. L. Pathological heterogeneity of angiographically occult vascular malformations of the brain. *Neurosurgery* 1993;**33**:547–54; discussion 54–55.

3. Rothbart, D., Awad, I. A., Lee, J., *et al.* Expression of angiogenic factors and structural proteins in central nervous system vascular malformations. *Neurosurgery* 1996;**38**:915–924; discussion 924–925.

4. Maraire, J. N. & Awad, I. A. Intracranial cavernous malformations: lesion behavior and management strategies. *Neurosurgery* 1995;**37**:591–605.

5. Al-Shahi Salman, R., Berg, M. J., Morrison, L. & Awad, I. A. Hemorrhage from cavernous malformations of the brain: definition and reporting standards. Angioma Alliance Scientific Advisory Board. *Stroke* 2008;**39**:3222–3230.

6. Beck, L., Jr. & D'Amore, P. A. Vascular development: cellular and molecular regulation. *FASEB J* 1997;**11**:365–373.

7. Del Curling, O., Jr., Kelly, D. L., Jr., Elster, A. D. & Craven, T. E. An analysis of the natural history of cavernous angiomas. *J Neurosurg* 1991;**75**:702–708.

8. de Souza, J. M., Domingues, R. C., Cruz, L. C., Jr., *et al.* Susceptibility-weighted imaging for the evaluation of patients with familial cerebral cavernous malformations: a comparison with t2-weighted fast spin-echo and gradient-echo sequences. *AJNR Am J Neuroradiol* 2008;**29**:154–158.

9. Jabbour, P., Gault, J. & Awad, I. A. What genes can teach us about human cerebrovascular malformations. *Clin Neurosurg* 2004;**51**:140–152.

10. Gault, J., Sarin, H., Awadallah, N. A., Shenkar, R. & Awad, I. A. Pathobiology of human cerebrovascular malformations: basic mechanisms and clinical relevance. *Neurosurgery* 2004;**55**:1–16; discussion 17.

11. Gunel, M., Awad, I. A., Finberg, K., *et al.* A founder mutation as a cause of cerebral cavernous malformation in Hispanic Americans. *New Engl J Med* 1996;**334**:946–951.

12. Chusid, J. G. & Kopeloff, L. M. Epileptogenic effects of pure metals implanted in motor cortex of monkeys. *J Appl Physiol* 1962;**17**:697–700.

13. Hoang, T. A. & Hasso, A. N. Intracranial vascular malformations. *Neuroimaging Clin N Am* 1994;**4**:823–847.

14. McCormick, P. W., Spetzler, R. F., Johnson, P. C. & Drayer, B. P. Cerebellar hemorrhage associated with capillary telangiectasia and venous angioma: a case report. *Surg Neurol* 1993;**39**:451–457.

15. Van Roost, D., Kristof, R., Wolf, H. K. & Keller, E. Intracerebral capillary telangiectasia and venous malformation: a rare association. *Surg Neurol* 1997;**48**:175–183.

16. Awad, I. A. On telangiectasia. *Am J Neurorad* 1996;**17**:1799–1800.

17. Abdulrauf, S. I., Kaynar, M. Y. & Awad, I. A. A comparison of the clinical profile of cavernous malformations with and without associated venous malformations. *Neurosurgery* 1999;**44**:41–46; discussion 46–47.

18. Awad, I. A. & Robinson, J. R. Comparison of the clinical presentation of symptomatic arteriovenous malformations (angiographically visualized) and occult vascular malformations. *Neurosurgery* 1993;**32**:876–878.

19. Mullan, S., Mojtahedi, S., Johnson, D. L. & Macdonald, R. L. Cerebral venous malformation-arteriovenous malformation transition forms. *J Neurosurg* 1996;**85**:9–13.

20. Petersen, T. A., Morrison, L. A., Schrader, R. M. & Hart, B. L. Familial versus sporadic cavernous malformations: differences in developmental venous anomaly association and lesion phenotype. *AJNR Am J Neuroradiol* 2009;**31**:377–382.

21. Aksoy, F. G., Gomori, J. M. & Tuchner, Z. Association of intracerebral venous angioma and true arteriovenous malformation: a rare, distinct entity. *Neuroradiology* 2000;**42**:455–457.

22. Chang, S. D., Steinberg, G. K., Rosario, M., Crowley, R. S. & Hevner, R. F. Mixed arteriovenous malformation and capillary telangiectasia: a rare subset of mixed vascular malformations. Case report. *J Neurosurg* 1997;**86**:699–703.

23. Wurm, G., Schnizer, M. & Fellner, F. A. Cerebral cavernous malformations associated with venous anomalies: surgical considerations. *Neurosurgery* 2005;**57**(1 Suppl):42–58.

24. Yanaka, K., Hyodo, A. & Nose, T. Venous malformation serving as the draining vein of an adjoining arteriovenous malformation. Case report and review of the literature. *Surg Neurol* 2001;**56**:170–174.

25. Labauge, P., Enjolras, O., Bonerandi, J. J., *et al.* An association between autosomal dominant cerebral cavernomas and a distinctive hyperkeratotic cutaneous vascular malformation in 4 families. *Ann Neurol* 1999;**45**:250–254.

26. Williamson, A., Patrylo, P. R., Lee, S. & Spencer, D. D. Physiology of human cortical neurons adjacent to cavernous malformations and tumors. *Epilepsia* 2003;**44**:1413–1419.

27. Kerrigan, J. F., Ng, Y. T., Chung, S. & Rekate, H. L. The hypothalamic hamartoma: a model of subcortical epileptogenesis and encephalopathy. *Semin Pediatr Neurol* 2005;**12**:119–131.

28. Morrell, F. Varieties of human secondary epileptogenesis. *J Clin Neurophysiol* 1989;**6**:227–275.

29. Eriksson, S. H., Nordborg, C., Rydenhag, B. & Malmgren, K. Parenchymal lesions in pharmacoresistant temporal lobe epilepsy: dual and multiple pathology. *Acta Neurol Scand* 2005;**112**:151–156.

30. Okujava, M., Ebner, A., Schmitt, J. & Woermann, F. G. Cavernous angioma associated with ipsilateral hippocampal sclerosis. *Eur Radiol* 2002;**12**:1840–1842.

31. Salanova, V., Markand, O. & Worth, R. Temporal lobe epilepsy: analysis of patients with dual pathology. *Acta Neurol Scand* 2004;**109**:126–131.

32. Cascino, G. D., Kelly, P. J., Sharbrough, F. W., *et al.* Long-term follow-up of stereotactic lesionectomy in partial epilepsy: predictive factors and electroencephalographic results. *Epilepsia* 1992;**33**:639–644.

33. Awad, I. A., Rosenfeld, J., Ahl, J., Hahn, J. F. & Luders, H. Intractable epilepsy and structural lesions of the brain: mapping, resection strategies, and seizure outcome. *Epilepsia* 1991;**32**:179–186.

34. Jooma, R., Yeh, H. S., Privitera, M. D. & Gartner, M. Lesionectomy versus electrophysiologically guided resection for temporal lobe tumors manifesting with complex partial seizures. *J Neurosurg* 1995;**83**:231–236.

35. Moore, J. L., Jr. Open and closed heart massage. *J Med Assoc Ga* 1962;**51**:239.

36. Dorsch, N. W. C. & McMahon, J. H. A. Intracranial cavernous malformations – natural history and management. *Crit Rev Neurosurg* 1998;**8**:154–168.

37. Kraemer, D. L. & Awad, I. A. Vascular malformations and epilepsy: clinical considerations and basic mechanisms. *Epilepsia* 1994;**35**(Suppl 6):S30–43.

38. Siegel, A. M., Roberts, D. W., Harbaugh, R. E. & Williamson, P. D. Pure lesionectomy versus tailored epilepsy surgery in treatment of cavernous malformations presenting with epilepsy. *Neurosurg Rev* 2000;**23**:80–83.

39. Stefan, H. & Hammen, T. Cavernous haemangiomas, epilepsy and treatment strategies. *Acta Neurol Scand* 2004;**110**:393–397.

40. Britton, J. W., Cascino, G. D., Sharbrough, F. W. & Kelly, P. J. Low-grade glial neoplasms and intractable partial epilepsy: efficacy of surgical treatment. *Epilepsia* 1994;**35**:1130–1135.

41. Spencer, D. D., Spencer, S. S., Mattson, R. H. & Williamson, P. D. Intracerebral masses in patients with intractable partial epilepsy. *Neurology* 1984;**34**:432–436.

42. Weber, J. P., Silbergeld, D. L. & Winn, H. R. Surgical resection of epileptogenic cortex associated with structural lesions. *Neurosurg Clin N Am* 1993;**4**:327–336.

43. Cappabianca, P., Alfieri, A., Maiuri, F., *et al.* Supratentorial cavernous malformations and epilepsy: seizure outcome after lesionectomy on a series of 35 patients. *Clin Neurol Neurosurg* 1997;**99**:179–183.

44. Cohen, D. S., Zubay, G. P. & Goodman, R. R. Seizure outcome after lesionectomy for cavernous malformations. *J Neurosurg* 1995;**83**:237–242.

45. Packer, R. J., Sutton, L. N., Patel, K. M., *et al.* Seizure control following tumor surgery for childhood cortical low-grade gliomas. *J Neurosurg* 1994;**80**:998–1003.

46. Rassi-Neto, A., Ferraz, F. P., Campos, C. R. & Braga, F. M. Patients with epileptic seizures and cerebral lesions who underwent lesionectomy restricted to or associated with the adjacent irritative area. *Epilepsia* 1999;**40**:856–864.

47. Rossi, G. F., Pompucci, A., Colicchio, G. & Scerrati, M. Factors of surgical outcome in tumoural epilepsy. *Acta Neurochir (Wien)* 1999;**141**:819–824.

48. Yeh, H. S., Tew, J. M., Jr. & Gartner, M. Seizure control after surgery on cerebral arteriovenous malformations. *J Neurosurg* 1993;**78**:12–18.

49. Zevgaridis, D., van Velthoven, V., Ebeling, U. & Reulen, H. J. Seizure control following surgery in supratentorial cavernous malformations: a retrospective study in 77 patients. *Acta Neurochir (Wien)* 1996;**138**:672–677.

50. Bengzon, A. R., Rasmussen, T., Gloor, P., Dussault, J. & Stephens, M. Prognostic factors in the surgical treatment of temporal lobe epileptics. *Neurology* 1968;**18**:717–731.

51. Dodrill, C. B., Wilkus, R. J., Ojemann, G. A., *et al.* Multidisciplinary prediction of seizure relief from cortical resection surgery. *Ann Neurol* 1986;**20**:2–12.

52. Smith, M. C. Multiple subpial transection in patients with extratemporal epilepsy. *Epilepsia* 1998;**39**(Suppl 4): S81–89.

53. Asanuma, H. Recent developments in the study of the columnar arrangement of neurons within the motor cortex. *Physiol Rev* 1975;**55**:143–156.

54. Morrell, F., Whisler, W. W. & Bleck, T. P. Multiple subpial transection: a new approach to the surgical treatment of focal epilepsy. *J Neurosurg* 1989;**70**:231–239.

55. Mountcastle, V. B. The columnar organization of the neocortex. *Brain* 1997;**120**:701–722.

56. Mountcastle, V. B. Modality and topographic properties of single neurons of cat's somatic sensory cortex. *J Neurophysiol* 1957;**20**:408–434.

57. Devinsky, O., Perrine, K., Vazquez, B., Luciano, D. J. & Dogali, M. Multiple subpial transections in the language cortex. *Brain* 1994;**117**:255–265.

58. Hufnagel, A., Zentner, J., Fernandez, G., *et al.* Multiple subpial transection for control of epileptic seizures: effectiveness and safety. *Epilepsia* 1997;**38**:678–688.

59. Sawhney, I. M., Robertson, I. J., Polkey, C. E., Binnie, C. D. & Elwes, R. D. Multiple subpial transection: a review of 21 cases. *J Neurol Neurosurg Psychiatry* 1995;**58**:344–349.

60. Shimizu, H., Suzuki, I., Ishijima, B., Karasawa, S. & Sakuma, T. Multiple subpial transection (MST) for the control of seizures that originated in unresectable cortical foci. *Jpn J Psychiatry Neurol* 1991;**45**:354–356.

61. Spencer, S. S. Corpus callosum section and other disconnection procedures for medically intractable epilepsy. *Epilepsia* 1988;**29**(Suppl 2):S85–99.

62. Spencer, S. S., Spencer, D. D., Williamson, P. D., *et al.* Corpus callosotomy for epilepsy. I. Seizure effects. *Neurology* 1988;**38**:19–24.

63. Wilson, D. H., Reeves, A., Gazzaniga, M. & Culver, C. Cerebral commissurotomy for control of intractable seizures. *Neurology* 1977;**27**:708–715.

64. Purves, S. J., Wada, J. A., Woodhurst, W. B., *et al.* Results of anterior corpus callosum section in 24 patients with medically intractable seizures. *Neurology* 1988;**38**:1194–1201.

65. Pilcher, W. H., Silbergeld, D. L., Berger, M. S. & Ojemann, G. A. Intraoperative electrocorticography during tumor resection: impact on seizure outcome in patients with gangliogliomas. *J Neurosurg* 1993;**78**:891–902.

66. Ben-Menachem, E., Hellstrom, K. & Verstappen, D. Analysis of direct hospital costs before and 18 months after treatment with vagus nerve stimulation therapy in 43 patients. *Neurology* 2002;**59**(6 Suppl 4):S44–47.

67. Murphy, J. V. Left vagal nerve stimulation in children with medically refractory epilepsy. The Pediatric VNS Study Group. *J Pediatr* 1999;**134**:563–566.

68. Schachter, S. C. Vagus nerve stimulation therapy summary: five years after FDA approval. *Neurology* 2002;**59**(6 Suppl 4):S15–20.

69. Schachter, S. C. & Wheless, J. W. The evolving place of vagus nerve stimulation therapy. *Neurology* 2002;**59**(6 Suppl 4):S1–2.

70. Benabid, A. L., Minotti, L., Koudsie, A., de Saint Martin, A. & Hirsch, E. Antiepileptic effect of high-frequency stimulation of the subthalamic nucleus (corpus luysi) in a case of medically intractable epilepsy caused by focal dysplasia: a 30-month follow-up: technical case report. *Neurosurgery* 2002;**50**:1385–1391; discussion 1391–1392.

71. Velasco, F., Velasco, M., Velasco, A. L., *et al.* Electrical stimulation of the centromedian thalamic nucleus in control of seizures: long-term studies. *Epilepsia* 1995;**36**:63–71.

72. Velasco, M., Velasco, F., Velasco, A. L., *et al.* Subacute electrical stimulation of the hippocampus blocks intractable temporal lobe seizures and paroxysmal EEG activities. *Epilepsia* 2000;**41**:158–169.

73. Haglund, M. M., Berger, M. S., Kunkel, D. D., *et al.* Changes in gamma-aminobutyric acid and somatostatin in epileptic cortex associated with low-grade gliomas. *J Neurosurg* 1992;**77**:209–216.

74. Requena, I., Arias, M., Lopez-Ibor, L., *et al.* Cavernomas of the central nervous system: clinical and neuroimaging manifestations in 47 patients. *J Neurol Neurosurg Psychiatry* 1991;**54**:590–594.

75. Hisada, K., Morioka, T., Nishio, S., *et al.* [Temporal lobe epilepsy associated with old intracerebral hemorrhage due to capillary telangiectasis in the temporal lobe: case report]. *No To Shinkei* 1999;**51**:729–735.

76. Huddle, D. C., Chaloupka, J. C. & Sehgal, V. Clinically aggressive diffuse capillary telangiectasia of the brain stem: a clinical radiologic-pathologic case study. *AJNR Am J Neuroradiol* 1999;**20**:1674–1677.

77. Awad, I. A., Robinson, J. R., Jr., Mohanty, S. & Estes, M. L. Mixed vascular malformations of the brain: clinical and pathogenetic considerations. *Neurosurgery* 1993;**33**:179–188; discussion 188.

78. Striano, S., Nocerino, C., Striano, P., *et al.* Venous angiomas and epilepsy. *Neurol Sci* 2000;**21**:151–155.

79. Tannier, C., Pons, M. & Treil, J. [Cerebral venous angiomas. 12 personal cases and review of the literature]. *Rev Neurol (Paris)* 1991;**147**:356–363.

80. Topper, R., Jurgens, E., Reul, J. & Thron, A. Clinical significance of intracranial developmental venous anomalies. *J Neurol Neurosurg Psychiatry* 1999;**67**:234–238.

81. Giombini, S. & Morello, G. Cavernous angiomas of the brain. Account of fourteen personal cases and review of the literature. *Acta Neurochir (Wien)* 1978;**40**:61–82.

Chapter 13

Surgery of spinal cavernous malformations

M. Yashar S. Kalani and Robert F. Spetzler

Over the past 50 years there have been significant advances in our understanding of angio- and vasculogenesis and in the treatment of malformations resulting from these processes gone awry. Vascular malformations are classified into three categories: aneurysmal, arteriovenous, or neoplastic. Given both their sporadic and familial distribution [1], their developmental-pathological link to capillary telangiectasias [2], and observed chromosomal abnormalities [3], cavernous malformations (CMs) could be regarded as neoplastic growths.

Spinal CMs are benign vascular hamartomas that consist of endothelium-lined vascular channels without intervening normal brain parenchyma. Surprisingly, these lesions do not significantly alter the vascular anatomy of the spinal cord. Spinal CMs are uncommon lesions, occurring infrequently in the vertebrae and occasionally extending into the extradural spinal canal [4]. Both intradural extramedullary [5,6] and isolated extradural [7,8] spinal CMs have been reported. Neither the origin nor the natural history of spinal CMs is well known. Recent genetic and family-linkage studies have implicated three genes involved in the proliferation and differentiation of angiogenic precursors and as members of the apopototic machinery in the pathological process.

In 1912 Schultze reported the first successful surgical removal of an intramedullary cavernous malformation of the spinal cord [9]. Since then advances in imaging and microsurgical technique have facilitated the diagnosis and treatment of these occult and sinister lesions. This chapter reviews pertinent pathology and addresses surgical approaches used for the treatment of spinal CMs. In the future, a better understanding of the molecular processes involved in the pathogenesis of these lesions may enable the use of less invasive modalities for the treatment of CMs.

Incidence

Spinal CMs were long considered exceptionally rare lesions. With the advent of magnetic resonance imaging (MRI), however, the diagnosis of spinal CMs increased. Based on current literature, spinal CMs account for 5 to 12% of all spinal vascular malformations and for 1 to 5% of all spinal epidural tumors [10,11]. Although spinal CMs have been identified in all age groups, symptomatic cases tend to manifest in early adulthood through middle age, with the highest number of cases diagnosed in the third to fourth decades of life [6,10,12]. Despite initial reports of a female-to-male distribution of 2:1, larger series now suggest that the gender distribution is 1:1 [13]. The reported prevalence of CMs is about 0.5% in the general population [14]. The incidence may be higher among pregnant women, who are more likely to present with hemorrhaging related to physiological changes associated with pregnancy, possibly because hormonal changes cause these lesions to grow [15].

The identification of one CM should increase suspicion for the presence of others in patients with otherwise unexplained neurological deficits. Reports of multiple CMs identified on imaging of the neuraxis suggest that may occur in 14 to 47% of cases [16,17].

Spinal CMs are not distributed equally throughout the spinal column: 54 to 77% are located in the thoracic, 20 to 30% in the cervical, and 5 to 10% in the lumbar segments; sacral lesions are exceptionally rare [12,13].

Origin of CMs

The exact mechanism underlying the pathogenesis of CMs is unknown. Histopathologically, spinal CMs (Fig. 13.1A) are indistinguishable from cerebral lesions (Fig. 13.1B). CMs can occur sporadically or as an

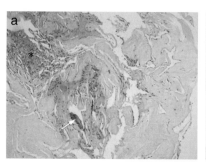
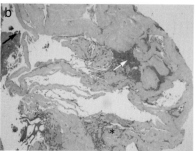

Figure 13.1. Low power (40× magnification) hematoxylin and eosin (H&E) stained sections of a spinal CM (A) and a cerebral CM (B) show that the histopathological features of the two lesions are identical. The sections show thin-walled sinusoids of endothelial cells associated with thrombosis (white arrow; pink stain), calcification (black arrow; dark blue stain), and hemosiderin deposits (brownish pigment within the cytoplasm of macrophages (*)). Used with permission from Barrow Neurological Institute. See color plate section.

autosomally dominant inherited familial condition. Familial forms of the disease have been attributed to mutations at three different loci implicated in regulating important processes such as proliferation and differentiation of angiogenic precursors (CCM1 on 7q21.2 and CCM2 on 7p15–p13) and a member of the apoptotic machinery (CCM3 on 3q25.2–q27) (Fig. 13.2) [18]. These processes are important for the generation, maintenance, and pruning of every vessel in the body. Therefore, it is unsurprising that the familial form of cerebral CMs usually presents with multiple malformations whereas sporadic cases usually exhibit solitary lesions [1,19]. Multi-locus analysis of familial CMs has shown that 40% of kindred are linked to the CCM1 and CCM3 loci each, and 20% are linked to CCM2 [18]. There is no reported difference in the clinical presentations or pathological features of the sporadic and familial forms. Only 10 to 20% of Caucasian patients with a cerebral CM have the familial form as compared to almost 50% of Hispanic patients [1,3]. Iatrogenic forms of SCMs have been attributed to trauma and radiation of the spine [20].

Clinical features

Most CMs probably go undiagnosed because small, asymptomatic lesions tend to be silent and are only discovered on postmortem examination. Symptomatic CMs usually manifest with myelopathy or hemorrhage. Although patients with spinal CMs may experience the acute onset of neurological dysfunction or progressive myelopathy over several years [21], the most common clinical presentation is slow progressive myelopathy [22]. The slow nature of disease progression may mimic a demyelinating process or Foix-Alajouanine syndrome and go undiagnosed for years [10].

The pathogenesis of both the acute and progressive myelopathies associated with spinal CMs is usually caused by hematomyelia. During the course of the

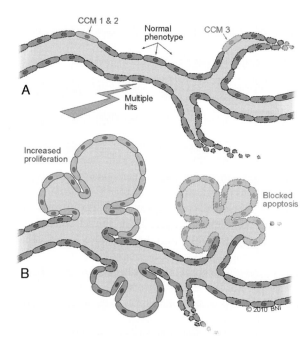

Figure 13.2. Although the origin of cavernous malformations is unknown, several mutations in important regulators of proliferation, differentiation, and the apoptotic machinery have been identified. Mutations regulating the decision of an endothelial cell to proliferate or differentiate (CCM1 and CCM2) cause unregulated growth of vasculature, while those involved in the apoptotic machinery (CCM3) interrupt the finely orchestrated pruning mechanism, further exacerbating the unregulated growth phenotype of this lesion. CM may form after exposure to radiation. Radiation may stimulate or block pathways similar to those in mutations identified in the familial cases, resulting in unregulated growth of endothelial cells and formation of CMs. Used with permission from Barrow Neurological Institute. See color plate section.

disease, small repeated episodes or one brisk episode of bleeding and hemorrhage causes a hemosiderin-stained gliotic capsule to form adjacent to the spinal cord. The combination of hemorrhage, subsequent clot formation, and the local pressure effects of the CM on the surrounding spinal cord lead to myelopathic symptoms. The progression of deficits may help distinguish spinal CMs from spinal arteriovenous malformations the symptoms of which are usually maximal at onset because of hemorrhage [23]. Once patients are symptomatic, progressive myelopathy is the typical course.

Spinal CMs can be incidental findings discovered on imaging of the neuraxis performed for another purpose. The mean size of spinal CMs is 16.3 mm with a range of 3 to 54 mm [13]. At our institution, we seldom treat asymptomatic patients with incidental lesions, preferring to monitor them with clinical examination and serial MR imaging. Patients with mild or spontaneously resolving symptoms may be followed expectantly with serial examinations to determine the need for intervention. The risk of irreversible neurological deficits after hemorrhage (estimated between 1.4% and 4.5% per year [12,24]) in these patients must be weighed against the risk of intervention in individual cases.

Gross total resection is the gold standard for the treatment of CMs. Since CMs are angiographically occult, endovascular therapy has no role in their treatment. Nor has radiation therapy shown efficacy as a treatment modality. The surgical resection of dorsally exophytic lesions is associated with the lowest risk of complications, followed by dorsal and ventral lesions. Surgical outcome primarily correlates with preoperative neurological status. Patients treated soon after the onset of symptoms exhibit more robust functional improvement within 3 years of treatment compared to patients whose treatment is delayed (76% vs. 52%) [12]. The optimal time for surgery is 4 to 6 weeks after hemorrhage [12].

Diagnostic imaging

Choosing the appropriate imaging modality is essential for both diagnosis and treatment planning. As mentioned, CMs are angiographically occult lesions, possibly from the lack of direct arterial input [25]; therefore, angiography and myelography are usually normal for these lesions. Although lacking sensitivity, computerized tomography (CT) may show evidence of an intramedullary lesion and spinal cord widening after contrast is administered [10,22].

MRI is the imaging modality of choice for the diagnosis of and surgical planning for spinal SCMs [26]. Indeed, the reported incidence of spinal CMs increased dramatically as MRI became a routine part

of the neurosurgical arsenal. MRI evaluation of spinal CMs frequently shows an iso- to hypointense lesion on T1-weighted images and a hyperintense "popcorn-like" lesion with a hypointense rim on T2-weighted images (Fig. 13.3). The hypointense rim visible on T2-weighted images is most likely attributable to the leakage of hemosiderin from repeated microhemorrhages [26]. Exceptions to these findings, however, are common. Both lesion(s) and hemorrhages evolve during the course of the acute bleed and chronic remodeling of the tissue. Therefore, the MRI appearance of CMs depends on the timing of this process. These variations include T1-weighted hyperintensity, T2-weighted hypointensity at the foci of hemorrhages 2 days to 2 weeks old, iso- and hypointense lesions on T2-weighted images from acute hemorrhage, increased T2-weighted signal in the spinal cord surrounding the lesion caused by edema and blood, and evolution from hyperintensity to hypointensity on T1- and T2-weighted images as the blood products are enzymatically processed and broken down [27]. Enhancement with gadolinium-DTPA can also vary across patients, resulting in features other than those deemed pathognomic for spinal CMs.

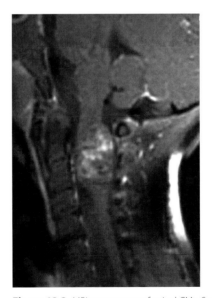

Figure 13.3. MRI appearance of spinal CMs. Sagittal T1-weighted MRIs reveal an iso- to hypointense lesion, while T2-weighted images show a hyperintense "popcorn-like" lesion with a hypointense rim. Since both the lesion(s) and hemorrhages evolve during the course of the acute bleed and chronic remodeling of the tissue, the MRI appearance of CMs can vary depending on the timing of this process. Used with permission from Barrow Neurological Institute.

Operative procedure

Preoperative considerations

The goals of surgery for spinal CMs are to resolve myelopathy, to halt progression of neurological deterioration, and to prevent hemorrhage of the CM resulting in neurological devastation. Before surgery, consent should be obtained from the patient. The consent process should explain the risks and benefits of treatments and alternatives (which may include no intervention at all) to patients. Patients should be educated about potential worsening of their deficits immediately after surgery. They should be informed that deficits typically improve over time and should be warned that a moderate course of postoperative rehabilitation will likely be necessary. Patient education at this point is critical to ease the anxiety of patients and family and to provide them with realistic expectations about the process of treatment and recovery.

Intraoperative monitoring

Intraoperative monitoring during spinal surgery is a valuable adjunct to help minimize complications. At our institution, spinal somatosensory evoked potentials (SSEPs) and motor evoked potentials (MEPs) are monitored in all patients. Baseline recordings are obtained so that intraoperative changes can be evaluated relative to the baseline. These monitoring techniques are applied before and after patients are positioned to prevent unwanted outcomes such as vascular compromise and spinal cord injury in patients with spondylosis. Postoperative neurological deficits do not always correlate with changes in the recorded waveforms.

Surgical technique

Surgery on the spinal column can be performed from an anterior (and anterolateral) or posterior (and posterolateral approach). Although each approach is useful, the surgeon must choose the surgical path that provides both decompression of the neural elements and adequate postoperative structural support. The best approach depends on a number of interrelated factors such as location of the lesion and the spinal level involved. Lesions at the extremes of the vertebral column pose a particular challenge. At the rostral extreme, transoral and mandible-splitting techniques may provide adequate anterior exposure. Caudally, combined anterior and posterior approaches may be used to achieve total sacrectomy for exposure of lesions. Given the morbidity and length of recovery associated with these aforementioned approaches, the preferred initial approach at the rostral and caudal extremes of the column is usually posterior. Indeed, in almost every case performed at our institution we have approached such lesions from the posterior approach.

The surgical techniques for removing spinal CMs are similar to those used to excise benign intramedullary spinal cord tumors. The exception is that spinal CMs may be more adherent to the contiguous spinal cord than benign tumors [27]. Because residual CMs often rehemorrhage and cause further myelopathy, complete excision should be the goal of surgery. Consequently, the bed of the CM in the spinal cord should be inspected thoroughly before closure.

A posterior approach with osteoplastic laminoplasty or laminectomy has been the approach of choice for most lesions treated at our institution. Osteoplastic laminoplasty and laminectomy are performed by making a keyhole laminotomy. A Midas Rex footplate is placed below the lamina, and drilling proceeds cephalad to remove the segment en bloc. The dura mater is opened sharply using microscissors and tacked to the adjacent soft tissues. Careful microscopic inspection of the dorsal surface of the spinal cord usually reveals a bluish discoloration (Fig. 13.4), which marks the location of the lesion. If the lesion or discoloration is not visible on visual inspection, intraoperative ultrasonography may be used to localize the lesion and to plan the myelotomy

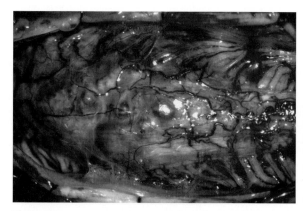

Figure 13.4. Intraoperative photograph of a spinal CM identified by its distinct bluish discoloration. Although these lesions may be readily identified using microscopic magnification, intraoperative ultrasonography may be needed to identify lesions without an exophytic component. Used with permission from Barrow Neurological Institute. See color plate section.

[28]. After the myelotomy is performed, the pia is gently tacked up to optimize the exposure. Monitoring SSEPs and MEPs helps prevent damage to normal tissue. During this maneuver, it is essential to maintain systemic blood pressure to avoid spinal cord ischemia.

CMs are resected using microsurgical techniques under the operating microscope. Care is taken to dissect sharply within the gliotic plane surrounding the lesion to avoid injury to normal spinal tissue. The use of electrocoagulation should be minimized, and hemosiderin-stained tissue should be preserved as much as possible. In most patients, a small amount of bleeding is encountered as the lesion is dissected free from the surrounding spinal cord parenchyma. Because of the low pressure of the lesion, bleeding is often minimal and readily controlled. As the lesion is removed, small pockets of clotted blood, vascular lumens, and "berry-like" projections, the remnants of recurrent prior hemorrhages, can be visualized.

Although smaller lesions can be resected en bloc (Fig. 13.5A), larger lesions, especially those that are enlarged by intracapsular hemorrhage, should first be decompressed internally and then dissected circumferentially (Fig. 13.5B). Failure to decompress such lesions first can cause undue trauma to the spinal cord [29]. Throughout the procedure total hemostasis must be achieved.

During the resection of intramedullary spinal CMs, cryptic venous malformations must be preserved. Their indiscriminant sacrifice can cause significant, permanent deficits [30]. Although a small individual venous channel may sometimes be coagulated safely, a more pronounced venous vessel around the CM should always be preserved (Fig. 13.6). In the senior surgeon's (RFS) experience with the resection of more than 50 intramedullary spinal cord CMs, only one patient suffered postoperative deficits, which were caused by the sacrifice of a midsized venous channel. When resection is completed, the lesion bed should be examined carefully to avoid leaving residual CM. Small residual branches of a primary venous malformation can mature and give rise to secondary or recurrent CMs.

After the final inspection, the dura mater is closed primarily using either 4–0 Nurolon or 6–0 Prolene sutures. In patients who undergo osteoplastic laminoplasty, the en bloc laminae segments are reaffixed to the spine using microfixation titanium plates or Surgilon sutures. The techniques described above minimize the operative risk and offer the best chance of total resection for most patients [31]. Patients who require additional surgery for residual CM should have their previous incisions reopened. The residual CM is then excised, and the dura is again closed with Prolene or Nurolon.

Postoperative management

Based on standard protocol, patients are assessed for extubation when their cough and gag reflexes are adequate. Postoperative swallowing should be evaluated in patients whose CM is located high in the cervical spinal cord and whose function could be at risk. Short-term tracheostomy may be considered when swallowing is suboptimal. Stable patients usually

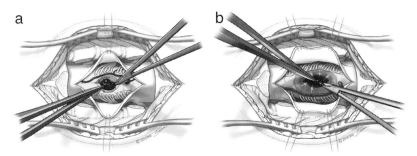

Figure 13.5. Schematic representation of the surgical technique used to resect spinal CMs, which are typically small, low-flow lesions with a mulberry-like appearance. The surgical technique used to remove these lesions is similar to that used to resect benign intramedullary spinal cord tumors. Using MRI guidance, the location of the lesion is identified. The dura is opened sharply over the lesion. The lesion is identified by its bluish discoloration. Care is taken to dissect sharply within the gliotic plane surrounding the lesion to avoid injury to normal spinal tissue. The use of electrocoagulation should be minimized, and hemosiderin-stained tissue should be preserved as much as possible. Although (A) smaller lesions are amenable to en bloc resection, (B) larger lesions should be decompressed internally and then dissected circumferentially to minimize trauma to the spinal cord. The lesion bed should be inspected carefully before closure to prevent leaving remnant spinal CM, which could give rise to recurrent disease. Used with permission from Barrow Neurological Institute. See color plate section.

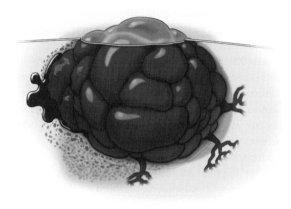

Figure 13.6. CMs are frequently associated with other vascular anomalies. During the resection of intramedullary spinal CMs, it is essential to identify and preserve any cryptic venous malformations. These cryptic malformations often serve as the primary blood supply for watershed regions adjacent to CMs, and their removal may result in ischemic damage to critical spinal tracts, resulting in permanent neurological devastation. Used with permission from Barrow Neurological Institute. See color plate section.

undergo MRI on postoperative day 1 both to obtain a baseline for comparison of future studies and to assess for the presence of residual lesion.

As discussed under "Diagnostic imaging", these lesions usually contain extensive areas of hemosiderin staining, which should not be removed during surgical resection. The presence of hemosiderin staining can mimic residual or recurrent CM and can make assessing the extent of resection difficult. Consequently, follow-up imaging should be obtained annually for at least the first 2 years after surgery to monitor for progression or recurrence of disease.

Despite postoperative MRIs consistent with a radiographic cure, recurrence rates as high as 5% have been reported years after resection of cerebral CMs [32]. This trend may reflect the presence of unrecognized residual lesion at surgery or a *de novo* lesion that formed after surgery. Patients should be followed on an outpatient basis at intervals of 1 week, 4 weeks, 6 months, 1 year, and 2 years or more frequently as needed or as determined by the physician. Symptomatic patients may need to be evaluated more frequently and closely. In asymptomatic patients with a negative MRI, the follow-up intervals can be increased at the surgeon's discretion.

Surgical outcomes

In expert hands, the surgical outcomes for patients with spinal CMs are excellent. In the senior author's experience with more than 40 spinal CMs, the functional outcome,

based on Frankel grade, of 91% of the patients remained the same or improved. Five (11%) patients developed new episodes of bleeding related to incomplete resection but improved after a second operation (Spetzler, R. F., unpublished data) as reported elsewhere in the literature [21,33]. Residual spinal CMs can rebleed and cause recurrent myelopathy; therefore, surgery should be performed before the next episode of hemorrhage. If symptoms recur in the absence of residual CM after surgery, local tethering of the spinal cord related to scar formation should be considered. Symptomatic spinal cord tethering can be detected on follow-up MRI, highlighting the need to repeat imaging for a few years after surgery.

Patients undergoing surgery for spinal CMs often experience transient neurological worsening during the immediate postoperative period, but most return to baseline or improve over time [31,34]. Resection effectively treats pain, with lasting improvements in almost half of the patients treated [35].

Conclusion

Spinal CMs represent a unique and challenging subset of vascular tumors of the central nervous system that are currently only amenable to surgical intervention. Previously considered exceedingly rare and occult, MRI has shown that these lesions are more common than once thought. As our knowledge base about the molecular pathogenesis of these lesions increases, it may be possible to combine expert microsurgical technique with small molecules and biologics to control and remedy these lesions.

References

1. Rigamonti, D., Hadley, M. N., Drayer, B. P., *et al.* Cerebral cavernous malformations. Incidence and familial occurrence. *New Engl J Med* 1988;**319**:343–347.

2. Rigamonti, D., Johnson, P. C., Spetzler, R. F., Hadley, M. N. & Drayer, B. P. Cavernous malformations and capillary telangiectasia: a spectrum within a single pathological entity. *Neurosurgery* 1991;**28**:60–64.

3. Denier, C., Goutagny, S., Labauge, P., *et al.* Mutations within the MGC4607 gene cause cerebral cavernous malformations. *Am J Hum Genet* 2004;**74**:326–337.

4. Guthkelch, A. N. Haemangiomas involving the spinal epidural space. *J Neurol Neurosurg Psychiatry* 1948;**11**:199–210.

5. Heimberger, K., Schnaberth, G., Koos, W., Pendl, G. & Auff, E. Spinal cavernous haemangioma (intradural-extramedullary) underlying repeated subarachnoid haemorrhage. *J Neurol* 1982;**226**:289–293.

6. Pagni, C. A., Canavero, S. & Forni, M. Report of a cavernoma of the cauda equina and review of the literature. *Surg Neurol* 1990;**33**:124–131.

7. Hillman, J. & Bynke, O. Solitary extradural cavernous hemangiomas in the spinal canal. Report of five cases. *Surg Neurol* 1991;**36**:19–24.

8. Padovani, R., Tognetti, F., Proietti, D., Pozzati, E. & Servadei, F. Extrathecal cavernous hemangioma. *Surg Neurol* 1982;**18**:463–465.

9. Schultze, F. Weiterer Beitrag zur Diagnose und operativen Behandlung von Geschwülsten der Rückenmarkshäute und des Rückenmarks. *Dtsch Med Wochenschr* 1912;**38**:1676–1679.

10. Cosgrove, G. R., Bertrand G., Fontaine Y. & Melanson, D. Cavernous angiomas of the spinal cord. *J Neurosurg* 1988;**68**:31–36.

11. Samii, M. & Klekamp, J. Surgical results of 100 intramedullary tumors in relation to accompanying syringomyelia. *Neurosurgery* 1994;**35**:865–873.

12. Zevgaridis, D., Medele, R. J., Hamburger, C., Steiger, H. J. & Reulen, H. J. Cavernous haemangiomas of the spinal cord. A review of 117 cases. *Acta Neurochir (Wien)* 1999;**141**:237–245.

13. Labauge, P., Bouly, S., Parker, F., *et al.* Outcome in 53 patients with spinal cord cavernomas. *Surg Neurol* 2008;**70**:176–181.

14. Labauge, P., Laberge, S., Brunereau, L., Levy, C. & Tournier-Lasserve, E. Hereditary cerebral cavernous angiomas: clinical and genetic features in 57 French families. Societe Francaise de Neurochirurgie. *Lancet* 1998;**352**:1892–1897.

15. Safavi-Abbasi, S., Feiz-Erfan, I., Spetzler, R. F., *et al.* Hemorrhage of cavernous malformations during pregnancy and in the peripartum period: causal or coincidence? Case report and review of the literature. *Neurosurg Focus* 2006;**21**:e12.

16. Santoro, A., Piccirilli, M., Frati, A., *et al.* Intramedullary spinal cord cavernous malformations: report of ten new cases. *Neurosurg Rev* 2004;**27**:93–98.

17. Vishteh, A. G., Zabramski, J. M. & Spetzler, R. F. Patients with spinal cord cavernous malformations are at an increased risk for multiple neuraxis cavernous malformations. *Neurosurgery* 1999;**45**:30–32.

18. Dashti, S. R., Hoffer, A., Hu, Y. C. & Selman, W. R. Molecular genetics of familial cerebral cavernous malformations. *Neurosurg Focus* 2006;**21**:e2.

19. Craig, H. D., Gunel, M., Cepeda, O., *et al.* Multilocus linkage identifies two new loci for a Mendelian form of stroke, cerebral cavernous malformation, at 7p15–13 and 3q25.2–27. *Hum Mol Genet* 1998;**7**:1851–1858.

20. Maraire, J. N., Abdulrauf, S. I., Berger, S., Knisely, J. & Awad, I. A. De novo development of a cavernous malformation of the spinal cord following spinal axis radiation. Case report. *J Neurosurg* 1999;**90** (2 Suppl):234–238.

21. Ogilvy, C. S., Louis, D. N. & Ojemann, R. G. Intramedullary cavernous angiomas of the spinal cord: clinical presentation, pathological features, and surgical management. *Neurosurgery* 1992;**31**:219–229.

22. Zentner, J., Hassler, W., Gawehn, J. & Schroth, G. Intramedullary cavernous angiomas. *Surg Neurol* 1989;**31**:64–68.

23. Harrison, M. J., Eisenberg, M. B., Ullman, J. S., *et al.* Symptomatic cavernous malformations affecting the spine and spinal cord. *Neurosurgery* 1995;**37**:195–204.

24. Sandalcioglu, I. E., Wiedemayer, H., Gasser, T., *et al.* Intramedullary spinal cord cavernous malformations: clinical features and risk of hemorrhage. *Neurosurg Rev* 2003;**26**:253–256.

25. Campeau, N. G. & Lane, J. I. De novo development of a lesion with the appearance of a cavernous malformation adjacent to an existing developmental venous anomaly. *AJNR Am J Neuroradiol* 2005;**26**:156–159.

26. Rigamonti, D., Drayer, B. P., Johnson, P. C., *et al.* The MRI appearance of cavernous malformations (angiomas). *J Neurosurg* 1987;**67**:518–524.

27. Thompson, B. G. & Oldfield, E. H. Spinal arteriovenous malformations. In H. R. Winn, ed., *Youmans Neurological Surgery*, 5th ed. (Philadelphia: Saunders, 2004), p. 2375.

28. Lunardi, P., Acqui, M., Ferrante, L. & Fortuna, A. The role of intraoperative ultrasound imaging in the surgical removal of intramedullary cavernous angiomas. *Neurosurgery* 1994;**34**:520–523.

29. Vishteh, A. G. & Spetzler, R. F. Radical excision of intramedullary cavernous angiomas. *Neurosurgery* 1999;**44**:428.

30. Vishteh, A. G., Sankhla, S., Anson, J. A., Zabramski, J. M. & Spetzler, R. F. Surgical resection of intramedullary spinal cord cavernous malformations: delayed complications, long-term outcomes, and association with cryptic venous malformations. *Neurosurgery* 1997;**41**:1094–1100.

31. Anson, J. A. & Spetzler, R. F. Surgical resection of intramedullary spinal cord cavernous malformations. *J Neurosurg* 1993;**78**:446–451.

32. Porter, R. W., Detwiler, P. W., Spetzler, R. F., *et al.* Cavernous malformations of the brainstem: experience with 100 patients. *J Neurosurg* 1999;**90**:50–58.

33. Tyndel, F. J., Bilbao, J. M., Hudson, A. R. & Colapinto, E. V. Hemangioma calcificans of the spinal cord. *Can J Neurol Sci* 1985;**12**:321–322.

34. Jallo, G. I., Freed, D., Zareck, M., Epstein, F. & Kothbauer, K. F. Clinical presentation and optimal management for intramedullary cavernous malformations. *Neurosurg Focus* 2006;**21**:e10.

35. Kim, L. J., Klopfenstein, J. D., Zabramski, J. M., Sonntag, V. K. & Spetzler, R. F. Analysis of pain resolution after surgical resection of intramedullary spinal cord cavernous malformations. *Neurosurgery* 2006;**58**:106–111.

Surgical treatment of cavernous malformations in children

Edward R. Smith and R. Michael Scott

Definition and histology

Cavernous malformations (CMs) are vascular lesions found in the central nervous system (CNS) and throughout the body. The nomenclature for these malformations can be confusing as they have been called cavernomas, cavernous angiomas, and cavernous hemangiomas. They have come to the attention of pediatric neurosurgeons because of their capacity to affect children through hemorrhage, seizure, focal neurological deficits, and headache.

CMs are composed of a compact mass of sinusoidal-type vessels contiguous with one another and with no intervening normal parenchyma. These well-circumscribed, unencapsulated masses are identified grossly as having a purple lobulated "mulberry" appearance (Fig. 14.1). Calcifications may be present, both grossly and microscopically. Cysts containing old hemorrhage products may be present and may help explain the controversial phenomenon of growth of these lesions; providing a substrate for neovascularization following hemorrhage. Surrounding tissue may be gliotic and stained from previous hemorrhage with green, yellow, or brown discoloration.

Epidemiology

CMs are relatively rare lesions, with an estimated prevalence of 0.4–0.5% in autopsy and MRI studies [1,2–4]. An incidence of 0.43 diagnoses per 100,000 people per year has been reported [5]. Symptomatic lesions manifest in all age groups. The peak incidence of presentation is usually in the third to fourth decade without a gender preponderance [4,6]. Affected children appear to be clustered in two age groups: infants and toddlers under the age of 3 years and children in early puberty; ages 12–16 years [7,8].

Most cases are sporadic (50–80%), i.e. they lack family history of CMs [1,4]. A single CM is found in 75% of sporadic cases and only 8–19% of familial cases [1,4]. In contrast, the presence of multiple CMs is strongly suggestive of familial CM: approximately 75% of all patients with multiple lesions ultimately are found to have affected relatives [9]. Only 10–25% of individuals with multiple lesions will be sporadic cases, with the remainder of patients with multiple CMs often attributed to secondary effects of radiation therapy [1,10–12].

Etiology

The cause of CMs remains under investigation. Recent advances have been made in the understanding of the contribution that specific mutations play in the development of these lesions. In particular, three genes have been associated with the formation of CMs: CCM1 (also known as *KRIT1*, found on chromosome 7q), CCM2 (also known as *malcaverin*, found on 7p), and CCM3 (also known as *Programmed Cell Death 10*, on 3p) [13–27]. Molecular studies of CCM1 have revealed that this binding protein (Krev-1/rap1a binding protein) is essential for normal embryonic vascular development and mutations in this gene, found in hereditary cases of CM, result in loss of function [28]. In patients with these CCM1 mutations, nearly all will have radiographic evidence of multiple CMs, but only about 60% of patients will develop symptoms [29].

Patients with familial CMs are prone to developing new lesions throughout their lifetime. Periodic MRI studies are recommended to follow patients known to be affected. Screening of family members, both genetically and radiographically, remains controversial, but may be helpful for genetic counseling and evaluating risk [30,31]. Other systems may be affected including

Cavernous Malformations of the Nervous System, ed. Daniele Rigamonti. Published by Cambridge University Press.
© Cambridge University Press 2011.

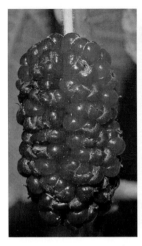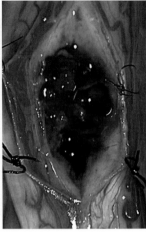

Figure 14.1. Comparison between a cavernous malformation (same case as depicted in MRI studies of spinal cord lesion in Fig. 14.3) and a mulberry. Note multiple lobules and variegated appearance of the lesion. See color plate section.

skin, eyes, and visceral organs, with CCM1 found as the most commonly mutated gene in these patients [32,33]. It is our practice to refer patients with multiple CMs to the genetics service for mutational testing and counseling.

Presentation

CMs may never cause symptoms and may be discovered only incidentally at autopsy or may be responsible for a variety of neurological complaints. The neurological signs and symptoms of symptomatic CMs correlate with the anatomic site of involvement and the age at presentation. CMs occur anywhere in the central nervous system (CNS), with symptomatic lesions most commonly presenting with hemorrhage, seizure, or focal neurological deficit [8,34–36]. Intracranial CMs cause symptoms by (relatively) low-pressure hemorrhages that exert a mass effect on the surrounding brain. The extravasation of blood into brain parenchyma creates a hemosiderin ring that may predispose susceptible tissue to seizure. Children with CMs may also have headache as a symptom, presumably secondary to mass effect or irritation of dural nociceptors from hemorrhage products.

Radiographic findings

Radiographic evaluation of suspected CM usually begins with computerized tomography (CT) or magnetic resonance imaging (MRI). CMs are often undetectable on angiography and are, therefore, grouped with the heterogeneous group of "angiographically occult vascular malformations"; there is general agreement that angiography is generally not indicated in their evaluation [37].

These lesions can range in size from microscopic to near-hemispheric, with an average size of about 5 cm in diameter in children [7].

The typical CT appearance is a well-defined collection of multiple, rounded densities showing minor contrast enhancement and without a mass effect. Often, there are calcifications [38]. Recent hemorrhage may or may not be present, depending on the clinical setting. MRI studies are distinctive; there is typically a "popcorn" appearance with an associated "bloom" on susceptibility imaging, suggesting hemosiderin deposition [8,39–41] (Fig. 14.2). Although the characteristics of CMs may vary considerably between children, attempts have been made to classify imaging findings and correlate them with pathology [1]. A grading system has been proposed that clusters CMs into four categories based on T1, T2, and susceptibility imaging characteristics [1].

Of particular note is the high rate of finding a developmental venous anomaly (DVA) in association with a CM (Fig. 14.2). They have been reported with frequencies approaching 100% in young children with CMs [7,42]. This finding is of particular relevance with regard to surgical therapy as these DVAs provide venous drainage to normal brain, and should be preserved at surgery if possible [43,44]. Certain authors have implicated DVAs in the etiology of cavernomas [45].

In a review of 163 previously published cases, 126 patients (76.8%) had supratentorial malformations, 34 (20.7%) were infratentorial, four (2.5%) were intraventricular, and four (2.5%) were multiple [46]. Calcifications were observed in 18 cases (11%). Among 31 patients studied by cerebral angiography, normal findings or an avascular mass were encountered. With the advent of MRI, increased imaging sensitivity has revealed a higher rate of patients with multiple CMs, with up to 21% of patients with CM found to have multiple lesions [35]. If multiple CMs are seen on imaging, then a familial or post-radiation etiology should be considered [47].

In patients presenting with acute hemorrhage, it may be difficult to ascertain the diagnosis. Strong consideration must be given to the possibility of an arteriovenous malformation (AVM), which is found more commonly than CM in children. In this particular clinical scenario (unlike general screening as previously discussed) angiography is extremely helpful in

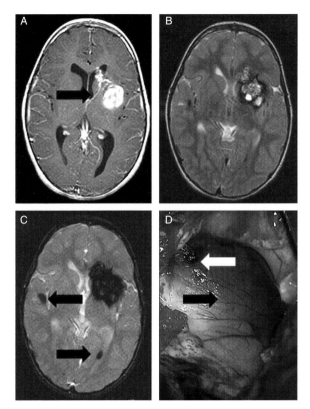

Figure 14.2. MRI appearance of cavernous malformations. (A) T1 post-contrast axial study of left frontal lesion; note irregular enhancement and presence of associated developmental venous malformation (arrow). (B) T2 images demonstrating "popcorn" appearance of lesion with multiple small cysts and darker rim of hemosiderin on periphery. (C) Susceptibility images reveal "bloom" of previous hemorrhages and highlight other lesions within this patient (arrows). (D) Operative correlation of radiographic studies with greenish, hemosiderin-stained surrounding tissue (black arrow) and darker, "mulberry"-like malformation (white arrow). See color plate section.

distinguishing between these entities. In children presenting with cystic or calcified lesions, the differential diagnosis may include tumors and susceptibility imaging may aid in identifying evidence of previous hemorrhage or other CMs.

Natural history and selection of treatment

Once a CM has been identified in a child, referral to a pediatric neurosurgeon is an appropriate first step. The surgeon must then weigh what is known about the risks of observation against the risks of intervention. The natural history of CMs can be difficult to predict. Depending on individual authors' definitions of hemorrhage, annual rates from CMs vary between

near undetectable and about 3% for lesions that are found incidentally and range between <4% and >23% for lesions that were found after a hemorrhage [1,34,48–50]. In general, hemorrhage from CMs is better tolerated with regard to mortality than from other high-flow lesions, such as AVMs. However, fatal hemorrhage from CM is a well-known entity, particularly if the lesion is in a high-risk location, such as the posterior fossa [34,51].

Of those children who have symptomatic hemorrhage, many can be at risk for temporal clustering of hemorrhages in a short period of time, with a rate of up to ~2% per lesion per month and 24% per year [49,52]. With repeated hemorrhage, the usual motif is that of progressive stepwise deficits. The child often presents with a profound decline in function at the time of hemorrhage, with subsequent partial recovery over several weeks to months, although the majority of children (63%) are unable to recover completely back to baseline [7,49,51,53–55]. With each subsequent hemorrhage, the ultimate level of function may decline (Fig. 14.3).

Given this natural history, several investigators have advocated early treatment of CMs in children, as their long life-span may favor a more aggressive approach [36,49,56,57]. Symptomatic lesions are considered for therapy. There has been debate regarding the utility of extirpation of asymptomatic lesions [58]. The decision to intervene is especially difficult in the patient who presents with symptoms and has multiple lesions. If the symptoms can be localized to a single lesion which is amenable to surgical resection, then that lesion should generally be removed [1,36]. Nevertheless, in the child with multiple CMs, the family should be informed that other lesions may appear and could potentially cause symptoms in the future.

Outcomes of surgical therapy have been remarkably good, with most series reporting a near 0% mortality rate and a 4–5% rate of new permanent deficits [53,58]. It is important to note that risks greatly increase in sensitive locations such as the brainstem, with rates of new, permanent postoperative deficits ranging from 12 to 25%, suggesting a need to approach lesions in these areas with caution [54,55].

For CMs located in high-risk locations, such as the brainstem or eloquent cortex, there is controversy regarding the potential role of radiation as a possible treatment option [53,54,59]. Radiosurgery has been reported to reduce the frequency of hemorrhage in these lesions from 17.3%/year to 4.5%/year [50,60].

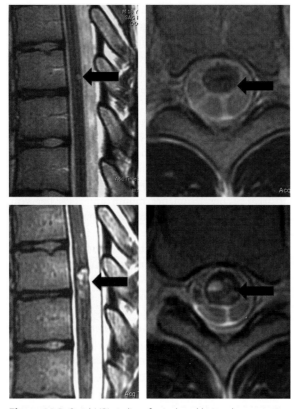

Figure 14.3. Serial MRI studies of spinal cord lesion demonstrating progressive enlargement with serial hemorrhages. These images were taken 6 months apart, with two distinct presentations of lower extremity sensory changes, weakness and urinary incontinence. Each time the child made a recovery from the presentation examination, but never returned to his neurological baseline and worsened with subsequent hemorrhages. (Operative photograph in Fig. 14.1.)

However, this decreased rate of hemorrhage comes at the cost of increased complications, including a 16% incidence of new permanent neurological deficit and a 3% mortality rate [60]. As such, its use must be balanced against the expected natural history of the lesion. When these data are viewed through the perspective of a child's expected long lifespan and are coupled with the poorly quantified long-term risk of secondary injury from radiation exposure, resection should be considered as first-line therapy whenever possible.

At our institution, it is our practice to surgically resect single CMs when they are located in non-eloquent cortex or spinal cord if they present with symptoms, documented radiographic enlargement, or hemorrhage (usually after a minimum of 4–6 weeks following hemorrhage in order to allow swelling

to resolve, unless there is urgency from significant mass effect). For lesions in eloquent cortex or in the brainstem, we will commonly decide to observe the lesion initially to determine whether it manifests a pattern of recurrent hemorrhage that would justify the risk of surgical intervention. If a subsequent hemorrhage occurs, then frequently we will undertake an operation. For deep lesions that are surgically inaccessible, we will usually observe and treat symptomatically, with very few ever referred for radiosurgery.

For patients with multiple lesions, we will refer them for genetic counseling. If no lesions are symptomatic, we will observe them with annual MRI studies. If individual lesions grow, become symptomatic, or manifest new hemorrhage on imaging, then we will subject that individual lesion to the algorithm detailed above.

Surgical technique

Surgical management of CMs in children is similar to that in adults [1,8,58,61]. In addition to the general principles of removing the entire lesion and preserving normal surrounding vasculature (especially associated DVAs), resection of a CM may include the removal of the surrounding hemosiderin ring, if the lesion is cortical, associated with seizures and in a low-risk location. In contrast, lesions in eloquent cortex, in the brainstem, or in the spinal cord should generally not have any non-lesional tissue resected in order to minimize injury to sensitive surrounding structures (Fig. 14.1).

At our institution, we have routinely employed frameless stereotaxy to aid in the localization of cranial lesions. This adjunct is particularly useful for deep lesions and we have found that placement of a catheter along the planned trajectory of approach, after opening the dura, is helpful as a guide to the lesion during dissection. We have also found the use of intraoperative ultrasound of immense value for real-time localization and assessment of extent of resection.

Postoperative issues

Close follow-up is indicated in patients who have undergone surgical resection of a CM. Cavernous malformations can recur if not excised *in toto* and the generation of new lesions has been documented, particularly in the setting of radiation-induced lesions and in familial cases [47,62]. In most patients, a postoperative MRI is ordered, usually 6 weeks to 6 months postoperatively, to assess the extent of resection and to serve as a new baseline for comparison with future studies. It is the practice in our institution to obtain follow-up imaging at 1-year intervals for 2–5 years postoperatively.

Patients with multiple CMs should have annual imaging to ascertain whether there is progression of any lesion since, in the pediatric population, there is a life-long risk for a lesion to bleed or grow, with surgery being subsequently required. It is less clear how to proceed with adults who have multiple lesions. Nevertheless, family members of patients with multiple lesions should be considered for screening studies. Candidates for screening include first-degree relatives with multiple CMs and/or family members with symptoms suggestive of intracranial disease (seizures, headaches or neurologic deficits).

Conclusion

The management of children with CMs requires a clear understanding of the natural history of these lesions and the risks of surgical intervention. Presentation is usually hemorrhage, seizure, focal neurological deficit, or headache. Diagnosis is best made with MRI. Patients with multiple lesions should be referred for genetic evaluation and counseling. Individuals with symptomatic, growing, or hemorrhagic malformations should be considered for surgical resection. Close follow-up after diagnosis and treatment is helpful to identify lesion progression or recurrence.

References

1. Zabramski, J. M., Wascher, T. M., Spetzler, R. F., et al. The natural history of familial cavernous malformations: results of an ongoing study. *J Neurosurg* 1994;**80**:422–432.

2. Hang, Z., Shi, Y. & Wei, Y. A pathological analysis of 180 cases of vascular malformation of brain. *Zhonghua Bing Li Xue Za Zhi* 1996;**25**:135–138.

3. Barnes, B., Cawley, C. M. & Barrow, D. L. Intracerebral hemorrhage secondary to vascular lesions. *Neurosurg Clin N Am* 2002;**13**:289–297.

4. Gault, J., Sarin, H. & Awadallah, N. A. Pathobiology of human cerebrovascular malformations: basic mechanisms and clinical relevance. *Neurosurgery* 2004;**55**:1–17.

5. Al-Shahi, R., Bhattacharya, J. J., Currie, D. G., et al. Prospective, population-based detection of intracranial vascular malformations in adults: the Scottish Intracranial Vascular Malformation Study (SIVMS). *Stroke* 2003;**34**:1163–1169.

6. Baumann, S. B., Noll, D. C., Kondziolka, D. S., et al. Comparison of functional magnetic resonance imaging with positron emission tomography and magnetoencephalography to identify the motor cortex in a patient with an arteriovenous malformation. *J Image Guid Surg* 1995;**1**:191–197.

7. Mottolese, C., Hermier, M., Stan, H., et al. Central nervous system cavernomas in the pediatric age group. *Neurosurg Rev* 2001;**24**:55–71:discussion 72–53.

8. Fortuna, A., Ferrante, L., Mastronardi, L., et al. Cerebral cavernous angioma in children. *Childs Nerv Syst* 1989;**5**:201–207.

9. Labauge, P., Laberge, S., Brunereau, L., et al. Hereditary cerebral cavernous angiomas: clinical and genetic features in 57 French families. Societe Francaise de Neurochirurgie. *Lancet* 1998;**352**:1892–1897.

10. Otten, P., Pizzolato, G. P., Rilliet, B., et al. 131 cases of cavernous angioma (cavernomas) of the CNS discovered by retrospective analysis of 24,535 autopsies. *Neurochirurgie* 1989;**35**:82–3, 128–31.

11. Siegel, A. M., Andermann, E., Badhwar, A., et al. Anticipation in familial cavernous angioma: a study of 52 families from International Familial Cavernous Angioma Study. IFCAS Group. *Lancet* 1998;**352**:1676–1677.

12. Siegel, A. M., Bertalanffy, H., Dichgans, J. J., et al. Familial cavernous malformations of the central nervous system. A clinical and genetic study of 15 German families. *Nervenarzt* 2005;**76**:175–180.

13. Zhang, J., Rigamonti, D., Dietz, H. C., et al. Interaction between krit1 and malcavernin: implications for the pathogenesis of cerebral cavernous malformations. *Neurosurgery* 2007;**60**:353–359.

14. Laurans, M. S., DiLuna, M. L., Shin, D., et al. Mutational analysis of 206 families with cavernous malformations. *J Neurosurg* 2003;**99**:38–43.

15. Laberge, S., Labauge, P., Marechal, E., et al. Genetic heterogeneity and absence of founder effect in a series of 36 French cerebral cavernous angiomas families. *Eur J Hum Genet* 1999;**7**:499–504.

16. Shenkar, R., Elliott, J. P., Diener, K., et al. Differential gene expression in human cerebrovascular malformations. *Neurosurgery* 2003;**52**:465–477; discussion 477–478.

17. Laberge-le Couteulx, S., Jung, H. H., Labauge, P., et al. Truncating mutations in CCM1, encoding KRIT1, cause hereditary cavernous angiomas. *Nat Genet* 1999;**23**:189–193.

18. Labauge, P., Enjorals, O., Bonerandi, J. J., et al. An association between autosomal dominant cerebral cavernomas and a distinctive hyperkeratotic cutaneous vascular malformation in 4 families. *Ann Neurol* 1999;**45**:250–254.

19. Dupre, N., Verlann, D. J., Hand, C. K., *et al.* Linkage to the CCM2 locus and genetic heterogeneity in familial cerebral cavernous malformation. *Can J Neurol Sci* 2003;**30**:122–128.

20. Craig, H. D., Günel, M., Cepeda, O., *et al.* Multilocus linkage identifies two new loci for a Mendelian form of stroke cerebral cavernous malformation at 7p15–13 and 3q25.2–27. *Hum Mol Genet* 1998;**7**:1851–1858.

21. Marchuk, D. A., Gallione, C. J., Morrision, L. A., *et al.* A locus for cerebral cavernous malformations maps to chromosome 7q in two families. *Genomics* 1995;**28**:311–314.

22. Gil-Nagel, A., Dubovsky, J., Wilcox, K. J., *et al.* Familial cerebral cavernous angioma: a gene localized to a 15-cM interval on chromosome 7q. *Ann Neurol* 1996;**39**:807–810.

23. Gunel, M., Awad, I. A., Finberg, K., *et al.* A founder mutation as a cause of cerebral cavernous malformation in Hispanic Americans. *New Engl J Med* 1996;**334**:946–951.

24. Gunel, M., Awad, I. A., Anson, J., *et al.* Mapping a gene causing cerebral cavernous malformation to 7q11.2-q21. *Proc Natl Acad Sci USA* 1995;**92**:6620–6624.

25. Dubovsky, J., Zabramski, J. M., Kurth, J., *et al.* A gene responsible for cavernous malformations of the brain maps to chromosome 7q. *Hum Mol Genet* 1995;**4**:453–458.

26. Chen, L., Tanriover, G., Yano, H., *et al.* Apoptotic functions of PDCD10/CCM3, the gene mutated in cerebral cavernous malformation 3. *Stroke* 2009;**40**:1474–1481.

27. Tanriover, G., Boylan, A. J., Diluna, M. L., *et al.* PDCD10, the gene mutated in cerebral cavernous malformation 3, is expressed in the neurovascular unit. *Neurosurgery* 2008;**62**:930–938.

28. Whitehead, K. J., Plummer, N. W., Adams, J. A., *et al.* Ccm1 is required for arterial morphogenesis: implications for the etiology of human cavernous malformations. *Development* 2004;**131**:1437–1448.

29. Hayman, L. A., Evans, R. A., Ferrell, R. E., *et al.* Familial cavernous angiomas: natural history and genetic study over a 5-year period. *Am J Med Genet* 1982;**11**:147–160.

30. Nannucci, S., Pescini, F., Poggesi, A., *et al.* Familial cerebral cavernous malformation: report of a further Italian family. *Neurol Sci* 2009;**30**:143–147.

31. Penco, S., Ratti, R., Bianchi, E., *et al.* Molecular screening test in familial forms of cerebral cavernous malformation: the impact of the Multiplex Ligation-dependent Probe Amplification approach. *J Neurosurg* 2009;**110**:929–934.

32. Sirvente, J., Enjolras, O., Wassef, M., *et al.* Frequency and phenotypes of cutaneous vascular malformations in a consecutive series of 417 patients with familial cerebral cavernous malformations. *J Eur Acad Dermatol Venereol* 2009;**23**:1066–1072.

33. Toll, A., Parera, E., Giménez-Arnau, A. M., *et al.* Cutaneous venous malformations in familial cerebral cavernomatosis caused by KRIT1 gene mutations. *Dermatology* 2009;**218**:307–313.

34. Aiba, T., Tanaka, R., Koike, T., *et al.* Natural history of intracranial cavernous malformations. *J Neurosurg* 1995;**83**:56–59.

35. Kim, D. S., Park, Y. G., Choi, J. U., *et al.* An analysis of the natural history of cavernous malformations. *Surg Neurol* 1997;**48**:9–17; discussion 17–18.

36. Frim, D. M. & Scott, R. M. Management of cavernous malformations in the pediatric population. *Neurosurg Clin N Am*1999;**10**:513–518.

37. Kesava, P. P. & Turski, P. A. MR angiography of vascular malformations. *Neuroimaging Clin N Am* 1998;**8**:349–370.

38. Bartlett, J. E. & Kishore, P. R. Intracranial cavernous angioma. *AJR Am J Roentgenol* 1977;**128**:653–656.

39. Rigamonti, D., Drayer, B. P., Johnson, P. C., *et al.* The MRI appearance of cavernous malformations (angiomas). *J Neurosurg* 1987;**67**:518–524.

40. Imakita, S., Nishimura, T., Yamada, N., *et al.* Cerebral vascular malformations: applications of magnetic resonance imaging to differential diagnosis. *Neuroradiology* 1989;**31**:320–325.

41. Sage, M. R., Blumbergs, P. C. Cavernous haemangiomas (angiomas) of the brain. *Australas Radiol* 2001;**45**:247–256.

42. Rigamonti, D., Hadley, M. N., Drayer, B. P., *et al.* Cerebral cavernous malformations. Incidence and familial occurrence. *New Engl J Med* 1988;**319**:343–347.

43. Lasjaunias, P., Terbrugge, K., Rodesch, G., *et al.* True and false cerebral venous malformations. Venous pseudo-angiomas and cavernous hemangiomas. *Neurochirurgie* 1989;**35**:132–139.

44. Ostertun, B. & Solymosi, L. Magnetic resonance angiography of cerebral developmental venous anomalies: its role in differential diagnosis. *Neuroradiology* 1993;**35**:97–104.

45. Wurm, G., Schnizer, M. & Fellner, F. A. Cerebral cavernous malformations associated with venous anomalies: surgical considerations. *Neurosurgery* 2005;**57**(1 Suppl):42–58.

46. Voigt, K. & Yasargil, M. G. Cerebral cavernous haemangiomas or cavernomas. Incidence, pathology, localization, diagnosis, clinical features and treatment. Review of the literature and report of an unusual case. *Neurochirurgia (Stuttg)* 1976;**19**:59–68.

47. Baumgartner, J. E., Ater, J. L., Ha, C. S., *et al.* Pathologically proven cavernous angiomas of the brain following radiation therapy for pediatric brain tumors. *Pediatr Neurosurg* 2003;**39**:201–207.

48. Moriarity, J. L., Clatterbuck, R. E. & Rigamonti, D. The natural history of cavernous malformations. *Neurosurg Clin N Am* 1999;**10**:411–417.

49. Porter, P. J., Willinsky, R. A., Harper, W., *et al.* Cerebral cavernous malformations: natural history and prognosis after clinical deterioration with or without hemorrhage. *J Neurosurg* 1997;**87**:190–197.

50. Kondziolka, D., Lunsford, L. D. & Kestle, J. R. The natural history of cerebral cavernous malformations. *J Neurosurg* 1995;**83**:820–824.

51. Fritschi, J. A., Reulen, H. J., Spetzler, R. F., *et al.* Cavernous malformations of the brain stem. A review of 139 cases. *Acta Neurochir (Wien)* 1994;**130**(1–4):35–46.

52. Barker, F. G., Amin-Hanjani, S., Butler, W. E., *et al.* Temporal clustering of hemorrhages from untreated cavernous malformations of the central nervous system. *Neurosurgery* 2001;**49**:15–24; discussion 24–25.

53. Scott, R. M., Barnes, P., Kupsky, W., *et al.* Cavernous angiomas of the central nervous system in children. *J Neurosurg* 1992;**76**:38–46.

54. Scott, R. M. Brain stem cavernous angiomas in children. *Pediatr Neurosurg* 1990–1991;**16**:281–286.

55. Porter, R. W., Detwiler, P. W., Spetzler, R. F., *et al.* Cavernous malformations of the brainstem: experience with 100 patients. *J Neurosurg* 1999;**90**:50–58.

56. Mazza, C., Scienza, R., Beltramello, A., *et al.* Cerebral cavernous malformations (cavernomas) in the pediatric age-group. *Childs Nerv Syst* 1991;**7**:139–46.

57. Giulioni, M., Acciarri, N., Padovani, R., *et al.* Surgical management of cavernous angiomas in children. *Surg Neurol* 1994;**42**:194–199.

58. Amin-Hanjani, S., Ogilvy, C. S., Ojemann, R. G., *et al.* Risks of surgical management for cavernous malformations of the nervous system. *Neurosurgery* 1998;**42**:1220–1227; discussion 1227–1228.

59. Di Rocco, C., Iannelli, A. & Tamburrini, G. Cavernous angiomas of the brain stem in children. *Pediatr Neurosurg* 1997;**27**:92–99.

60. Amin-Hanjani, S., Ogilvy, C. S., Candia, G. J., *et al.* Stereotactic radiosurgery for cavernous malformations: Kjellberg's experience with proton beam therapy in 98 cases at the Harvard Cyclotron. *Neurosurgery* 1998;**42**:1229–1236; discussion 1236–1238.

61. Di Rocco, C., Iannelli, A. & Tamburrini, G. Surgical management of paediatric cerebral cavernomas. *J Neurosurg Sci* 1997;**41**:343–347.

62. Larson, J. J., Ball, W. S., Bove, K. E., *et al.* Formation of intracerebral cavernous malformations after radiation treatment for central nervous system neoplasia in children. *J Neurosurg* 1998;**88**:51–56.

Resection of cavernous malformations of the brainstem

Helmut Bertalanffy, Jan-Karl Burkhardt, Ralf Alfons Kockro, Oliver Bozinov and Johannes Sarnthein

Introduction

Cavernous malformations of the brainstem differ from those in other locations in terms of clinical picture, bleeding rate, and operability. A typical feature of brainstem cavernous malformations is their significant clinical impact. Frequently, even small lesions or relatively small hematomas may cause severe neurological deficits due to the compact arrangement of fiber tracts and cranial nerve nuclei within the brainstem. Conversely, large hematomas within the pons may occasionally cause only mild symptoms when the hematoma develops slowly over many hours or days. The reason for this lies in the fact that hemorrhages from brainstem cavernomas usually occur within the lesion itself. In most instances a kind of lesion capsule is present in the periphery of the cavernoma that facilitates smooth expansion, with the intralesional hematoma gaining volume in a fashion similar to inflating a balloon. Thus, long tracts and cranial nerve nuclei within the brainstem are slowly distorted and displaced, but not irreparably damaged. Concomitantly, intrinsic vessels of the brainstem are gradually compressed with the consequence of a locally reduced perfusion. Larger cavernous malformations may cause additional perilesional edema within the brainstem, and this may worsen the functional disturbance. On MRI, this morphological situation can be recognized quite well, but the images reflect just an instant situation that can dramatically change over time. The dynamic component, e.g. the speed of symptom evolution, must therefore be taken into account as well.

The following is a description of the most important aspects related to the management of brainstem cavernomas and reflects our current attitude in dealing with these challenging vascular lesions.

Review of the literature

Cerebral cavernous malformations and particularly brainstem cavernomas were rarely diagnosed before the introduction of MRI into clinical practice [1]. Alternative imaging modalities such as CT scan often missed their appearance, especially in small and non-hemorrhagic cavernomas [2]. These vascular lesions were grouped together with others such as venous malformations, small AVMs, capillary telangiectasias or mixed lesions which could not be detected in angiography and were therefore named as angiographically occult vascular malformations (AOVM) [3–4].

In 1928 Walter Dandy described for the first time the successful neurosurgical resection of a cerebral cavernous malformation located in the pontomedullary junction [3]. Subsequently, surgery for symptomatic brainstem cavernomas was initiated in more and more specialized neurosurgical centers. Especially in the past two decades, larger surgical series were published with increasing frequency; Fritschi et al. summarized the results of 93 surgical cases in 1994 [5], Porter et al. a series of 86 cases in 1999 [11], Samii et al. analyzed 36 cases in 2001 [6], Wang et al. reported the remarkable number of 137 patients in 2003 [7], Ferroli et al. had 52 cases in 2005 [8], Li et al. 37 [9] and Hauck et al. 44 cases in 2009 [10], respectively, and de Oliviera et al. treated 45 cases in 2010 [12]. Our own experience is currently based on more than 140 patients who underwent surgery and approximately 70 patients who were treated conservatively for a symptomatic brainstem cavernoma.

In each case, the indication for surgery was decided individually based on radiological characteristics, the exact location of the brainstem cavernoma and the

Cavernous Malformations of the Nervous System, ed. Daniele Rigamonti. Published by Cambridge University Press.
© Cambridge University Press 2011.

patient's clinical history [4,12–13]. A great variety of surgical approaches were used according to the surgeon's experience and preferences. Quite unanimously, the following goals of surgery were defined in patients presenting with a brainstem cavernoma: (1) removing the lesion completely to avoid rebleeding [4]; (2) avoiding resection of the surrounding hemosiderin-loaded gliotic tissue, and (3) leaving an associated venous malformation or developmental venous anomaly (DVA) intact to prevent venous congestion and venous infarction in this region [4,12–13]. Despite the complexity of these lesions, good results were reported; for instance, in the series of Porter et al., 88% of 86 surgically treated patients remained unchanged or improved compared to their preoperative clinical condition [11]. Likewise, Wang et al. reported favorable results with 72.3% of 137 surgically treated patients who improved or were alike compared to their preoperative status [7].

Clinical manifestation

Brainstem cavernomas can cause a great variety of symptoms [4,10,14–15]. Some of them may appear as well-known neurological disorders such as diplopia, ataxia, motor weakness, sensory deficits, etc. In other instances, patients may complain of rather unspecific problems such as fatigue, unusual visual disturbances or others. Generally, the occurrence and the severity of neurological disorders depend mainly upon the site of the cavernous malformation and, as we have frequently seen, to a lesser degree on the lesion's size [4,16–17]. Occasionally, even small lesions of the midbrain or medulla may cause symptoms much more severe than those induced by a huge pontine lesion. On an earlier occasion we have pointed out that symptoms can remain constant over a longer period of time, may gradually worsen or, conversely, improve [4]. Each situation must be evaluated differently. As cavernomas are dynamic lesions, they may change morphologically without detectable reason. Even highly experienced neurosurgeons cannot exactly predict the behavior of cavernomas over time. Moreover, it remains difficult to exactly interpret the clinical importance of various fluctuating symptoms such as brief vertigo or facial or truncal sensory disturbances that may appear suddenly but do not persist longer than a few minutes. In rare instances, though, when large hemorrhages develop over several hours, devastating neurological deficits may appear.

Hemorrhage rate and impact on decision-making

Quite a number of clinical and epidemiological investigations have dealt with the problem of hemorrhage rate in brainstem cavernomas [4,18–20]. Many authors have noted that the natural history of brainstem cavernomas is different from that of other locations because this subgroup of cavernous malformations has a much higher tendency towards bleeding. However, when discussing the bleeding rate from a cavernous malformation, a bleeding event similar to hemorrhages from other vascular malformations of the brain is suggested, and in many instances the clinical significance of the bleeding event may be overestimated. The presence of hemosiderin around the lesion is the consequence of transendothelial diapedesis of erythrocytes, but, otherwise, it is definitely not evidence of gross hemorrhage. Intralesional bleeding produces a lesion expansion, while a true gross hemorrhage beyond the lesion into the brainstem parenchyma is rather rare. A better knowledge of the natural history of brainstem cavernomas in general, and a more or less accurate estimation in a single case in particular, plays a major role in the process of decision-making regarding the choice of therapy. As a general rule in a brainstem cavernoma that has bled at least once, the malformation should be regarded as a potential threat to the patient. Thus, in many cases, the clinical significance of a hemorrhage from a brainstem cavernoma should not be underestimated. Moreover, multiple bleeding episodes increase the likelihood of a persistent neurological deficit. As we have pointed out elsewhere [4], the simple annual bleeding rate alone does not sufficiently characterize the clinical significance of a brainstem cavernoma and does not fully inform the patient about the risk of future morbidity or even mortality caused by this lesion. We have learned over the years that no general rule exists that could be applied in the majority of patients harbouring cavernous malformation of the brainstem. Instead, each patient should be regarded individually and management should be tailored to the specific case.

Associated venous malformations

It is generally believed that cerebral cavernous (CCM) and venous malformations (CVM) share a common origin and pathogenetic mechanism [21–24]. Guclu and co-workers studied the literature and found

200 families with CCMs who underwent mutational analysis in all three CCM genes [25]. According to these authors there was one family with members affected by both CCM and CVM. They concluded that CVM is a benign developmental anomaly that should be managed separately from CCM.

In clinical practice, there is coexistence between CVM and CCM in approximately 20 – 30% of cases [4]. While a similar percentage of our own patients had an associated venous malformation within the brainstem or its vicinity, a large intraaxial CVM (Fig. 15.1A, B) was present in only a few of them. In other individuals, a large CVM was found in the adjacent cerebellum. In the majority of patients with coexistence of both malformations, the CCM and the CVM were in close vicinity to each other, and parts of the CVM corresponded to draining veins of the CCM. Rarely, the brainstem cavernoma and the intrinsic brainstem CVM were entirely separated from each other.

As a general rule, we have learned that not the venous malformation itself but the CCM is the source of hemorrhage [4,26]. Accordingly, we do not attempt to entirely eliminate the CVM, for instance by directly coagulating the vein, because a significant portion of the healthy brainstem parenchymal tissue may be drained

via this CVM [10]. However, tributaries of the CVM that are identified intraoperatively as draining veins of the cavernoma are usually coagulated and divided during surgery [4]. Interestingly, we could observe that after total removal of a brainstem cavernoma, a residual venous malformation within or adjacent to the cavernoma cavity may play a causative role in the occurrence of a postoperative re-bleeding, although this may not be the case in all instances. At present, it is difficult to exactly define the clinical importance of adjacent remnants of the venous malformation that can be identified on postoperative MRI.

Multiplicity

Multiple intracranial cavernous malformations (Fig. 15.1C) occur in 10 – 21% of patients [21,27–31]. In hereditary disease, up to 93% of patients may harbor two or more intracranial lesions [32–33]. We have encountered the following situations in patients with multiple lesions: (1) a solitary lesion within the brainstem and concomitantly one or more additional lesions in a location other than the brainstem; (2) two or more simultaneous lesions within the brainstem that are not in direct contact with each other; (3) one or more silent

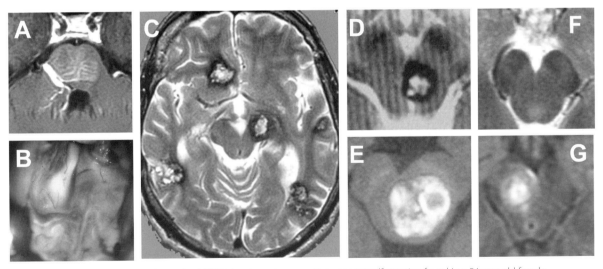

Figure 15.1. (A) T1-W contrast-enhanced axial MRI showing a large pontine venous malformation found in a 54-year-old female. (B) Intraoperative view of the surface of the rhomboid fossa in a 30-year-old male showing a large superficial venous malformation (CVM). The patient underwent surgery for removal of a cavernous malformation (not seen in this image) that was located more superiorly and had no direct contact to this CVM. (C) T2-W axial MRI showing multiple intracerebral cavernous malformations including a lesion within the left midbrain tegmentum. (D) T2-W axial MRI taken in a 55-year-old female furnishes evidence of a small cavernous malformation within the left part of the midbrain tectum. (E) More than 2 years later this lesion clearly increased in size, mostly due to intrinsic proliferative activity. (F) T2-W axial MRI taken at the level of the midbrain in a 31-year-old female who suffered from hereditary disease. Multiple cerebral cavernous malformations were found in this patient but none was initially located within the brainstem. (G) Two years later the patient presented with a left-sided hemiparesis caused by a hemorrhagic *de novo* cavernous malformation within the right midbrain tegmentum. See color plate section.

intraaxial lesions with a new (*de novo*) brainstem lesion occurring in the same patient at a later stage. Each of these situations required a particular management strategy.

While the disease may be cured in patients harboring a solitary lesion by totally removing the malformation, the problem is more complex in patients with multiple cavernomas. So far we have limited our management to treating only the symptomatic lesion(s) when surgery has been considered indicated as usual [4]. These patients underwent regular follow-up examinations. Other individuals required multiple surgical procedures depending on the clinical course and the estimated aggressivity of the remaining cavernous malformation.

Lesion growth

An increase in the lesion's volume may frequently be observed after repeated intralesional hemorrhages but should be differentiated from a true proliferative lesion growth (Fig. 15.1D,E). A high-resolution MRI may usually allow one to clearly distinguish between these situations. A true neoplastic-like growth is rather rare, but has been documented in at least three of our patients. There is no general consensus over how to manage such growing lesions, particularly if lesion growth develops slowly over years without producing new symptoms. We now believe that if a proliferative lesion growth has been unequivocally documented in a cavernous malformation of the brainstem, surgery should be seriously considered as an option because the size of the cavernoma may influence the surgical outcome [12,14,34–35]. Nevertheless, we do not propagate this as a general rule, as the indication for surgery also depends upon a number of other criteria that are discussed below.

De novo formation

A *de novo* formation is the occurrence of a CCM at a site of the brain that showed a normal aspect on previous MR images (Fig. 15.1F,G). The importance of small hemosiderin spots that can occasionally be detected on gradient-echo sequences is poorly understood. In some of our patients, such a black spot later developed into a true cavernous malformation that even caused significant brain hemorrhage. It is unknown whether such *de novo* lesions behave more aggressively in terms of bleeding rate. The exact underlying pathogenetic mechanism or the stimulus that leads to a

de novo formation of a cavernoma is unknown as well. While the risk of appearance of a new lesion in a patient with nonhereditary disease and a solitary lesion seems to be extremely low, *de novo* malformations occur more frequently in patients with multiple lesions and/or hereditary disease [4]. For this reason, regular MRI follow-up examinations should be performed at least in the latter patient group.

Management of brainstem cavernomas

General aspects

Patients who harbor a cavernous malformation of the brainstem may present in various clinical situations: (1) in the acute stage of bleeding with progressive symptoms; (2) in the subacute stage with or without specific symptoms; (3) in the late stage with mild or without any symptoms; (4) as an asymptomatic individual with the incidental finding of a brainstem cavernous malformation, the MRI having been performed for unrelated reasons.

In each of these situations, the following important questions arise:

(1) Are we really dealing with a cavernous malformation of the brainstem?
  This question should be properly answered by high-quality MR images; occasionally, the suspicion of a cavernous malformation cannot be confirmed on control MRI.
(2) Is there a need for urgent early treatment or is it acceptable to adopt a wait-and-see policy?
  As a first step, except for emergency cases, patients may be closely monitored both clinically and radiologically in order to learn more about the specific natural history and to better estimate the aggressiveness of the underlying cavernous malformation;
(3) What is the optimal therapy at first glance? Some patients may not require immediate action and can be observed both clinically and radiologically.

When surgery seems to be the better alternative, one can choose between the following possibilities:

- perform immediate surgery;
- recommend surgery, but giving the patient sufficient time to re-consider the situation and take a decision free of time pressure, particularly in

individuals who are not yet fully convinced of the need for surgery;

- recommend surgery, but only if worsening of symptoms occurs within the following days or weeks; otherwise continue with observation (Fig. 15.2);
- treat an associated problem (e.g. occlusive hydrocephalus).

To find the safest option for the patient not only in the short but especially in the long term can be quite difficult and requires great experience. All aspects related to the decision-making process should be explained in detail to the patient and his relatives. Frequent questions posed by patients who choose observation instead of surgery are for instance how often MRI checks should be performed and how to behave during the waiting period in terms of social life, sports etc. Others would like to know whether stereotactic radiosurgery is a valid treatment option.

We usually do not recommend significant restrictions of social life; it is suggested, though, to refrain from anticoagulant medication and extreme sports.

As for radiosurgery, despite recent claims that stereotactic radiosurgery reduces the rebleeding rate for CCMs located in so-called high-surgical-risk areas of the brain [36], we consider this treatment option inadequate for truly preventing re-hemorrhage in brainstem

cavernomas according to our own observations. We are following up more than 70 non-surgical patients who harbor a deep-seated CCM with regular MRI checks. The vast majority of these patients remain free of hemorrhage and symptoms over a long period of time, some individuals up to more than two decades. None of these patients underwent stereotactic radiosurgery.

Patient selection

Selecting a patient as a surgical candidate is one of the most important but also one of the most challenging aspects of brainstem cavernoma management. Criteria on which the decision-making is based are mere estimates that may vary widely from neurosurgeon to neurosurgeon (or neurologist). These criteria are the rate of rebleeding, the expected clinical course with conservative management and the success and complication rates in case of surgery. Moreover, many patients may be significantly influenced by the opinion of other doctors or by their own internet search.

At the beginning, we try to estimate the risk of clinical worsening (risk of rebleeding, increasing hematoma, increasing perilesional edema etc.). Then we estimate the general operability, the expected success rate and the specific risks of surgery and, concomitantly, think about possible surgical approaches, making an initial choice for the best access route.

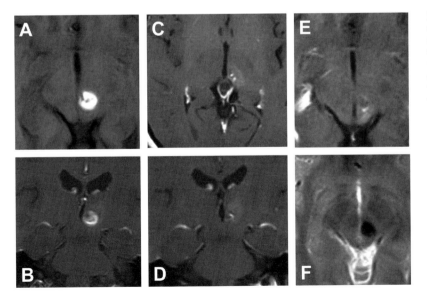

Figure 15.2. Axial non-enhanced (A) and coronal contrast-enhanced T1-W MRI (B) of a 41-year-old patient who presented with headache and diplopia, showing a recent mesencephalic hemorrhage extending into the thalamus. No surgical treatment was indicated, and the patient was followed-up clinically and neuroradiologically. (C, D) Two months after the hemorrhagic event the patient's symptoms have resolved and the intraparenchymal hemorrhage has almost disappeared. A small venous malformation is seen in the area of the previous hemorrhage. (E, F) At 12 months after the onset of symptoms, contrast-enhanced images show the persisting small CVM and some hemosiderin deposits. Clinically no further bleeding occurred, and the patient was managed with repeated follow-up controls over several years.

Timing of surgery

Basically, there are three situations related to the timing of surgery;

(1) surgery in the acute stage as an urgent or even emergency procedure;
(2) surgery in the subacute stage;
(3) surgery in the interval, not directly related to a bleeding episode.

Approximately a quarter of our patients underwent surgery in the acute stage. Figure 15.3 shows an example of extensive brainstem hematoma caused by a pontine cavernous malformation. Surgery in the acute stage has at least two advantages. On the one hand, evacuating a large and in most instances fluid intraaxial hematoma provides a cavity that serves as a working space for further microsurgical manipulation within the brainstem and facilitates removal of the remaining lesion. On the other hand, this early evacuation of the hematoma immediately improves the impaired microcirculation of the brainstem and may even lead to rapid resolution of the perilesional intraparenchymal edema (Fig. 15.3). The latter may correlate with a dramatic clinical improvement, as we have experienced in many of our cases. In our opinion, the recommendation to avoid surgery in the acute stage found in the older literature is not valid any more. The decision to operate in the acute stage is made on both clinical and MRI findings (e.g. rapid clinical deterioration).

Operating upon an intraaxial cavernous malformation with an intralesional hematoma in the subacute stage, for instance 2–4 weeks after the last hemorrhagic episode, is another option that can be applied in patients with less dramatic symptoms or only mild clinical worsening. In such cases it makes sense not to postpone surgery too long due to at least two major disadvantages: one is that after the intralesional hematoma has been resorbed, the working space within the brainstem is rather limited; the other is that, several weeks or even months after the hemorrhagic episode, a tight scar forms within the malformation that firmly adheres to the surrounding parenchymal tissue of the brainstem. Surgical evacuation requires more mechanical manipulation in such cases and bears the risk of local tissue damage.

It must be mentioned, though, that many patients do not present in the acute stage because initially they were managed conservatively elsewhere. We would therefore recommend neurologists or other doctors who first see such symptomatic patients directly after an acute hemorrhage has occurred to send these patients to an experienced neurosurgeon or ask for his opinion in the early stage, particularly if patients are presenting in poor clinical condition.

Brainstem cavernoma and pregnancy

It is widely believed that pregnancy is associated with an increased risk of hemorrhage in cerebral cavernous malformations [37–39]. Despite the lack of clear

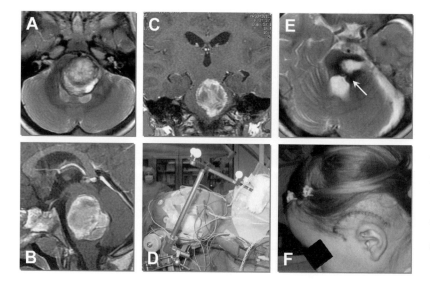

Figure 15.3. T2-W axial (A) and T1-W contrast-enhanced MRI in sagittal (B) and coronal plane (C), taken in a 3.5-year-old girl who presented with right-sided hemiparesis, unable to walk alone. The images demonstrate a large intrapontine cavernous malformation with an extensive intralesional hematoma. Surgery was performed in the acute stage, and the lesion was accessed from laterally via a left-sided subtemporal transtentorial approach with the patient in the supine position (D). Total removal of the cavernoma is demonstrated on postoperative MRI, and the parenchymal tissue dorsal to the resection cavity (arrow) has remained intact (E). The postoperative photograph of this girl shows the skin incision in the left temporal region (F). See color plate section.

evidence and larger series supporting this assumption, it is still unknown which hormones or other factors play a distinctive role in this event [40]. However, exacerbation of symptoms and an increase in lesion size is more often present in pregnant than in not pregnant CCM patients [39,41].

With regard to the localization, little is known about brainstem cavernomas and their correlation to pregnancy. Only 11 patients harboring a brainstem cavernoma during pregnancy were described in the literature [11,13,41] and, hence, there are no clear recommendations for their management. Most patients were treated conservatively, and surgery was not performed during pregnancy. Porter *et al.* mentioned the largest group, namely seven pregnant patients, of whom only one was treated surgically [11]. We have successfully operated on three symptomatic patients with successful removal of their brainstem cavernomas; one underwent surgery during pregnancy, the other two directly after delivery. The decision to perform an emergency procedure or to choose a non-surgical management is, therefore, rather based on individual criteria such as the patient's condition, progression of symptoms, trimester of pregnancy and the appearance of the lesion on MR images.

Goals of surgery

A brainstem cavernoma is always a potential threat to the patient due to the risk of symptomatic bleeding, sometimes with devastating consequences. Consequently, the main goal of surgery is eliminating the risk of bleeding. Moreover, to prevent recurrent hemorrhage in the future, the lesion must be removed totally without leaving any remnants of the malformation behind. This goal has to be explained clearly to the patient before scheduled surgery, in a fashion that this purpose and the associated risk of temporary morbidity are well understood. In the acute stage of patients who rapidly deteriorate, the goal of surgery is not only eliminating the risk of rebleeding but also to interrupt the present course with progressive deterioration and, ultimately, to improve the neurological condition.

For many of our patients suffering from brainstem cavernoma, the knowledge of the presence of a threatening vascular malformation within the brainstem and the knowledge that a potential hemorrhage cannot be readily controlled constitutes a heavy psychological burden. Eliminating this threatening situation and

enabling the patient to resume a normal life is another major goal of surgery.

Preoperative planning

Once the decision for surgery has been made, the procedure must be carefully planned. For this purpose it is recommendable to use all available information, which includes the following:

- clinical data with precise description of onset of symptoms in order to recognize which structures of the brainstem have been initially involved;
- previous MR images if available that may show the site of an initial perhaps much smaller bleeding than later;
- a complete set of current MR images that ideally should not be older than a few days before the scheduled surgery;
- if possible, diffusion tensor imaging with reconstruction of long-tract fibers within the brainstem that may add valuable information;
- knowledge of co-morbidity, particularly of clinically silent coagulopathy that must be treated adequately before and even during surgery (as required in some of our patients);

It is important to meticulously analyze the MR images while paying particular attention to the following aspects:

- What amount of the lesion is composed by hematoma and what amount by the malformation itself?
- Are there calcifications present within the lesion?
- What is the relationship between the lesion and the surface of the brainstem?
- Is there a perilesional edema within the brainstem?
- Is the lesion surrounded by hemosiderin-loaded gliotic tissue or does the lesion, at least in some portions, show direct contact with the brainstem parenchymal tissue?
- What is the shape of the lesion? Is it more spherical or perhaps egg-shaped with a longitudinal diameter? If so, what is the direction of this longitudinal diameter (information important for the access trajectory)?
- Are there any anatomical variations present, for instance at the site of the skull base or in structures surrounding the brainstem such as the cerebellum or temporal lobe?

- Is there an associated venous malformation? If so, what is the anatomical relationship between CCM and CVM?
- What is the exact vascular pattern of structures surrounding the brainstem (cerebellum, temporal lobe) particularly with regard to bridging veins?

From the morphological point of view the following aspects are of utmost importance:

- the exact location within the three components of the brainstem (midbrain, pons or medulla);
- the size of the lesion;
- the lesion's composition (small lesion with large hematoma, cavernoma without intralesional hematoma, cavernoma with intralesional calcification, etc.);
- the relationship of the lesion to the surface of the brainstem (totally intrinsic, close to the anterior or anterolateral surface, close to the surface of the rhomboid fossa but subependymal, exophytic, etc.).

From the view point of planning the surgical procedure, it is important to know that each surgical approach may expose only a certain part of the brainstem. One has to anticipate exactly the surgical window offered by each approach, with special attention to individual anatomical details concerning the brainstem itself and the surrounding structures (temporal lobe, cerebellum, superficial veins, cranial nerve rootlets, and choroid plexus).

Another aspect is the viewing trajectory offered by each surgical approach. As some lesions may have a longitudinal orientation, it is important to choose the surgical approach according to this orientation in order to allow visualization of all portions of the lesion without the necessity for significant and risky retraction of surrounding brain structures or the brainstem itself.

Neuroradiological imaging

While CT scans may provide valuable information with respect to the bony anatomy of the skull base (including air cells or the profile of the petrous bone), and digital subtraction angiography may be helpful for visualizing the exact venous drainage, the hallmark of surgical planning is centered on MR imaging. A combination of gradient- and spin-echo T1- and T2-weighted imaging series enables one to establish the exact location and size of the lesion as well as its spatial relationships to possible entry zones into the brainstem. High-resolution T2 steady state

(CISS or FIESTA) sequences allow for visualization of cranial nerves which indicate the position of their respective nuclei or point to specific subsurface structures like the cortico-spinal tract in close vicinity to the entry zone of the sixth cranial nerve. Contrast-enhanced time of flight series may delineate associated venous malformations. More recently diffusion tensor imaging (DTI) has been developed to visualize the course of ascending and descending fiber tracts in the brainstem. The cortico-spinal tract can be visualized quite reliably on most MR imaging post-processing consoles, even in close vicinity to intraaxial lesions, and also the sensory fibers of the medial lemniscus may be delineated in a good number of cases [42–43]. Depicted as 3D structures in combination with triplanar T1 and T2 MRI studies, the courses of white matter tracts provide crucial information when determining the optimal surgical route towards a lesion. Furthermore, knowing the course and proximity of relevant tracts next to specific portions of the lesion may help in refining the dissection and resection methods in order to avoid damage to immediately adjacent fibers. Moreover, postoperative MRI may reveal changes in the course of fibers after cavernoma removal and verifies the degree of resection. At our center, we have been using the Dextroscope [44–45], a virtual reality visualization and planning platform that allows display of three-dimensionally fused MRI and CT imaging series, in order to plan the surgical resection of a brainstem cavernoma. The simultaneous 3D display of skull base (derived from CT), brainstem surface and cavernoma silhouette (MRI), vasculature (MRA/MRV) and fiber tracts (DTI) enables spatial comprehension of anatomical relationships as well as simulation of surgical viewpoints to anticipate the intraoperative scenario. This allows for discussing and defining suitable surgical strategies (Fig. 15.4).

Neuronavigation

Intraoperative navigation with image guidance systems provides useful information during all stages of surgery – from skin incision to cavernoma dissection. Most importantly, it enables operating along the planned trajectory towards the target, assessing the proximity of crucial anatomical structures and identifying possible cavernoma remnants. DTI-derived white matter tracts have been integrated into the navigational set-up, allowing the combined 2D/3D display of MRI planes, lesion contour and white matter tracts [46].

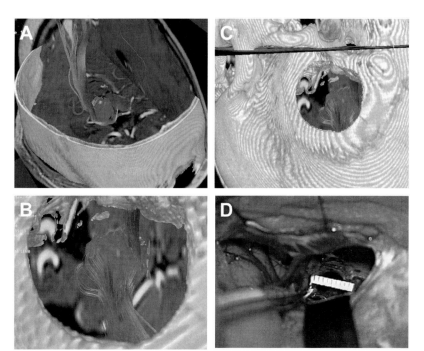

Figure 15.4. Visualization of the corticospinal tract, medial lemniscus and cavernoma within the right midbrain and upper pons in a 38-year-old male (same patient as shown in Fig. 15.6). (A) View from superiorly, anteriorly and laterally showing the tracts located lateral to the cavernoma. The multi-modality 3D data set consists of a tri-planar MRI; the cavernoma was segmented from the MRI, the skull from CT scans, and the fiber tracts derived from DTI. (B, C) Surgical perspective through a simulated temporal craniotomy. Note the corticospinal tract along the anterior margin of the cavernoma and the sensory fibers along its dorsal portion. The surgical corridor was chosen between both tracts. (D) Intraoperative photograph showing the subtemporal approach and cavernoma exposure through a small vertical brainstem opening in the planned position. The vein of Labbé and tributaries at the base of the temporal lobe have been dissected free and spared throughout the procedure. See color plate section.

Since conventional image guidance depends on preoperative imaging, the effect of brain shift is well recognized. However, in the area of the brainstem and skull base, especially when dealing with rather small targets, the brain distortion usually lies within a predicable range. It can be further minimized by avoiding soft tissue retractors and unnecessary large bone openings.

In 2001, Mamat *et al.* first described intraoperative fiber tracking using a 0.5 T scanner [47]. Within the following years this technique has also been implemented on intraoperative 1.5 T scanners, and faster tractography algorithms now allow updating the navigation system with intraoperatively acquired white matter tracts [46]. Although this technique has been used more often in supratentorial tumor surgery, it is expected that intraoperative MR imaging, particularly white matter tract visualization, will play an increasingly important role in brainstem surgery in the near future.

Apart from the rather time-consuming and costly high-field intraoperative MRI, ultrasound is emerging as an intraoperative navigational alternative, especially when used in combination with navigation systems [48–50]. Probably due to concentrated hemosiderin in and around the lesion, cavernomas tend to show strong echogenicity and are therefore suitable targets for visualization with ultrasound techniques [51–52].

The resolution and signal-to-noise ratio of current ultrasound technology are increasingly approaching those of MRI, especially with the onset of matrix array probes, high-frequency imaging and advanced image-processing methods. In the area of the brainstem, the application of ultrasound is still somewhat limited by the deep-seated position of the lesions, the small size of craniotomy and, hence, the poor accessibility of the target with the ultrasound beam [52]. However, recently introduced real-time 3D ultrasound techniques and the decreasing size of the ultrasound probes are promising advances to establish ultrasound as a straightforward, flexible and yet reliable and high-resolution imaging technique.

Surgical procedure

General aspects

Once the decision has been made to operate upon a cavernous malformation of the brainstem, several points are of utmost importance.

- To ensure that the risk of further bleeding has been completely eliminated, the malformation should be completely removed without leaving a residual portion behind.

- The exposure of the brainstem should be designed in a fashion that not only the superficial but also the deep portions of the cavernous malformations can be reached properly and without hazardous brain retraction.
- Great care must be paid to choose the best site for approaching the lesion, according not only to the gross external anatomical configuration but also to the intrinsic brainstem anatomy.

The surgical strategy for removal of a brainstem cavernoma comprises three different aspects: (1) selecting the optimal surgical approach that allows for exposing a specific part of the brainstem either anteriorly, laterally or posteriorly and also enables the surgeon to reach all portions of the cavernous malformation without jeopardizing the structures around the brainstem; (2) selecting the appropriate entry zone into the brainstem according to specific morphological aspects of the cavernoma, the brainstem, the vascular pattern on the surface of the brainstem and the presence of cranial nerve rootlets; (3) applying a special microsurgical technique to dissect between cavernoma and surrounding brainstem tissue in a fashion that, on the one hand, the cavernoma can be removed completely, and on the other hand, the brainstem is manipulated as little as possible.

Anesthesia and monitoring

Surgical details should be discussed with the anesthetist before commencing the procedure, so that the anesthetist can be prepared for intervention if required. To avoid interfering venous congestion, the venous pressure should be kept as low as possible. Sometimes, when manipulating within the brainstem, patients may show a vagal reaction with sudden bradycardia that may require the administration of atropine.

Electrophysiological monitoring is mandatory in every surgery involving the brainstem. We perform continuous monitoring of sensory and motor pathways (SSEP, MEP) as well as monitoring of auditory evoked potentials. Depending on the location within the brainstem, cranial nerve EMG proved to be most helpful. When surgery is performed via the floor of the fourth ventricle, mapping of the rhomboid fossa is mandatory.

Positioning of the patient

We have used a number of surgical approaches to expose the brainstem. Accordingly, patients have been placed in the prone, concorde, in the lateral park bench position, in the supine as well as in the sitting positions. The head is flexed and turned when using the lateral suboccipital approach, and flexed without rotation when using the suboccipital midline approach. The selection of the optimal approach in each patient is based upon several factors such as the patient's age, general physical constitution, co-morbidity and anatomical details. As a general rule, the sitting position is avoided in obese and in elderly individuals.

Selection of the surgical approach

A great variety of surgical approaches are available to reach any part of the brainstem [4,6–10,12–15,19–20,53–60]. However, each surgical approach provides exposure of only a limited portion of the brainstem, rendering a careful selection of the approach an important prerequisite for the success of the surgery. In our experience, a few principles concerning the surgical approaches to the brainstem have proven beneficial. The approach should provide direct access to the cavernous malformation with minimal retraction of surrounding structures such as temporal lobe, cerebellum, cranial nerves, cisternal arteries and veins. It may appear that the shortest distance to the lesion should dictate the site of access into the brainstem. Approaching an intrinsic brainstem cavernoma through the floor of the fourth ventricle is a well-established procedure and is indicated in many instances (Fig. 15.5). However, direct access through the rhomboid fossa should be avoided in cases in which a lateral approach would allow for an equally good exposure of the lesion, even if the distance to the cavernoma may be longer than through the rhomboid fossa. The reason is that the parenchymal structures of the brainstem below the rhomboid fossa are more sensitive than structures in the lateral portion of the pons and medulla. Another principle is to avoid complex skull base approaches, particularly transpetrosal access routes, since they are time-consuming and bear additional risks. Such approaches may simply be unnecessary. A lateral pontine cavernoma or even anterolateral lesions can easily be reached without using a combined transpetrosal approach as propagated by some neurosurgeons. As a general principle we always preserve bridging veins of the brain and cerebellum, and the approach is designed accordingly.

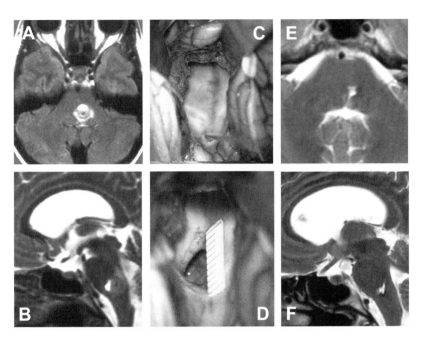

Figure 15.5. Preoperative T1-W axial (A) and T2-W sagittal MRI (B) of a 36-year-old female who presented with internuclear ophthalmoplegia. Surgery was performed via the floor of the fourth ventricle with the patient placed in the sitting position. The rhomboid fossa showed a slight yellowish discoloration and excavation in the midline (C). The lesion was exposed through a midline incision below the facial colliculus (D). Total removal of the lesion is demonstrated on postoperative T2-W MRI in axial (E) and sagittal plane (F). See color plate section.

Surgical approaches to the midbrain

To access mesencephalic cavernomas we have used the following approaches: the anterior interhemispheric subfrontal approach, the cranioorbitozygomatic approach with resection of the anterior clinoid process and transsylvian exposure, the subtemporal approach, the supracerebellar lateral approach, and the combined occipital transtentorial approach. Each of these approaches is chosen according to the relationship between cavernoma and midbrain tegmentum or midbrain tectum. When using the subtemporal approach (Fig. 15.6), a lumbar CSF drain is placed prior to surgery that facilitates elevation of the temporal lobe. Depending upon the venous pattern of temporal lobe drainage, separating the vein of Labe and tributaries from the temporal lobe may be necessary so that the veins can be left in place while gently elevating the temporal lobe. Usually, the tentorial edge is split behind the entry point of the trochlear nerve, and the cut edges of the tentorium are fixed laterally with fibrin glue. This approach exposes the superior portion of the pons and the lateral part of the midbrain (Fig. 15.6). Both the trochlear and the oculomotor nerves can be visualized and spared. The supracerebellar paraculminal approach exposes the tectal region and the dorsolateral aspect of the midbrain and is also suitable for pontomesencephalic cavernomas.

Lesions extending into the dorsal thalamus can be accessed with this approach as well. However, the caudal extension of exposure is limited to a level approximately at the junction between the superior and middle thirds of the pons. If the lesion extends even further caudally, the combined supracerebellar and occipital transtentorial approach may serve as an alternative.

Surgical approaches to the pons

Cavernomas of the pons may be totally intrinsic and located below the surface of the brainstem (Fig. 15.5). In other instances they may reach the surface or even bulge exophytically out of the brainstem, either anterolaterally, laterally or posteriorly into the fourth ventricle (Fig. 15.7). They may be confined to the pons or may extend superiorly into the midbrain and inferiorly into the medulla. The most suitable approaches to expose pontine cavernomas are the subtemporal transtentorial approach, the lateral supracerebellar approach, the retrosigmoid approach with exposure of the CP angle, the far-lateral transcondylar approach for caudal lesions, and the midline telovelar approach to exposure lesions via the rhomboid fossa. For the reasons mentioned above, it is safer to expose an intrinsic cavernoma from laterally than traversing the floor of the fourth ventricle (Fig. 15.8). Important

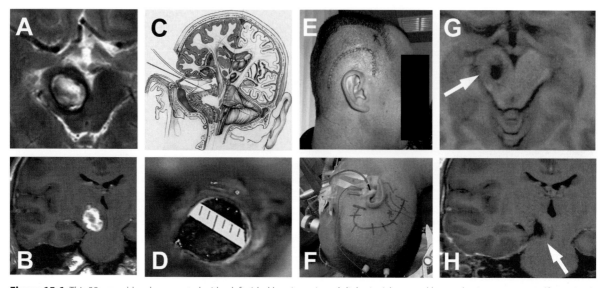

Figure 15.6. This 38-year-old male presented with a left-sided hemiparesis and diplopia. A large and hemorrhagic cavernous malformation is seen in the depth of the right midbrain tegmentum on T2-W axial (A) and T1-W coronal MRI (B). The lesion was exposed via a right-sided subtemporal route, as illustrated by Peter Roth (C). The opening on the surface of the brainstem (approximately 7 mm) remained smaller than the initial diameter of the lesion (D). The skin incision on the right temporal region can be seen both on the postoperative photograph of the patient (E) and marked on the skin in the operating room (F). Total removal of the lesion without damage of the temporal lobe or the brainstem is demonstrated on postoperative MRI in axial (G) and coronal plane (H). The arrows point to the resection cavity. No additional neurological deficits occurred postoperatively. See color plate section.

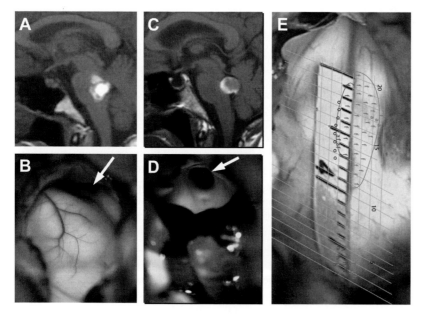

Figure 15.7. (A) Sagittal T1-W non-enhanced MRI showing a large intraaxial cavernous malformation with fresh intralesional hematoma. The lesion is bulging subependymally into the fourth ventricle and has been approached via the rhomboid fossa using the telovelar exposure. (B) The intraoperative photograph taken in this patient shows the left side of the upper rhomboid fossa below the aqueduct (arrow) bulging into the fourth ventricle. (C) Sagittal T1-W MRI showing a similar lesion in another patient. More than half of the cavernous malformation is bulging exophytically into the fourth ventricle. This lesion was also exposed via the telovelar midline approach. (D) The intraoperative photograph demonstrates that the lesion broke into the fourth ventricle through the ependyma of the rhomboid fossa. Superiorly, the aqueduct is visible (arrow). (E) Mapping the rhomboid fossa using a millimeter scale placed in longitudinal direction. The measurement in the caudal-cranial direction commenced at the obex. The area of facial nerve response is marked with "f" and is encircled on both sides. Obviously, this area clearly differs between the left and right side. See color plate section.

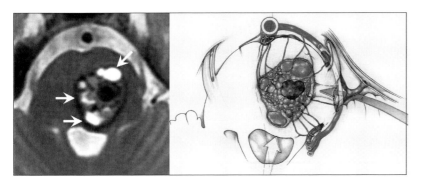

Figure 15.8. Left: axial non-enhanced T1-W MRI of a male showing a large pontine cavernoma at the level of the trigeminal root. The lesion contains several areas of fresh hematoma cavities (arrows). Right: the artistic illustration by Peter Roth highlights the various parts of which the lesion is composed: multiple caverns, several hematoma cavities and the vascular supply. Although access via the rhomboid fossa would have yielded the shortest distance to the lesion (white arrow), the malformation was approached and totally removed from laterally (green arrow). See color plate section.

structures below the surface of the rhomboid fossa are the posterior longitudinal fascicle, the fibers of the facial nerve, and the sixth nerve nucleus. These structures can easily be damaged by surgical manipulation that is avoided when using a lateral access route. As can be seen on postoperative MRI, the parenchymal tissue in the dorsal aspect of the pons remains intact when the rhomboid fossa is not traversed (Fig. 15.3).

Surgical approaches to the medulla

Cavernomas located in the lowest part of the brainstem within the medulla are exposed either from dorsally via a midline suboccipital craniotomy and telovelar exposure, or from laterally and anterolaterally using the far-lateral transcondylar approach. With such exposures medullary lesions can readily be visualized, but surgical manipulation within the medulla must be very cautious as the anatomical structures are more densely packed than within the pons. Anatomical orientation is facilitated by the specific shape and outer aspect of the medulla where the pyramidal tracts, the olive, the lower rhomboid fossa, and the rootlets of cranial nerves I, X, X, XI, and XII can easily be identified.

Selection of the entry zone into the brainstem

In principle, three different situations are encountered.

(1) Cavernomas that are located totally intraaxially below the surface of the brainstem and without direct relationship to the brainstem surface may show a normal appearance. Selecting the appropriate entry zone in such lesions is certainly one of the most challenging steps of the procedure.

(2) Intrinsic lesions may reach the surface of the brainstem, which may bulge due to an underlying hematoma (Fig. 15.7B). In some cases the lesion may not necessarily be visible; in others a small area of the cavernoma may be recognizable under the pial or ependymal surface in any brainstem region.

(3) Certain lesions are partially exophytic, with one portion of the lesion lying within the parenchymal tissue and the other being located either in the cisternal space or within the fourth ventricle (Fig. 15.7D). In the latter cases, the entry point into the brainstem is pre-defined as the lesion itself has already created an opening that can be used to remove the lesion. When the surface of the brainstem is bulging, we try to open the brainstem in an area where the lesion is suspected to be closest to the surface. However, the exact entry zone is chosen according to adjacent pial arteries and veins of the brainstem, and with respect to associated venous malformations, the presence of cranial nerves or, at the level of the rhomboid fossa, according to the location and extent of the facial colliculus (Fig. 15.5D). We found that the area of the facial colliculus varies widely in the same patient between the left and right side (Fig. 15.7E), and interindividually between patients. Electrophysiological mapping of the facial colliculus is, therefore, mandatory in all cases.

If possible, even in large lesions, the opening of the brainstem should not exceed 10 millimeters (Figs. 15.5D and 15.6D). The brainstem parenchymal tissue can be gently spread with bipolar forceps, instead of incising the brainstem with microscissors. The rationale behind this technique is the fact that even superficial fibers of the brainstem can be slowly dilated while keeping them intact throughout the surgical manipulation. In cases in which a large intralesional hematoma can be aspirated, it is not difficult to maintain the opening on the surface of the brainstem smaller than the initial diameter of the lesion.

Microsurgical dissection technique

From the morphological point of view, cavernous malformations are very heterogeneous lesions wherever they might be located. The difficulty in brainstem cavernomas lies mainly in the fact that only a very limited surgical field is available, most of the times at a significant depth. Moreover, only a small portion of the cavernoma may be directly within the visual field of the surgeon. Other portions must be brought into the surgeon's sight by gentle traction using the bipolar forceps and the suction tube. The first step is always identifying a dissection plane between lesion and brainstem parenchymal tissue. By following this plane in four directions, the cavernoma is gradually shrunk with bipolar coagulation at low current intensity and thus separated from the surrounding brainstem. In contrast to some tumors with a homogeneous surface, cavernous malformations are composed of various tissue materials that may require different microsurgical manipulation. Some portions of the cavernoma consist of soft caverns that can be coagulated to decrease the volume of the lesion. The lesion may also contain several hematoma cavities of various sizes that may be opened and their contents aspirated to further decrease the lesion's volume. In other portions of the lesion a tight scar may be present where the lesion firmly adheres to the adjacent parenchyma. This may be the site of the initial hemorrhage since hemosiderin deposits may be more accentuated here. In certain areas of the lesion tiny arterial feeders from the brainstem parenchyma penetrate the cavernoma capsule (Fig. 15.8); in other areas draining veins may be present, often related to an adjacent venous malformation. Both arteries and veins need to be precisely coagulated and sharply cut with microscissors. Using small cottonoids can be helpful to separate the isolated parts of the lesion from the surrounding parenchymal tissue. As the surgical field lies in a deep location and the microscope is focused on this field, care must be paid to concomitantly observe the superficial parts of the brain. For this reason, introducing and removing the instruments (bipolar forceps, suction tube, microscissors) into the deep-seated surgical field is always carried out with slow and gentle movements.

Clinical results

In recent years, the number of reports describing good results after removal of brainstem cavernomas has gradually increased. The evaluation method, however, is quite heterogeneous, and the criteria for assessing the postoperative outcome vary from one author to another. There are no standardized criteria for uniformly evaluating the postoperative outcome after removal of a brainstem cavernoma. This makes it difficult to compare results and patient populations from various published reports. Clinical evaluation should include the patient's immediate postoperative clinical status, new neurological morbidity and complications, and the assessment of completeness of lesion removal as estimated at the end of surgery and according to the postoperative MRI. Using the Karnofsky rating scale gives a more detailed description of the postoperative outcome [4].

As for our series, in addition to the neurological status we also evaluated the patient's quality of life in our first 71 consecutive patients using the Short Form-36 questionnaire (SF-36). The Karnofsky Performance Status Scale improved in 44 out of 71 surgically treated patients (62%), remained unchanged in 19 (27%) and deteriorated in eight individuals (11%). In the SF-36 score the Mental Component Summary improved with surgery. Moreover, 58 individuals (82%) declared a clear subjective benefit from surgery.

In the whole population comprising more than 130 surgically treated patients, 36% improved in the early postoperative period, 33% remained unchanged while 31% deteriorated. In the latter group approximately three-quarters (74%) developed only temporary neurological deficits. In the long term, 89% of our patients either improved or remained in the same neurological condition as preoperatively. Nine percent of the patients experienced new and permanent deficits.

Complications

Postoperative morbidity in brainstem surgery may be caused by direct surgical manipulation, by local vascular factors or, as we have occasionally encountered, by hematological factors such as an associated coagulopathy [4,20]. Neurological complications may include a great number of deficits, among them various degrees of internuclear ophthalmoplegia, worsening of motor deficits, third, sixth, seventh, eleventh and twelfth nerve palsies, gaze disturbances, facial, truncal and extremity numbness, dysphagia, dysarthria, gait ataxia, and spasticity. Such complications can be considered an acceptable postoperative morbidity if they resolve more or less completely in a reasonable period of time, usually within a few weeks or months. If the deficits persist, such as a complete oculomotor nerve paresis found in three of our patients, they should be accounted as permanent and undesired complications.

Unfortunately, a 65-year-old female with a previous history of breast cancer, who harbored a large medullary cavernoma, died 4 weeks after surgery, accounting for a mortality rate of 0.7%. Although her neurological condition was good after surgery and a full neurological recovery was expected, she needed a tracheostoma in the early postoperative period. Soon after placement, an infection developed at the site of the tracheostoma that eventually led to intractable sepsis.

Rebleeding

Hemorrhage after microsurgical removal of a brainstem cavernoma is a highly undesired event [10,20]. Considering that the main goal of surgery is removal of the vascular malformation in order to avoid future bleedings, surgery is rendered unsuccessful in the case of a significant rebleeding. Indeed, if a lesion has been removed completely and no pathological vessels or portions of the cavernoma have been left behind, it is unlikely that re-hemorrhage will occur. On the other hand, as cavernomas are dynamic lesions and *de novo* formation is possible, there is no absolute guarantee of having eliminated the risk of rebleeding in 100% of cases. In our surgical series, postoperative rebleeding occurred in six patients, accounting for a rebleeding rate of 4.4%. In only one patient the cavernoma cavity was filled with a fresh hemorrhage immediately after surgery, as detected a few hours after the procedure on control CT scans. Immediate evacuation of the hematoma revealed no obvious remnants of the vascular malformation. However, in the periphery of the cavernoma cavity, residual parts of a venous malformation were visible and were suspected to be the source of rebleeding. In the other five patients, re-hemorrhage occurred between 1 week and 4 years postoperatively. Particularly in two patients who were pregnant when the symptomatic hemorrhage occurred, small portions of the malformation were not detected at initial surgery. Both patients required re-exploration, and the

cavernoma remnants were found during the second procedure. The clinical course after this second procedure was uneventful in both patients.

Conclusions

Patients harboring a brainstem cavernoma require careful clinical and neuroradiological evaluation, particularly if the lesion has produced a clinically significant hemorrhage. The propensity for bleeding of a brainstem cavernoma may be higher than in cavernomas of other locations. Occasionally, hemorrhage from a cavernous malformation of the brainstem may cause severe, even life-threatening symptoms. Curative therapy by microsurgery is possible with excellent outcome. However, establishing a correct indication for surgery requires great experience. Not all patients who have suffered an initial hemorrhage from a brainstem cavernoma are good candidates for surgery. A subgroup of patients may clearly benefit from a wait-and-see policy. Modern diagnostic and therapeutic methods such as fiber tracking, special planning software, electrophysiological monitoring, neuronavigation and precise microsurgical techniques, including the selection of the optimal approach and entry zone into the brainstem, may add to the success of surgery. With such a strategy, the vast majority of patients can be managed successfully.

References

1. Rigamonti, D., Drayer, B. P., Johnson, P. C., *et al.* The MRI appearance of cavernous malformations (angiomas). *J Neurosurg* 1987;**67**:518–524.

2. Bertalanffy, H., Gilsbach, J. M., Eggert, H. R. & Seeger, W. Microsurgery of deep-seated cavernous angiomas: report of 26 cases. *Acta Neurochir (Wien)* 1991;**108**:91–99.

3. Dandy, W. E. Venous abnormalities and angiomas of the brain. *Arch Surg* 1928;**17**:715–793.

4. Bertalanffy, H., Benes, L., Miyazawa, T., *et al.* Cerebral cavernomas in the adult. Review of the literature and analysis of 72 surgically treated patients. *Neurosurg Rev* 2002;**25**:1–53; discussion 54–55.

5. Fritschi, J. A., Reulen, H. J., Spetzler, R. F. & Zabramski, J. M. Cavernous malformations of the brain stem. A review of 139 cases. *Acta Neurochir (Wien)* 1994;**130**:35–46.

6. Samii, M., Eghbal, R., Carvalho, G. A. & Matthies, C. Surgical management of brainstem cavernomas. *J Neurosurg* 2001;**95**:825–832.

7. Wang, C. C., Liu, A., Zhang, J. T., Sun, B. & Zhao, Y. L. Surgical management of brain-stem cavernous malformations: report of 137 cases. *Surg Neurol* 2003;**59**:444–454; discussion 454.

8. Ferroli, P., Sinisi, M., Franzini, A., *et al.* Brainstem cavernomas: long-term results of microsurgical resection in 52 patients. *Neurosurgery* 2005;**56**:1203–1212; discussion 1212–1214.

9. Li, H., Ju, Y., Cai, B. W., *et al.* Experience of microsurgical treatment of brainstem cavernomas: report of 37 cases. *Neurol India* 2009;**57**:269–273.

10. Hauck, E. F., Barnett, S. L., White, J. A. & Samson, D. Symptomatic brainstem cavernomas. *Neurosurgery* 2009;**64**:61–70; discussion 71.

11. Porter, R. W., Detwiler, P. W., Spetzler, R. F., *et al.* Cavernous malformations of the brainstem: experience with 100 patients. *J Neurosurg* 1999;**90**:50–58.

12. de Oliveira, J. G., Lekovic, G. P., Safavi-Abbasi, S., *et al.* Supracerebellar infratentorial approach to cavernous malformations of the brainstem: surgical variants and clinical experience with 45 patients. *Neurosurgery* 2010;**66**:389–399.

13. Garrett, M. & Spetzler, R. F. Surgical treatment of brainstem cavernous malformations. *Surg Neurol* 2009;**72**(Suppl 2):S3–9; discussion S10.

14. Ohue, S., Fukushima, T., Kumon, Y., Ohnishi, T. & Friedman, A. H. Surgical management of brainstem cavernomas: selection of approaches and microsurgical techniques. *Neurosurg Rev* 2010;**33**:315–22; discussion 323–324.

15. Huang, A. P., Chen, J. S., Yang, C. C., *et al.* Brain stem cavernous malformations. *J Clin Neurosci* 2010;**17**:74–79.

16. Kupersmith, M. J., Kalish, H., Epstein, F., *et al.* Natural history of brainstem cavernous malformations. *Neurosurgery* 2001;**48**:47–53; discussion 54.

17. Ziyal, I. M. & Ozgen, T. Natural history of brainstem cavernous malformations. *Neurosurgery* 2001;**49**:1023–1024.

18. Al-Shahi Salman, R., Berg, M. J., Morrison, L. & Awad, I. A. Hemorrhage from cavernous malformations of the brain: definition and reporting standards. Angioma Alliance Scientific Advisory Board. *Stroke* 2008;**39**:3222–3230.

19. Sola, R. G., Pulido, P., Pastor, J., Ochoa, M. & Castedo, J. Surgical treatment of symptomatic cavernous malformations of the brainstem. *Acta Neurochir (Wien)* 2007;**149**:463–470.

20. Gross, B. A., Batjer, H. H., Awad, I. A. & Bendok, B. R. Brainstem cavernous malformations. *Neurosurgery* 2009;**64**:E805–818; discussion E818.

21. Bertalanffy, H., Kuhn, G., Scheremet, R. & Seeger, W. Indications for surgery and prognosis in patients with cerebral cavernous angiomas. *Neurol Med Chir (Tokyo)* 1992;**32**:659–666.

22. Miyagi, Y., Mannoji, H., Akaboshi, K., Morioka, T. & Fukui, M. Intraventricular cavernous malformation associated with medullary venous malformation. *Neurosurgery* 1993;**32**:461–464; discussion 4.

23. Rigamonti, D. & Spetzler, R. F. The association of venous and cavernous malformations. Report of four cases and discussion of the pathophysiological, diagnostic, and therapeutic implications. *Acta Neurochir (Wien)* 1988;**92**:100–105.

24. Sasaki, O., Tanaka, R., Koike, T., *et al.* Excision of cavernous angioma with preservation of coexisting venous angioma. Case report. *J Neurosurg* 1991;**75**:461–464.

25. Guclu, B., Ozturk, A. K., Pricola, K. L., *et al.* Cerebral venous malformations have distinct genetic origin from cerebral cavernous malformations. *Stroke* 2005;**36**:2479–2480.

26. Topper, R., Jurgens, E., Reul, J. & Thron, A. Clinical significance of intracranial developmental venous anomalies. *J Neurol Neurosurg Psychiatry* 1999;**67**:234–238.

27. Voigt, K. & Yasargil, M. G. Cerebral cavernous haemangiomas or cavernomas. Incidence, pathology, localization, diagnosis, clinical features and treatment. Review of the literature and report of an unusual case. *Neurochirurgia (Stuttg)* 1976;**19**:59–68.

28. Otten, P., Pizzolato, G. P., Rilliet, B. & Berney, J. [131 cases of cavernous angioma (cavernomas) of the CNS, discovered by retrospective analysis of 24,535 autopsies]. *Neurochirurgie* 1989;**35**:82–83, 128–131.

29. Del Curling, O., Jr., Kelly, D. L., Jr., Elster, A. D. & Craven, T. E. An analysis of the natural history of cavernous angiomas. *J Neurosurg* 1991;**75**:702–708.

30. Kim, D. S., Park, Y. G., Choi, J. U., Chung, S. S. & Lee, K. C. An analysis of the natural history of cavernous malformations. *Surg Neurol* 1997;**48**:9–17; discussion 18.

31. Kondziolka, D., Lunsford, L. D. & Kestle, J. R. The natural history of cerebral cavernous malformations. *J Neurosurg* 1995;**83**:820–824.

32. Labauge, P., Brunereau, L., Levy, C., Laberge, S. & Houtteville, J. P. The natural history of familial cerebral cavernomas: a retrospective MRI study of 40 patients. *Neuroradiology* 2000;**42**:327–332.

33. Clatterbuck, R. E., Moriarity, J. L., Elmaci, I., *et al.* Dynamic nature of cavernous malformations: a prospective magnetic resonance imaging study with volumetric analysis. *J Neurosurg* 2000;**93**:981–986.

34. Batra, S., Lin, D., Recinos, P. F., Zhang, J. & Rigamonti, D. Cavernous malformations: natural

history, diagnosis and treatment. *Nat Rev Neurol* 2009;**5**:659–670.

35. Haque, R., Kellner, C. P. & Solomon, R. A. Cavernous malformations of the brainstem. *Clin Neurosurg* 2008;**55**:88–96.

36. Lunsford, L. D., Khan, A. A., Niranjan, A., *et al.* Stereotactic radiosurgery for symptomatic solitary cerebral cavernous malformations considered high risk for resection. *J Neurosurg* 2010.

37. Aiba, T., Tanaka, R., Koike, T., *et al.* Natural history of intracranial cavernous malformations. *J Neurosurg* 1995;**83**:56–59.

38. Dias, M. S. & Sekhar, L. N. Intracranial hemorrhage from aneurysms and arteriovenous malformations during pregnancy and the puerperium. *Neurosurgery* 1990;**27**:855–865; discussion 865–866.

39. Safavi-Abbasi, S., Feiz-Erfan, I., Spetzler, R. F., *et al.* Hemorrhage of cavernous malformations during pregnancy and in the peripartum period: causal or coincidence? Case report and review of the literature. *Neurosurg Focus* 2006;**21**:e12.

40. Pozzati, E., Acciarri, N., Tognetti, F., Marliani, F. & Giangaspero, F. Growth, subsequent bleeding, and de novo appearance of cerebral cavernous angiomas. *Neurosurgery* 1996;**38**:662–669; discussion 669–670.

41. Flemming, K. D., Goodman, B. P. & Meyer, F. B. Successful brainstem cavernous malformation resection after repeated hemorrhages during pregnancy. *Surg Neurol* 2003;**60**:545–547; discussion 547–548.

42. Nimsky, C., Ganslandt, O., Hastreiter, P., *et al.* Preoperative and intraoperative diffusion tensor imaging-based fiber tracking in glioma surgery. *Neurosurgery* 2005;**56**:130–137; discussion 138.

43. Nimsky, C., Ganslandt, O., Hastreiter, P., *et al.* Intraoperative diffusion-tensor MR imaging: shifting of white matter tracts during neurosurgical procedures – initial experience. *Radiology* 2005;**234**:218–225.

44. Kockro, R. A., Stadie, A., Schwandt, E., *et al.* A collaborative virtual reality environment for neurosurgical planning and training. *Neurosurgery* 2007;**61**:379–391; discussion 391.

45. Stadie, A. T., Kockro, R. A., Reisch, R., *et al.* Virtual reality system for planning minimally invasive neurosurgery. Technical note. *J Neurosurg* 2008;**108**:382–394.

46. Nimsky, C., Ganslandt, O. & Fahlbusch, R. Implementation of fiber tract navigation. *Neurosurgery* 2007;**61**:306–317; discussion 317–318.

47. Mamata, Y., Mamata, H., Nabavi, A., *et al.* Intraoperative diffusion imaging on a 0.5 Tesla interventional scanner. *J Magn Reson Imaging* 2001;**13**:115–119.

48. Woydt, M., Horowski, A., Krone, A., Soerensen, N. & Roosen, K. Localization and characterization of intracerebral cavernous angiomas by intra-operative high-resolution colour-duplex-sonography. *Acta Neurochir (Wien)* 1999;**141**:143–152.

49. Sure, U., Benes, L., Bozinov, O., *et al.* Intraoperative landmarking of vascular anatomy by integration of duplex and Doppler ultrasonography in image-guided surgery. *Surg Neurol* 2005;**63**:133–142.

50. Sure, U., Gatscher, S., Alberti, O., Witte, J. & Bertalanffy, H. Image-guided duplex and Doppler ultrasound for microsurgery of cerebral AVMs. *Zentralbl Neurochir* 2000;**61**:47–48.

51. Bertalanffy, H., Benes, L., Miyazawa, T., *et al.* Cerebral cavernomas in the adult. Review of the literature and analysis of 72 surgically treated patients. *Neurosurg Rev* 2002;**25**:1–55.

52. Bozinov, O., Burkhardt, J. K., Fischer, C., *et al.* Advantages and limitations of intraoperative 3D ultrasound in neurosurgery. *Acta Neurochir Suppl (Wien)* 2011;**109**:191–196.

53. Ohue, S., Fukushima, T., Friedman, A. H., Kumon, Y. & Ohnishi, T. Retrosigmoid suprafloccular transhorizontal fissure approach for resection of brainstem cavernous malformation. *Neurosurgery* 2010;**66**:306–312; discussion 312–313.

54. Ramirez-Zamora, A. & Biller, J. Brainstem cavernous malformations: a review with two case reports. *Arq Neuropsiquiatr* 2009;**67**:917–921.

55. Recalde, R. J., Figueiredo, E. G. & de Oliveira, E. Microsurgical anatomy of the safe entry zones on the anterolateral brainstem related to surgical approaches to cavernous malformations. *Neurosurgery* 2008;**62**:9–15; discussion 17.

56. Feiz-Erfan, I., Horn, E. M. & Spetzler, R. F. Transanterior perforating substance approach to the thalamomesencephalic junction. *Neurosurgery* 2008;**63**:ONS69–72; discussion ONS72.

57. Bruneau, M., Bijlenga, P., Reverdin, A., *et al.* Early surgery for brainstem cavernomas. *Acta Neurochir (Wien)* 2006;**148**:405–414.

58. Deshmukh, V. R., Albuquerque, F. C., Zabramski, J. M. & Spetzler, R. F. Surgical management of cavernous malformations involving the cranial nerves. *Neurosurgery* 2003;**53**:352–357; discussion 357.

59. Vinas, F. C., Gordon, V., Guthikonda, M. & Diaz, F. G. Surgical management of cavernous malformations of the brainstem. *Neurol Res* 2002;**24**:61–72.

60. Sarma, S. & Sekhar, L. N. Brain stem cavernoma excised by subtemporal-infratemporal approach. *Br J Neurosurg* 2002;**16**:172–177.

Principles for managing cavernous malformations in eloquent locations

Uğur Türe and Ahmet Hilmi Kaya

Introduction

Cerebral cavernous malformations (cavernomas) are one of the four types of cerebrovascular malformations. The other three are arteriovenous malformations, capillary telangiectases, and venous malformations [1]. A sporadic and a hereditary form of cavernous malformations have been described [2]. These lesions are well-circumscribed, consisting of closely packed and enlarged capillary-like vessels. They do not contain intervening parenchyma and, histologically, the vascular channels (which resemble dilated capillaries) are lined by a single layer of vascular endothelium surrounded by a layer of dense fibrous tissue [3,4].

Cavernous malformations account for 5% to 10% of vascular malformations in the central nervous system. Eighty percent are located supratentorially, with a mostly superficial preference, and these histopathologically benign lesions occur in 0.1% to 0.9% of the population [5–8].

The most prominent clinical features of cerebral cavernous malformations are seizure, hemorrhage and progressive neurological deficits [3,9]. Seizures occur in about 30% of patients with cavernous malformations. Overt annual bleeding rates range from 0.7% to 3.1% and hemorrhage may cause severe morbidity and mortality in young patients [3,9,10]. Nearly 20% of cerebral cavernous malformations appear with focal neurological deficits, which are most likely related to occult bleeding episodes inside the cavernous malformation that cause its enlargement (mainly active cavernous malformations). Inactive lesions may be detected incidentally without signs or symptoms. The clinical manifestations of a cavernous malformation are related to its location: cavernous malformations located in more restricted areas, such as the thalamus or brainstem, tend to display more neurological signs than those in the hemispheric location.

Cavernous malformations arising in special parts of the central nervous system such as the motor cortex, the thalamus, and the brainstem may exhibit a different clinical picture and create a different surgical challenge. Such cavernous malformations are referred to by different terms, such as cavernous malformations in eloquent cortex, deep-seated cavernous malformations, and others [11]. The adjective "eloquent" originates from fourteenth-century Middle English, Anglo-French and Latin, and means "marked by forceful and fluent expression". It is usually used to describe a person's quality of speech [12]. When the term is used to describe an area of the brain, it implies the more expressive areas. But non-parenchymal areas such as vascular territories (for example, that of the perforators) and cranial nerves also play indispensable roles in expressive function, but using the terms eloquent or non-eloquent for these areas is not well accepted. The motor cortex and the pyramidal tract may be described as eloquent areas, but the same description cannot be used for the hippocampus. However, the hippocampus, with its neighboring neurovascular elements in the perimesencephalic cistern and its deep location under the opercular areas and sylvian vascular territories, presents considerable difficulty during surgery. Therefore, surgery in some brain areas not designated eloquent also risks injury because of neighboring neurovascular structures and the hidden location of these areas in a compact volume. Considering these many conflicts in these specific areas, a more suitable term might be eloquent location rather than eloquent area or cortex. Consequently, eloquent locations may include motor, speech and visual cortical areas with their white matter pathways such as the pyramidal tract, superior longitudinal fasiculus and optic radiation; limbic and paralimbic areas such as the subcallosal area, amygdala, hippocampus, parahippocampal gyrus, cingulate gyrus and insula; central nuclei such as the thalamus, hypothalamus and basal ganglia; the whole brainstem including the midbrain, pons and medulla oblongata; and deep cerebellar nuclei and cerebellar peduncles. In short, with respect to function, neighboring anatomy and surgical difficulty, most of the central nervous system can be considered eloquent locations (Figs. 16.1a–c).

Rationale for surgery

Indications for surgical intervention in patients with cerebral cavernous malformations include seizure, symptomatic hemorrhage, a progressive neurological deficit, and intractable, well-localized headache related to the lesion [6,13,14]. Seizure is an important indication and various studies stress that "earlier surgical intervention has better seizure control in [patients with] cerebral cavernous malformations" [10,15]. There is little controversy in deciding to operate on patients with progressive neurological deficits or a large hemorrhage that causes significant mass effect and threatens the patient's life. Recently, there has been an increasing recognition of "growing cavernous malformations": these lesions show progressive enlargement on serial neuroradiological examinations, and even though they may not be symptomatic, they might be considered candidates for surgical resection [14–18]. A cavernous malformation-related headache that is intractable to medical treatment may also be considered an indication for surgical intervention [14].

When a cavernous malformation is in an eloquent location, besides all the indications described above, additional factors become relevant. These factors can be categorized as clinical or surgical.

Clinically, some cavernous malformations in eloquent locations display a distinctly different course. Supratentorial cavernous malformations that are encountered incidentally, are clinically silent, or are in multiple locations can be observed conservatively. However, when in eloquent locations, hemorrhage related to an incidental cavernous malformation may result in a devastating clinical outcome. For this reason, we believe surgery should be considered more often for cavernous malformations in eloquent locations. Patients with a cavernous malformation predominantly in the limbic and paralimbic areas with epilepsy require specific evaluation. Such lesions should be evaluated in conjunction with an epileptologist, and extended

resection might be added to lesionectomy. However, usually lesionectomy with excision of the hemosiderin rim offers good results for patients with epilepsy.

Brainstem cavernous malformations seem to hemorrhage more often and re-bleeding is more devastating than in supratentorial cavernous malformations [9,10,19,20]. We strictly recommend early surgery for brainstem cavernous malformations with hemorrhage, especially in the acute phase, because it allows easier excision due to the hemorrhagic cleavage around the cavernous malformation. This cleavage prevents injury to the neighboring structures during excision and, in the chronic phase, the cavernous malformation adheres to neighboring structures and presents more surgical difficulties. In our experience, preoperative neurological deficits tend to decrease promptly after surgery in patients with brainstem cavernous malformations who were admitted with hemorrhage and operated on during the acute phase of bleeding.

Surgically, other factors are important in patients with cavernous malformations in eloquent locations. First, the deep location of most of the areas mentioned necessitates an appropriate orientation to the lesion without disturbance of the overlying cerebral tissue, white matter, the intracranial course of the cranial nerves, and the vascular territories. Second, cavernous malformations in these areas require fine microneurosurgical access to the margin and excision without injury to neighboring tissues. Thus, the ideal surgical trajectory, from skin incision to the margin of the lesion, should be planned according to these two key factors. For example, a pontine cavernous malformation may have more than one surgical trajectory toward the surface of the pons, either lateral or posterior, but the trajectory chosen must be the least invasive alternative. Apart from the use of fine microneurosurgical techniques and an orientation to the cisternal and regional anatomy, other considerations, such as the orientation to white matter and the compartmental anatomy, are also important. Third, important preoperative and intraoperative tools, such as preoperative fiber tractography [21,22], intraoperative monitoring [23,24], and intraoperative ultrasonography [25], are invaluable aids in choosing the best route to these risky areas.

Based on the factors described above, we do not always agree with the general idea of approaching a brainstem cavernous malformation from the nearest point on the pial surface. First, the nearest trajectory to the cavernous malformation from the surface is not

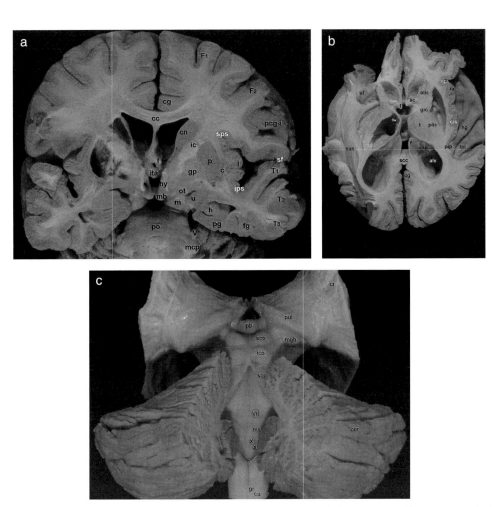

Figure 16.1. In order to demonstrate some of the eloquent locations in which cavernous malformations may be located, cadaver brains are shown. The anatomical locations of the cavernous malformations from the cases presented in this chapter can be seen in these images. (a) Coronal section of a cadaver brain through the foramen of Monro, anterior view. The putamen, globus pallidus and caudate nucleus of the right hemisphere are removed using the fiber dissection technique to reveal the internal capsule. Various eloquent locations of the brain are demonstrated. Note the close relationship of the superior periinsular sulcus with the internal capsule. (b) Axial section of a cadaver brain through the foramen of Monro, superior view. Right-sided the putamen, globus pallidus, and caudate nucleus are dissected away to demonstrate the anterior limb of the internal capsule and the lateral extension of the anterior commissure. Together with left-sided putamen, globus pallidus, caudate nucleus and thalamus, the left frontal, temporal, and insular cortex are removed in order to demonstrate the lateral extension of the anterior commissure joining to the sagittal stratum. The anterior and posterior limbs of the internal capsule are also illustrated. Asterisk denotes the mammillothalamic tract of Vicq d'Azyr. (c) Posterior view of the brainstem and thalamus with neighboring corona radiata of cadaver specimen is shown. Vermis of the cerebellum dissected away, therefore the floor of the fourth ventricle is exposed. Bilateral cerebral hemispheres are also removed but part of the corona radiata near the thalamus is preserved. Abbreviations: ac, anterior commissure; alic, anterior limb of internal capsule; alv, atrial portion of lateral ventricle; aps, anterior periinsular sulcus; c, claustrum; cc, corpus callosum; cer, cerebellum; cg, cingulate gyrus; chp, choroid plexus; cis, central insular sulcus; cn, caudate nucleus; cr, corona radiata; cu, cuneate fasciculus; f, fornix; F1, superior frontal gyrus; F2, middle frontal gyrus; fg, fusiform gyrus; gic, genu of internal capsule; gp, globus pallidus; gr, gracile fasciculus; h, hippocampus; hg, Heschl gyrus; hy, hypothalamus; i, insula; ia, insular apex; ic, internal capsule; ico, inferior colliculus; ips, inferior periinsular sulcus; ita, interthalamic adhesion; m, midbrain; mb, mamillary body; mcp, middle cerebellar peduncle; mgb, medial geniculate body; ms, medullary striae of fourth ventricle; o, obex; ot, optic tract; p, putamen; pb, pineal body; pcg-i, inferior portion of precentral gyrus; pg, parahippocampal gyrus; pip, posterior insular point; plic, posterior limb of internal capsule; po, pons; pul, pulvinar of thalamus; sas, sagittal stratum; scc, splenium of corpus callosum; sco, superior colliculus; scp, superior cerebellar peduncle; sf, sylvian fissure; sps, superior peri-insular sulcus; t, thalamus; T1, superior temporal gyrus; T2, middle temporal gyrus; T3, inferior temporal gyrus; tpl, temporal planum; u, uncus; uf, uncinate fasciculus. Roman numbers in circles indicate the nuclei of the corresponding cranial nerves. See color plate section.

163

always the safest route, a fact we have discovered during intraoperative neuromonitoring. Second, the nearest trajectory can be used in the lowest portion of the brainstem, the medulla oblongata; the upper parts do not allow such a prospect. For example, a cavernous malformation in the upper pons may have its nearest margin at the base of the fourth ventricle, but its main bulk may be located more inferiorly. A surgical trajectory under the vermis toward the upper part of the fourth ventricular base that turns inferiorly after reaching the nearest margin would be hazardous. A more inferior approach to the cavernous malformation, confirmed by monitoring, may be more suitable.

Navigational support, although frequently advised by the literature [26], is not recommended by us in the surgery of these risky cavernous malformations if navigational support means "dissection toward the lesion solely according to the guide of the instrument without considering the overlying or neighboring neural tissue". Although navigation is helpful in cranial-base surgery, it is not a real-time method because cerebrospinal fluid drainage and surgical positions distort the parenchymal position of the lesion, especially in eloquent locations, with possible disorientation during surgery. If the lesion can be reached through arachnoidal dissection, a parenchymal trajectory should be avoided. Nonetheless, with the current status of microanatomical definition in neurosurgery, all of these critical areas are approachable. The best neuronavigation is an ideal combination of the surgeon's neuroanatomical orientation and knowledge and a host of anatomical landmarks in the patient. Cavernous malformations without any sign on the pial surface may be difficult to localize, but the surgeon's own description of the exact anatomical location according to preoperative neuroradiological findings and the use of intraoperative ultrasonography should supply the security needed during the operation.

The use of stereotactic radiosurgery (SRS) is controversial in the treatment of such cavernous malformations. Despite some optimism based on current findings [27,28], SRS cannot be considered highly effective or safe because either the bleeding rates or seizure activity do not disappear after SRS. In addition, SRS has its own complication rates [29].

As neurosurgeons we must accept that every part of the brain is eloquent, but we use the term "eloquent location" specifically to denote regions with the potential for unfavorable clinical results postoperatively. Other regions that do not usually manifest unfavorable clinical signs may actually have them, but we cannot see or properly evaluate them. Accepting that the whole brain is eloquent prevents unnecessary retraction and resection. So, regardless of whether the location is eloquent or not, our surgical aim is always to try to preserve the nervous system as much as possible.

Specific eloquent locations of cavernous malformations

Motor cortex, speech cortex and visual cortex with their white matter pathways

The precentral gyrus, namely the motor cortex, belongs to the posterior part of the frontal lobe. It lies between the medial surface of the frontal lobe above the cingulate gyrus and the sylvian fissure. During its course on the lateral aspect of the cerebral surface, it turns anteroinferiorly toward the sylvian fissure. It is limited anteriorly by the precentral sulcus and posteriorly by the central sulcus. At its most medial edge, it usually connects to the postcentral gyrus, forming the paracentral lobule. At its most lateral edge, the central sulcus usually does not enter the sylvian fissure and, at this point, the precentral gyrus and the postcentral gyrus unite to form the subcentral gyrus, which lies in the medial aspect of the frontoparietal operculum [30]. At the level of the superior sagittal sinus, the central sulcus is found about 2 cm anterior to the midpoint of an imaginary line from the nasion to the inion, and from this point courses anterolaterally to the sylvian fissure in an imaginary line reaching towards the midpoint of the zygomatic arch [31]. The central sulcus is generally in one piece, but the precentral sulcus is usually separated by the superior, middle or inferior frontal gyri [32–34].

With the use of preoperative MRI, all details related to a cavernous malformation in or near the motor cortex can be obtained. Its general location in the precentral gyrus, such as near the interhemispheric fissure or opercular area, around the sylvian fissure, or at the midpoint can be determined with preoperative evaluation. This general localization is usually enough to plan the craniotomy, and verifying the margin closest to the cortical surface in different sections of the MRI is also important. Surface MRI sections can also be used to evaluate the venous territory and sulcal pattern at the cortex. The rest of the intervention, however, depends mostly on intraoperative ultrasound and intraoperative monitoring, such as SEP, MEP, cortical mapping, the phase-reversal technique to

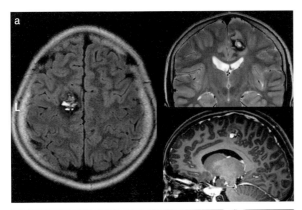

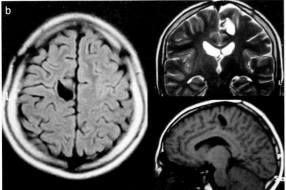

Figure 16.2. (a) A 13-year-old male complaining of a severe headache, which started 2 months earlier and gradually increased, was examined by MRI. Flair axial, T2-weighted coronal and post-contrast T1-weighted sagittal images show a heterogeneous mass having a reticulated core of high and low signal intensities in the left (L) posterior medial portion of the superior frontal gyrus just anterior to the motor cortex, which was compatible with a diagnosis of cavernous malformation. (b) The lesion was removed totally including the adjacent hemosiderin rim using an anterior interhemispheric approach, preserving the superior cerebral (bridging) veins as well as the rest of the superior frontal gyrus.

verify the central sulcus, and subcortical stimulation. Resecting the hemosiderin rim around the cavernous malformation is advantageous for controlling seizures, but in these restricted areas, its resection must be accompanied by fine subcortical stimulation to delineate the pyramidal tract. With these adjuncts, the safest surgical corridor to the cavernous malformation, either transfissural or transsulcal routes, can be used (Fig. 16.2a,b).

A cavernous malformation in the speech cortex may involve the posterior part of the inferior frontal gyrus (pars triangularis and pars opercularis), namely Broca's area; the posterior part of the superior temporal gyrus, or Wernicke's area; the supramarginal and angular gyri (inferior parietal lobule); and the superior longitudinal fasciculus interconnecting these areas in the dominant hemisphere [35,36]. Each part of these speech areas is localized around the sylvian fissure and its sulcal architecture supplies important information to these locations. The horizontal ramus and ascending ramus of the sylvian fissure border the pars triangularis. The ascending ramus of the sylvian fissure and the precentral sulcus border the pars opercularis. On the other hand, the posterior part of the superior temporal gyrus (Wernicke's area) is limited superiorly by the posterior ramus of the sylvian fissure and inferiorly by the superior temporal sulcus. The inferior parietal lobule is formed by a combination of the supramarginal and angular gyri. The supramarginal gyrus inferior to the intraparietal sulcus is located around the posterior ascending ramus of the sylvian fissure, while just posteriorly the angular gyrus is located around the distal part of the superior temporal sulcus.

The visual cortex is located at the medial surface of the occipital lobe around the calcarine fissure, and this fissure practically separates the inferiorly located lingual gyrus (medial temporo-occipital gyrus) of the occipital lobe from the superiorly located cuneus. In addition, after blending with the parieto-occipital sulcus at the tip of the cuneus, the calcarine fissure extends anteriorly toward the parahippocampal gyrus, dividing it into two parts. The visual cortex also extends anteriorly along the anterior calcarine fissure [32,33]. A cavernous malformation may involve the visual pathways from the calcarine sulcus to the optic nerve through optic radiation, the lateral geniculate body, or the optic tract and chiasm.

The location of a cavernous malformation in speech and visual areas must be topographically defined through preoperative radiological evaluation. Supplementary techniques such as surface MRI, functional MRI, intraoperative monitoring, intraoperative ultrasonography, and verification of the optic pathways and superior longitudinal fasciculus with fiber tractography aid in a successful surgical intervention. Some surgeons prefer to use an awake craniotomy for patients with a cavernous malformation in the speech cortex, but we do not use this approach for these well-circumscribed lesions.

Limbic and paralimbic areas

Mediobasal temporal region

The mediobasal temporal region (MTR) is actually the portion of the limbic lobe which also includes the

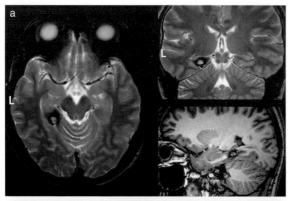

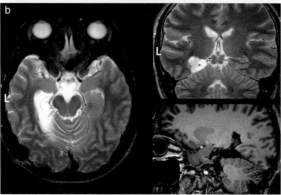

Figure 16.3. (a) This 31-year-old male had a generalized tonic-clonic seizure 8 months earlier. Since then he had seizures once a month and recurrent daily episodes of absence seizures even after prompt anti-epileptic drug medication. He was neurologically intact. T2-weighted axial and coronal and T1-weighted sagittal MRI images revealed a well-defined, lobulated lesion with a reticulated core of heterogeneous signal intensity in the left (L) sided posterior hippocampus and parahippocampal gyrus. (b) The lesion was excised totally by a left paramedian supracerebellar-transtentorial approach in semi-sitting position with extended removal of hippocampus for better seizure control. Postoperative MRI images show that the rest of the temporal lobe is preserved. No seizures were seen in the postoperative follow-up period.

cingulate gyrus, the subcallosal area and the insula. The MTR includes allocortical and mesocortical structures such as the piriform cortex, amygdala, hippocampus, and the parahippocampal gyrus [37]. This long structure extends around the midbrain from the piriform cortex to the isthmus cinguli. Because of its elongated architecture, it is useful to classify the MTR into three sections [38]. This division defines the amygdala, the uncus, the anterior portion of the parahippocampus, and the head of the hippocampus as the anterior part of the MTR. The middle portions of the parahippocampal gyrus and the hippocampus constitute the middle part of the MTR. The posterior part of

the MTR includes the tail of the hippocampus and parahippocampal gyrus up to the isthmus cinguli and anterior portion of the lingual (medial temporo-occipital) gyrus posteroinferiorly.

A variety of surgical approaches to the MTR have been described. These include the transcortical-transventricular approaches [39], the pterional-transsylvian approach [40–43], the subtemporal approach [44], the petrosal approach [37], the supratentorial infraoccipital approach [45], and the posterior interhemispheric approach to the posterior mediobasal temporal region [40,41]. We use the pterional-transsylvian approach for cavernous malformations in the anterior portion of the MTR such as the amygdala, head of the hippocampus and parahippocampal gyrus but we prefer the paramedian supracerebellar transtentorial approach for lesions located in the middle and posterior portions of the MTR. Yaşargil [46] developed the supracerebellar transtentorial approach to remove a posterior hippocampal cavernous malformation without injuring the optic radiation. Later, the supracerebellar transtentorial approach was revitalized by Yonekawa and colleagues [47] for approaching the posterior portion of the MTR. Over the past 2 years, the paramedian supracerebellar transtentorial approach has been utilized frequently by the senior author and used to resect not only the posterior portion but also the middle and anterior portions of the MTR. This approach is unique because it directly exposes the mediobasal temporal region without interfering with the parenchyma and preserves the white matter (Fig. 16.3a,b).

Cingulate gyrus

The cingulate gyrus lies on the medial side of the hemisphere surrounding the corpus callosum from the subcallosal area to the inferior portion of the splenium, turning inferolaterally to meet the parahippocampal gyrus at the level of the isthmus cinguli. For removing cavernous malformations along the whole length of the cingulate gyrus the anterior, middle or posterior interhemispheric approaches are the best routes.

Opening the interhemispheric fissure anteriorly is difficult because both cingulate gyri adhere to each other under the falx. Preserving the gyrus is important during dissection of these adherent gyri because the other gyrus may be severed due to hemorrhage of the cavernous malformation. Identifying the pericallosal arteries is also important. During dissection of the middle portion of the interhemispheric fissure, the bridging veins may prevent surgical access. Delineating the bridging veins preoperatively with computed tomographic venography may help discern the ideal location for the craniotomy, and arachnoidal dissection around bridging veins for mobilization is also helpful.

Insula

The insula has a pyramidal shape and is hidden by the frontal, parietal and temporal operculas at the base of the sylvian fissure. A detailed anatomy and the vascular supply of the insula have been described previously by the senior author [30,48]. The insula is bordered by the opercular area and peri-insular sulci, which include the anterior peri-insular sulcus beneath the orbitofrontal operculum, the superior peri-insular sulcus beneath the frontoparietal operculum, and the inferior peri-insular sulcus beneath the temporal operculum. The limen insula is at the lateral limit of the sylvian vallecula and acts as an entrance to the insula. The central insular sulcus is an important landmark on the insula, extending from the superior peri-insular sulcus to the limen insula, and it divides the insula into anterior and posterior parts. This sulcus mostly corresponds to the central sulcus of Rolando. The posterior insula is generally composed of two long gyri, the anterior and the posterior, which are separated by the post-central insular sulcus. The anterior part of the insula is composed of the anterior, middle and posterior short insular gyri, as well as the accessory and tranverse gyri in its anteroinferior region.

The lateral opercular neighborhood of the insula is important from the surgical point of view; eloquent locations such as Broca's and the precentral gyrus are included in these opercular regions overlying the insula. Meticulous dissection and maximal efforts are required when exposing the insula through the transsylvian route.

The medial neighborhood of the central portion of the insula includes the extreme capsule, the claustrum, the external capsule, the lentiform nuclei (putamen and globus pallidus), and the internal capsule from lateral to medial. However, insular cortex close to the peri-insular sulci is separated from the internal capsule only by the extreme capsule.

One of the most important factors in successful surgery of insular cavernous malformations relates to preserving the lateral lenticulostriate arteries arising from the M1 segment and preserving the M2 main trunks of the middle cerebral artery [6,8,49]. The middle cerebral artery is the most complex of all cerebral vessels and is closely related to the insular region. The M1 segment of the middle cerebral artery (the sphenoidal segment) extends inside the sylvian vallecula toward the insular apex and bifurcates at the level of the limen insula. Lateral lenticulostriate arteries (LLAs) arise primarily from this segment to supply the putamen, the globus pallidus, the head and body of the caudate nucleus, the internal capsule, the adjacent corona radiata, and the lateral portion of the anterior comissure. After arising from the inferomedial aspect of the M1 segment, LLAs extend toward the anterior perforated substance (APS) and turn in an acute angle superiorly through the APS in a fan-like manner to reach their target areas. Therefore, not only is the proximal course of the LLAs related to the insula anteroinferiorly, but their distal course is also closely related to the insula medially. The M2 segment (insular segment) of the middle cerebral artery corresponds to branches of the M1 overlying the insula up to the level of the peri-insular sulci. These segments are the most important source of the insular branches and 85% to 90% of these branches are short insular arteries supplying the insular cortex and extreme capsule. Ten percent are medium-sized arteries that supply up to the claustrum and external capsule, and 5% are long branches supplying as far as the corona radiata. The M3 segment (opercular segment) extends from the peri-insular sulci towards the cortical surface at the exit of the sylvian fissure. During its course over the insula, parallel but in a direction opposite to the M2 segments, it supplies the regions of the superior or inferior peri-insular sulci in 25% of cases.

Opening the sylvian fissure is a critical part of surgery of insular cavernous malformations. This opening should be wide enough to avoid unnecessary retraction of the operculi. Opening the sylvian fissure along its full length orients the surgeon with various landmarks on the insula. Especially, opening of the posterior aspect of the sylvian fissure could be challenging because the transverse parietal gyri and transverse temporal gyri (Heschl gyri) intermingle. The surgeon's exact preoperative description of the lesion in the insula based on fine neuroradiological examination is also critical. This description allows appropriate orientation toward the lesion according to surface anatomical landmarks of the insula (Fig. 16.4a,b). Additionally, intraoperative ultrasonography helps disclose the lesion. Great effort must be taken under high magnification so as not to injure deeply coursing vessels. Preoperative fiber tractography can help to

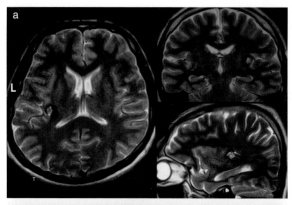

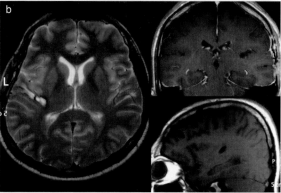

Figure 16.4. (a) A 25-year-old male presented with a 4-year history of limbic seizures. The T2-weighted MRI shows a left (L) sided posterior insular cavernous malformation located exactly at the posterior insular point. (b) The lesion was totally excised with the neighboring hemosiderin rim using a left-sided pterional transsylvian approach without damaging frontoparietal and temporal operculi. Seizure control was acheived.

verify the intimate relationship between the lesion and the internal capsule.

Deep nuclei (hypothalamus, thalamus and basal ganglia) and internal capsule

The thalamus is a large mass of gray matter with a rostral limit at the interventricular foramen and a caudal limit at the posterior commissure and aqueduct. From the surgical point of view, this ovoid mass has different surfaces: the ventrolateral, superior, medial, and posterior. The ventrolateral surface of the thalamus is hidden by the internal capsule anterolaterally and the mesencephalic subthalamic structures anteroinferolaterally to the thalamus. This surface is not free and is not an appropriate trajectory for surgery. On the other hand, the superior surface freely faces the lateral ventricle, the medial surface faces the third ventricle, and

the posterior surface (pulvinar of thalamus) faces medial to the quadrigeminal cistern and lateral to the atrium of the lateral ventricle, since the fornix lies between them. These three surfaces predispose the thalamus to surgical intervention. The insula, especially its posterior portion, sits more lateral to the posterior limb of the internal capsule that borders the anterolateral part of the ventrolateral thalamus. When the exact location of a cavernous malformation in the thalamus is verified by neuroimaging, the next step is to plan the route to this lesion via the most appropriate of the three free surfaces. Fiber tractography clearly discloses the anatomical relationship of the cavernous malformation and the internal capsule.

The approaches suitable for reaching the thalamus include the anterior interhemispheric transcallosal approach, either ipsilaterally [34,50–52] or contralaterally [53] for the superior and medial surfaces of the thalamus; the infratentorial supracerebellar approach [54] for the medial side of the posterior surface; the posterior interhemispheric parasplenial approach [8,40] for the lateral side of the posterior surface.

The anterior interhemispheric approach satisfactorily unveils the superior surface of the thalamus. This approach allows great flexibility for exploring the lateral ventricle and the patient does not need postoperative anticonvulsants because the incision is through the corpus callosum and not the cortex. The third ventricle can also be reached through the same approach via the foramen of Monro through the lateral ventricle, which in turn discloses the medial surface of the thalamus.

The posterior interhemispheric parasplenial approach, introduced by Yaşargil [40], exposes the subsplenial, pineal, parapineal, and pulvinar portions of the thalamus. Through an incision in the precuneal region, the atrial surface of the pulvinar of the thalamus can be identified.

For cavernous malformations mainly located in the medial aspect of the pulvinar, the paramedian infratentorial supracerebellar approach is useful [40,51,54,55]. With this approach, the pulvinar thalami are centered between the internal cerebral vein and basal vein of Rosenthal (Fig. 16.5a–d).

A cavernous malformation in the basal ganglia involves three main nuclei, namely the caudate nucleus, putamen, and globus pallidus. The last two, the putamen and globus pallidus, are combined and together form the lentiform nucleus. The anterior limb of the internal capsule is the key anatomical structure for such

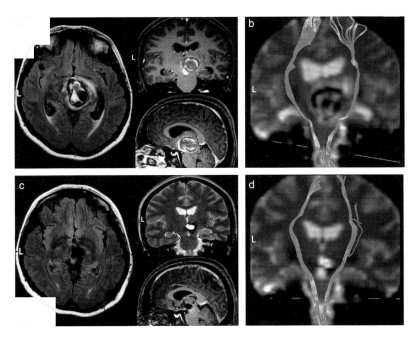

Figure 16.5. (a) A 39-year-old female with a history of sudden onset of left hemiparesis 45 days prior to admission was referred to our clinic. Flair axial and postcontrast T1-weighted MRI study revealed right-sided midbrain-thalamus cavernous malformation. (b) Pre-operative fiber tractography in coronal view revealed that the right-sided pyramidal tract was anterolaterally dislocated by the lesion. (c) The lesion was excised using a right-sided supracerebellar approach in semi-sitting position. Postoperative MRI shows a pure lesionectomy was achieved without damage to neighboring structures. (d) Postoperative fiber tractography demonstrated the pyramidal tract returned to its original location. See color plate section, panels b and d.

a classification, and the lentiform nuclei lies lateral to the internal capsule and medial to the insula. Thus, for a cavernous malformation in the lentiform nuclei the transylvian-transinsular approach as outlined above is suitable. The anterior short insular gyri are the primary entrance to the lentiform nuclei but, in particular, the more inferior part of this anterior insular lobe is closest to the globus pallidus. Intraoperative ultrasonography is very helpful for localizing a cavernous malformation under the insula, and preoperative fiber tractography also helps delineate the intimate relationship of the cavernous malformation to the internal capsule. All the regular rules for meticulous dissection to preserve the perforators must be applied.

The second major part of the basal ganglia, the head of the caudate nucleus, lies medial to the anterior limb of the internal capsule at the lateral base of the frontal horn of the ventricle. The most appropriate approach to cavernous malformations at this location is the anterior interhemispheric transcallosal approach.

Cavernous malformations of the lentiform nuclei differ greatly, both clinically and surgically, from those of the caudate nucleus. First, caudate nucleus cavernous malformations tend to be clinically silent after hemorrhage, whereas hemorrhage of lentiform nuclei cavernous malformations may lead to devastating clinical signs. Surgical morbidity is also higher with lentiform nuclei cavernous malformations due to their close

relation with the lateral lenticulostriate arteries and the genu and posterior limb of the internal capsule in comparison to caudate nucleus cavernous malformations.

Based on these factors, a cavernous malformation in the internal capsule may require either the transsylvian or interhemispheric approach, depending upon its location. Most lesions in the anterior or posterior limbs can be approached via the transsylvian route. A lesion in the genu necessitates a deep parenchymal trajectory from the surface of the insula, but the anterior interhemispheric transcallosal approach reaches the genu lateral to the conjunction of the caudate nucleus and the thalamus at the base of the lateral ventricle. Cavernous malformations located in the internal capsule have a predilection for the most anterior or most posterior portions [34].

Brainstem

Brainstem cavernomas are described comprehensively in Chapter 15; please refer to Chapter 15.

Ventricles

Intraventricular cavernous malformations may be truly intraventricular, attaching to ependyma or choroid plexus of the ventricle or at least with an intraparenchymal component [56]. So, a paraventricular structure such as the caudate nucleus from its head

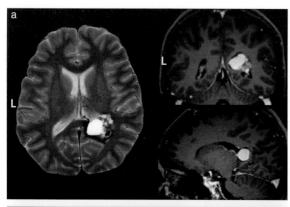

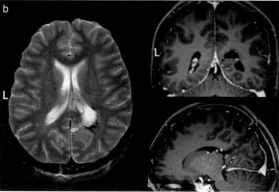

Figure 16.6. A 30-year-old female with 1-year history of numbness on her left side which was worsening day by day. An MRI scan was performed and a cavernous malformation located in the atrium of the right lateral ventricle was seen. (b) A posterior interhemispheric-precuneal approach was performed in order to remove the lesion without damaging optic pathways.

to tail through its body, thalamus, hypothalamus, brainstem, vermis may host the cavernous malformation intraventricularly, but ependymal lining of the same anatomical structures may also host the cavernous malformation at the same location. There is no need to emphasize that the surgical approach to most of the intraventricular locations can be comparatively followed throughout this chapter, such as the frontal horn of the lateral ventricle under the heading "head of caudate nucleus"; body of the lateral ventricle under the heading "body of caudate nucleus" and "thalamus"; the temporal horn of the lateral ventricle under the heading "hippocampus"; the third ventricle under the heading "thalamus and hypothalamus"; and lastly the fourth ventricle under the heading "brainstem". However, it is worth noting two additional ventricular locations descriptively. One of them is the posterior third ventricular region and the other is the

atrium of the lateral ventricle. Posterior third ventricular cavernous malformations may usually be approached by infratentorial supracerebellar or posterior interhemispheric approaches [57]. On the other hand, the atrium of the lateral ventricle is one of the surgically most difficult locations for cavernous malformations and different approaches have been proposed. A superior parietal occipital approach, a posterior middle temporal gyrus approach, and lateral temporoparietal approaches through the cortical trajectories toward the atrium may be preferred but have high risks of apraxia, acalculia, aphasia, dyslexia and impaired recognition of emotion and visual field deficits [57]. But, to the best of our knowledge, for exposure of the atrium of the lateral ventricle, a posterior interhemispheric precuneal approach [40] is the preferable approach, and we perform this approach in cavernous malformations located in the atrium of the lateral ventricle (Fig. 16.6a,b).

It must be emphasized that all the critical locations summarized throughout this chapter have intimate relationships with fiber tracts such as pyramidal tracts, sensorial fibers, and optic radiations. There is no doubt that fiber tractography and neuromonitoring have crucial roles in the definition of these fasicular structures, but knowledge of the anatomical background related to fiber dissection techniques [58] has also aided in outlining these fasicular structures.

Conclusion

Cavernous malformations are benign vascular lesions with the potential for morbidity and mortality because of hemorrhage, especially in eloquent locations. With detailed neuroanatomical knowledge, microneurosurgical techniques, and technological modalities, the risk related to surgical intervention is no longer major. In turn, significantly encouraging results can often indicate that a more aggressive approach will succeed. Surgery improves the unfavorable prognosis more in these patients than in those with more superficially located lesions. For cavernous malformations in eloquent locations, surgery is still the most effective treatment modality.

References

1.   McCormick, W. The pathology of vascular ("arteriovenous") malformations. *J Neurosurg* 1966;24:807–816.

2. Günel, M., *et al.* Genetic heterogeneity of inherited cerebral cavernous malformation. *Neurosurgery* 1996;**38**:1265–1271.

3. Zabramski, J. M., *et al.* The natural history of familial cavernous malformations: results of an ongoing study. *J Neurosurg* 1994;**80**:422–432.

4. Rigamonti, D., *et al.* Cerebral cavernous malformations. Incidence and familial occurrence. *New Engl J Med* 1988;**319**:343–347.

5. Haque, R., Kellner, C. & Solomon, R. Cavernous malformations of the brainstem. *Clin Neurosurg* 2008;**55**:88–96.

6. Bertalanffy, H., Gilsbach, J., Eggert, H. & Seeger, W. Microsurgery of deep-seated cavernous angiomas: report of 26 cases. *Acta Neurochir (Wien)* 1991;**108**:91–99.

7. Samii, M., Eghbal, R., Carvalho, G. & Matthies, C. Surgical management of brainstem cavernomas. *J Neurosurg* 2001;**95**:825–832.

8. Yaşargil, M. G. *Microneurosurgery*, vol. 3B. (New York: Georg Thieme, 1988).

9. Kondziolka, D., Lunsford, L. D. & Kestle, J. R. The natural history of cerebral cavernous malformations. *J Neurosurg* 1995;**83**:820–824.

10. Robinson, J., Awad, I. & Little, J. Natural history of the cavernous angioma. *J Neurosurg* 1991;**75**:709–714.

11. Zimmerman, R., Spetzler, R., Lee, K., Zabramski, J. & Hargraves, R. Cavernous malformations of the brain stem. *J Neurosurg* 1991;**75**:32–39.

12. http://www.merriam-webster.com/dictionary/eloquent (accessed 24 December 2009).

13. Bertalanffy, H., *et al.* Cerebral cavernomas in the adult. Review of the literature and analysis of 72 surgically treated patients. *Neurosurg Rev* 2002;**25**:1–53.

14. Bortolotti, C., Nannavecchia, B., Lanzino, G., Perrini, P. & Andreoli, A. Supratentorial cavernous malformations. In G. Lanzino and R. F. Spetzler, eds., *Cavernous Malformations of Brain and Spinal Cord* (New York: Thieme, 2008), pp. 65–70.

15. Awad, I., Robinson, J. J., Mohanty, S. & Estes, M. Mixed vascular malformations of the brain: clinical and pathogenetic considerations. *Neurosurgery* 1993;**33**:179–188; discussion 188.

16. Jung, K., *et al.* Cerebral cavernous malformations with dynamic and progressive course: correlation study with vascular endothelial growth factor. *Arch Neurol* 2003;**60**:1613–1618.

17. Pozzati, E., Giuliani, G., Nuzzo, G. & Poppi, M. The growth of cerebral cavernous angiomas. *Neurosurgery* 1989;**25**:92–97.

18. Sure, U., *et al.* Biological activity of adult cavernous malformations: a study of 56 patients. *J Neurosurg* 2005;**102**:342–347.

19. Porter, R., *et al.* Cavernous malformations of the brainstem: experience with 100 patients. *J Neurosurg* 1999;**90**:50–58.

20. Wang, C. C., Liu, A., Zhang, J. T., Sun, B. & Zhao, Y. L. Surgical management of brain-stem cavernous malformations: report of 137 cases. *Surg Neurol* 2003;**59**:444–454.

21. Chen, X., Weigel, D., Ganslandt, O., Buchfelder, M. & Nimsky, C. Diffusion tensor imaging and white matter tractography in patients with brainstem lesions. *Acta Neurochir (Wien)* 2007;**149**:1117–1131; discussion 1131.

22. Kovanlikaya, I., *et al.* Assessment of the corticospinal tract alterations before and after resection of brainstem lesions using Diffusion Tensor Imaging (DTI) and tractography at 3T. *Eur J Radiol* 2009; Epub ahead of print.

23. Kothbauer, K., Deletis, V. & Epstein, F. Intraoperative monitoring. *Pediatr Neurosurg* 1998;**29**:54–55.

24. Deletis, V. What does intraoperative monitoring of motor evoked potentials bring to the neurosurgeon? *Acta Neurochir (Wien)* 2005;**147**:1015–1017.

25. Regelsberger, J., Lohmann, F., Helmke, K. & Westphal, M. Ultrasound-guided surgery of deep seated brain lesions. *Eur J Ultrasound* 2000;**12**:115–121.

26. Tirakotai, W., *et al.* Image-guided transsylvian, transinsular approach for insular cavernous angiomas. *Neurosurgery* 2003;**53**:1299–1304; discussion 1304–1295.

27. Liu, K., *et al.* Gamma knife surgery for cavernous hemangiomas: an analysis of 125 patients. *J Neurosurg* 2005;**102**(Suppl):81–86.

28. Liscák, R., Vladyka, V., Simonová, G., Vymazal, J. & Novotny, J. J. Gamma knife surgery of brain cavernous hemangiomas. *J Neurosurg* 2005;**102**(Suppl):207–213.

29. Karlsson, B., Kihlström, L., Lindquist, C., Ericson, K. & Steiner, L. Radiosurgery for cavernous malformations. *J Neurosurg* 1998;**88**:293–297.

30. Türe, U., Yaşargil, D., Al-Mefty, O. & Yaşargil, M. Topographic anatomy of the insular region. *J Neurosurg* 1999;**90**:720–733.

31. Rhoton, A. J. The cerebrum. Anatomy. *Neurosurgery* 2007;**61**:37–118; discussion 118–119.

32. Ribas, G., Yasuda, A., Ribas, E., Nishikuni, K. & Rodrigues, A. J. Surgical anatomy of microneurosurgical sulcal key points. *Neurosurgery* 2006;**59**:ONS177–210; discussion ONS210–171.

33. Ono, M., Kubik, S. & Abernathey, C. D. *Atlas of Cerebral Sulci* (Stuttgart: Thieme, 1990).

34. Yaşargil, M. G. *Microneurosurgery*, vol. 4A (Stuttgart: Thieme 1994).

35. Snell, R. S. *Clinical Neuroanatomy*. (New York: Lippincott-Raven, 1997).

36. Standring, S. *Gray's Anatomy* (New York: Elsevier, 2005).

37. Türe, U. & Pamir, M. Small petrosal approach to the middle portion of the mediobasal temporal region: technical case report. *Surg Neurol* 2004;**61**:60–67; discussion 67.

38. de Oliveira, E., *et al.* Anatomic principles of cerebrovascular surgery for arteriovenous malformations. *Clin Neurosurg* 1994;**41**:364–380.

39. Oliver., A. Temporal resections in the surgical treatment of epilepsy. In W. H. Theodore, ed., *Surgical Treatment of Epilepsy* (Amsterdam: Elsevier, 1992), pp. 175–188.

40. Yaşargil, M. G. *Microneurosurgery*, vol. 4B (Stuttgart: Thieme, 1996).

41. Yaşargil, M., *et al.* Tumours of the limbic and paralimbic systems. *Acta Neurochir (Wien)* 1992;**118**:40–52.

42. Yaşargil, M., Wieser, H., Valavanis, A., von Ammon, K. & Roth, P. Surgery and results of selective amygdala-hippocampectomy in one hundred patients with nonlesional limbic epilepsy. *Neurosurg Clin N Am* 1993;**4**:243–261.

43. Yaşargil, M. G., Teddy, P. J. & Roth, P. Selective amygdalohippocampectomy: operative anatomy and surgical technique. In L. Symon *et al.*, eds., *Advances and Technical Standards in Neurosurgery*, vol. 12 (New York: Springer, 1985).

44. Hori, T., *et al.* Retrolabyrinthine presigmoid transpetrosal approach for selective subtemporal amygdalohippocampectomy. *Neurol Med Chir (Tokyo)* 1999;**39**:214–224; discussion 224–215.

45. Smith, K. & Spetzler, R. Supratentorial-infraoccipital approach for posteromedial temporal lobe lesions. *J Neurosurg* 1995;**82**:940–944.

46. Voigt, K. & Yaşargil, M. Cerebral cavernous haemangiomas or cavernomas. Incidence, pathology, localization, diagnosis, clinical features and treatment. Review of the literature and report of an unusual case. *Neurochirurgia (Stuttg)* 1976;**19**:59–68.

47. Yonekawa, Y., *et al.* Supracerebellar transtentorial approach to posterior temporomedial structures. *J Neurosurg* 2001;**94**:339–345.

48. Türe, U., Yaşargil, M., Al-Mefty, O. & Yaşargil, D. Arteries of the insula. *J Neurosurg* 2000;**92**:676–687.

49. Heffez, D. Stereotactic transsylvian, transinsular approach for deep-seated lesions. *Surg Neurol* 1997;**48**:113–124.

50. Bernstein, M., Hoffman, H., Halliday, W., Hendrick, E. & Humphreys, R. Thalamic tumors in children. Long-term follow-up and treatment guidelines. *J Neurosurg* 1984;**61**:649–656.

51. Cuccia, V. & Monges, J. Thalamic tumors in children. *Childs Nerv Syst* 1997;**13**:514–520; discussion 521.

52. Villarejo, F., *et al.* Radical surgery of thalamic tumors in children. *Childs Nerv Syst* 1994;**10**:111–114.

53. Lawton, M., Golfinos, J. & Spetzler, R. The contralateral transcallosal approach: experience with 32 patients. *Neurosurgery* 1996;**39**:729–734; discussion 734–725.

54. Steiger, H., Götz, C., Schmid-Elsaesser, R. & Stummer, W. Thalamic astrocytomas: surgical anatomy and results of a pilot series using maximum microsurgical removal. *Acta Neurochir (Wien)* 2000;**142**:1327–1336; discussion 1336–1327.

55. Ozek, M. & Türe, U. Surgical approach to thalamic tumors. *Childs Nerv Syst* 2002;**18**:450–456.

56. Pechstein, U., Zentner, J., Van Roost, D. & Schramm, J. Surgical management of brain-stem cavernomas. *Neurosurg Rev* 1997;**20**:87–93.

57. Konovalov, A., *et al.* Brainstem cavernoma. *Surg Neurol* 2000;**54**:418–421.

58. Hakuba, A., Liu, S. & Nishimura, S. The orbitozygomatic infratemporal approach: a new surgical technique. *Surg Neurol* 1986;**26**:271–276.

Radiosurgery of cavernous malformations: the Pittsburgh experience

Douglas Kondziolka, L. Dade Lunsford, Hideyuki Kano and John C. Flickinger

Cavernous malformations (CM) are relatively common, angiographically occult vascular malformations of the brain [1–5]. The vast majority are thought to be congenital [6–8]. The association with developmental venous anomalies (DVA) is well recognized [4,9–12]. Many occur in cortical or subcortical locations that can safely be removed when symptomatic [13–16]. Other malformations are deeply located or in functional brain regions [17,18].

Over the last 25 years, we have improved our understanding of their imaging appearance, and natural history [2,9,11,19–24]. Typical presentations include seizures (40–50%), hemorrhages (10–25%), or focal neurological deficits (20%), and many have headache [18,25,26]. The annual hemorrhage rate is estimated to be 0.1–2.5% per lesion-year and 0.25–16.5% per patient-year. In our initial natural history study we reported that the hemorrhage risk was elevated in patients with prior hemorrhages [27,28] and exceeded a 30% annual risk once two symptomatic events had occurred. The role of resection in previously unruptured brainstem malformations has been advocated but is controversial [29].

The role of radiosurgery has remained controversial despite recommendations that SRS should be reserved for hemorrhagic malformations in high-risk locations [21,26,30]. We think this is mainly due to the lack of an imaging test that confirms cure. Nevertheless, for patients with hemorrhagic malformations in high-risk locations, it may be the best alternative.

Clinical patient population

In this analysis, we studied the outcomes of 103 CM patients who underwent gamma knife radiosurgery between 1988 and 2005. The mean patient age was 39 years (range 5–79). Sixty-six patients (64%) had sustained two symptomatic hemorrhages, and 35 (34%)

had more than two such events (range 3–12). A hemorrhage was defined as detection of a new neurological deficit associated with imaging evidence of new blood consistent with a typical CM appearance. Two patients (1.9%) had a single hemorrhage associated with significant neurological deterioration (Table 17.1); these patients represent the only exceptions to our selection protocol. Eight (8%) had related seizures. A partial resection had been performed in 17 patients (16.5%). Brain locations included brainstem ($n = 66$), thalamus or basal ganglia ($n = 27$), or deep lobar areas ($n = 10$) (Table 17.1). Seven patients had associated developmental venous anomalies (DVA) detected by angiography or MRI.

Radiosurgical technique

Our technique of stereotactic radiosurgery (SRS) has been described in previous reports [26,30]. Patients under the age of 12 years ($n = 5$) underwent SRS with frame application under general anesthesia. CT was used for stereotactic radiosurgery dose planning in all patients before the year 1990 ($n = 26$). Contrast-enhanced 3D volume acquisition MR imaging using SPGR (spoiled gradient-recalled acquisition in steady state) sequence (1–1.5 mm thick slices) was performed. Variable echo multiplanar and long relaxation time sequences were obtained to define the hemosiderin signal surrounding the CM.

Single or multiple isocenter (range 2–14) radiosurgery dose plans were used to target the CCM margins. The peripheral isodose line was placed so that the target volume was the mixed signal change within the T2-defined hemosiderin ring. The mean number of isocenters was 3.3. The mean target volume was 1.31 ml (range 0.12–7.6 ml). The mean marginal dose was 16 Gy

---

Table 17.1 Patient demographics for cavernous malformation patients (n = 103)

	No. of patients	Percent (%)
Sex		
Male	57	55.34
Female	46	44.60
Signs and symptoms		
One bleed	2	1.90
Two bleeds	66	64.10
Three or more bleeds	35	34.00
Associated seizures (partial or generalized)	8	7.76
Locations		
Brainstem (medulla, pons, midbrain)	66	64.10
Basal ganglia/thalamus	27	26.20
Lobar	10	9.70
Prior management		
Microsurgical excision	17	16.50
Proton beam irradiation and SRS	1	0.97
Follow-up after SRS		
2–5 years	54	52.43
>5–10 years	33	32.00
>10–20 years	16	15.53

SRS = stereotactic radiosurgery.

(range 12–20 Gy) and the mean maximum dose was 30 Gy (range 21.7–40 Gy). Radiosurgery was performed with the cobalt-60 Gamma Knife (Elekta AB, Stockholm, Sweden).

Follow-up assessments

We obtained imaging follow-up beginning 6 months after radiosurgery and then at annual intervals for several years, then approximately every 2–3 years if the patient was stable. A new hemorrhage was defined as a new blood density in association with a new neurological symptom or sign. The hemorrhage rate was calculated using the following equation: annual hemorrhage rate = total number of hemorrhages in all patients / total number of patient-years observed. Hemorrhage rates were compared before and after SRS using a paired t-test.

Serial imaging

Follow-up imaging after SRS revealed regression of the targeted volume in 59 (57%) and no change in size in 44 (43%) CM. Nineteen (18%) patients developed delayed increased T2 signal changes surrounding the target volume which we attributed to adverse radiation effects (ARE). Fourteen of these 19 had associated symptoms or signs and five were asymptomatic.

Hemorrhage before and after radiosurgery

Before radiosurgery, the hemorrhage rate was calculated from the number of hemorrhages in the interval between the first symptomatic, image-defined hemorrhage and the date of SRS. Two (1.9%) of 103 CCM patients died during follow-up. One patient with a brainstem lesion had a fatal hemorrhage 7 months after SRS. A second patient with a brainstem CM died from unknown causes 29 months after SRS. There were 511 patient-years of observation for a mean observation time of 5 years per patient (range 0.17–31 years) prior to SRS. During this time, 269 hemorrhages were observed, a mean of 2.61 per patient. After the exclusion of the first hemorrhage (269 − 103 = 166), the annual hemorrhage rate was 33% (166 hemorrhages in 511 patient-years of observation).

After radiosurgery, the observation period was calculated from the date of radiosurgery until the last imaging follow-up, surgical removal, or death. There were a total of 582 patient-years of follow-up, providing a mean follow-up period of 5.7 years per patient (range 0.6–19.2 years). We noted 26 hemorrhages during this time. Thus, we found a mean hemorrhage rate of 0.25 per patient and a total annual hemorrhage rate of 4.5%. We confirmed a significant ($p < 0.0001$) reduction (33% versus 4.5%) in this annual bleed rate after ($p < 0.0001$).

Within the first 2 years after SRS, 22 hemorrhages were identified in 204 patient-years of follow-up, defining an annual hemorrhage rate of 10.8% during this early period. Four hemorrhages were detected afterwards (378.4 patient-years follow-up, for an annual hemorrhage rate of 1.1%). We confirmed a significant ($p < 0.0001$) reduction in the annual hemorrhage rate once 2 years had passed after SRS.

In the 86 patients who had SRS as primary management of their CCM, 21 (20.4%) rebled after SRS. Four of these patients underwent a resection because of this hemorrhage. Five of 17 (29.4%) patients who had SRS after a prior partial surgical resection rebled and four of these patients underwent an additional surgical resection. This difference was significant ($p = 0.01$).

Seizure outcomes

Six of eight patients with partial or generalized seizures achieved seizure control off medications after radiosurgery. One patient had seizure control but required continued medication. One patient had seizure worsening associated with new T2 signal change and required prolonged oral corticosteroid administration. This sample size is not large enough to draw any firm conclusions on the role of radiosurgery in this setting.

The role of radiosurgery

In 1988 we theorized that SRS could play a role in the management of high-risk CCM. We thought that the CCM vessels could respond to SRS in a similar way as the vessels of an arteriovenous malformation. We believed that this response could only be identified by a reduction in long-term bleeding rates and that SRS might become a clinically useful approach if it was safe enough and actually reduced bleeding rates.

By 1995, we had collected enough data to test our hypotheses. We reported our initial SRS experience in 47 patients with cavernous malformations [26]. At a mean follow-up period of 3.6 years, there was a significant reduction of hemorrhage risk, especially after a 2-year latency period [26]. In our next report of 82 patients, the annual hemorrhage rate was 12.3% per year for the first 2 years followed by 0.76% per year from 2 to 12 years [30]. The results showed a significant reduction in the risk of hemorrhage. Reports from other centers have also demonstrated favorable patient outcomes (Table 17.2).

Table 17.2 Prior reports on cavernous malformation radiosurgery

Authors	Year	No. of pts.	Mean follow-up (months)	Annual hemorrhage rate (%)			ARE (%)
				Before SRS	After SRS < 2 yr	After SRS > 2 yr	
Amin-Hanjani et al. [13]	1998	73	65	17.3	NA	4.5	20.6
Chang et al. [1]	1998	95	65	NA	9.4	1.6	7.0
Karlsson et al. [28]	1998	22	78	NA	10–12	5.0	27
Kida et al. [7]	1999	80	27	31.8	7.3	8.8	21
Pollock et al. [12]	2000	17	51	24.8	8.8	2.9	59
Kim et al. [31]	2002	22	38.3	35.5	1.55	NA	27
Liscak et al. [10]	2005	107	48	2	NA	1.6	27
Liu et al. [21]	2005	125	64	NA	10.3	3.3	13.1
García-Muñoz et al. [32]	2007	17	NA	34.4	NA	7.2	13.3
Present study	2009	103	67.8	32.48	10.8	1.06	11.65

ARE = adverse radiation effects; SRS = stereotactic radiosurgery.

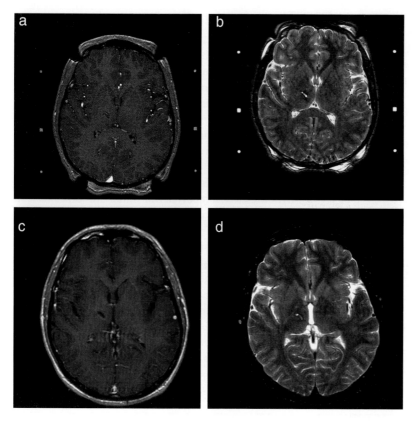

Figure 17.1. A 16-year-old male experienced bleeding from a right thalamic cavernous malformation 2 months before radiosurgery. He developed a left hemiparesis and slurred speech with later improvement. Axial T1-weighted contrast-enhanced MR image shows a weakly enhancing right thalamic cavernous malformation at SRS (volume 0.5 cm^3, margin dose 16 Gy) (a). Axial T2-weighted MR image is shown (b). Three years later and without new symptoms, the malformation shows no contrast uptake (c). The T2 appearance is shown (d).

Chang *et al.* [1] reported 57 patients with CM in deep brain locations. They reported an annual pre-radiosurgery hemorrhage rate of 9.4% which lessened to 1.6% after 3 years. ARE were observed in 7% of patients. Amin-Hanjani and colleagues [13] reported 95 patients with 98 CMs who received stereotactic Bragg-peak proton beam therapy. They found that the annual hemorrhage rate dropped from 17.3% to 4.5% after a latency period of 2 years but that 16% developed permanent neurological deficits and 3% died. Pollock *et al.* [12] reported a lower hemorrhage rate after SRS in 17 patients (from 40% to 2.9% after a latency interval of 2 years) but also found a high risk for ARE (59%). Their median margin dose of 18 Gy may have been too high, leading to toxicity in the adjacent hemosiderin-stained brain. Kim *et al.* [31] in a small report of 22 patients found that the annual bleed rate lessened from 36% to 4%, and that six had evidence of morbidity. Liu *et al.* [21] reported 125 patients whose hemorrhage rate was reduced from 10.3% to 3.3% after 2 years. García-Muñoz *et al.* [32] reported 15 patients with a reduction in the annual hemorrhage rate from 35% to 7%. Surgeons continue

to debate whether the value of radiosurgery is worth the chance of continued hemorrhage during the latency interval for the vascular response.

As a result, some institutions maintain reservations over the use of radiosurgery for hemorrhagic CCMs. The initial experience from the Karolinska Hospital in Stockholm noted concerns related to risk of reactive edema [22]. Analysis of this experience and a prior report [33] indicates that some patients had associated developmental venous anomalies (DVA) which are inappropriate vascular targets for SRS, some received a high radiation dose, and many were targeted with computed tomography.

Radiobiological effects on cavernous malformations

The radiobiological effect on a cavernous malformation has not been well established. It is possible that endothelial-lined channels undergo a proliferative hyalinization leading to eventual luminal closure. This hypothesis is supported by limited histopathological analysis of cavernous malformations after radiosurgery.

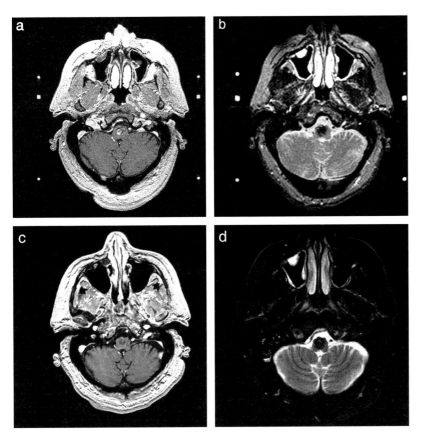

Figure 17.2. A 55-year-old woman sustained two hemorrhages over a 3-year period from a cavernous malformation in the medulla. She developed left-body sensory dysfunction and incoordination. Axial T1-weighted contrast-enhanced MR image shows the cavernous malformation in the medulla (volume 0.6 cm^3, margin dose 14 Gy) (a). Axial T2-weighted MR image is shown (b). No further hemorrhages were noted. Axial T1-weighted MR image shows no contrast enhancement at the site of the cavernous malformation 7 years after radiosurgery (c). Axial T2-weighted MR image shows the hemosiderin-stained tissue at the target site (d). Her symptoms remained unchanged.

Gewirtz et al. [20] reported histopathological changes in their series of 11 patients who underwent resection after SRS. They found that the lesions were not completely thrombosed but showed a combination of vessel fibrosis, fibrinoid necrosis, and ferrugination. Obviously they were removed because of some clinical problem and not because the surgeon thought the lesion was completely obliterated. Nyary et al. [23] studied a surgically resected thalamic CCM, 1 year after 40 Gy irradiation. They noted endothelial cell destruction and significant fibrosis in the connective stroma. We think that CCM may respond similarly to other vascular malformations with delayed narrowing of the vascular channels.

Summary

Since no imaging modality is satisfactory to define the CM response to radiosurgery, only clinical outcomes can be used to measure effectiveness. Our radiosurgical selection protocol places emphasis on patients with deep seated CMs in areas of critical brain function,

and who have had two or more bleeds confirmed by worsening neurological function and new MRI evidence of bleeding. At our multidisciplinary conference, all patients are judged to have excessive risks for a microsurgical approach based on their lack of contact with a pial or ependymal surface. This study cannot confirm the theory that temporal clustering of bleeding events from CMs occurs [34].

Most patients with a cavernous malformation remain without symptoms and have an annual hemorrhage incidence of approximately 1% per year or less. After two or more confirmed bleeds, the annual risk rises significantly. We have found no evidence to support the theory that multiple bleeds cluster in time and then spontaneously cease, a feature that again may reflect the selection and referral bias of our patients. We cannot refute the hypothesis that some CCMs may bleed repeatedly for some interval and then cease to bleed. We think our data support the role of SRS for properly selected hemorrhagic CM located in critical brain regions. Successful radiosurgery appears to reduce rebleeding rates – from more than 32% per year after two prior bleeds to 1% per year, a rate similar to that seen in CCM discovered incidentally.

References

1. Chang, S. D., Levy, R. P., Adler, J. R., Jr., *et al.* Stereotactic radiosurgery of angiographically occult vascular malformations: 14-year experience. *Neurosurgery* 1998;**43**:213–220; discussion 220–211.

2. Larson, J. J., Ball, W. S., Bove, K. E., Crone, K. R. & Tew, J. M., Jr. Formation of intracerebral cavernous malformations after radiation treatment for central nervous system neoplasia in children. *J Neurosurg* 1998;**88**:51–56.

3. Maraire, J. N. & Awad, I. A. Intracranial cavernous malformations: lesion behavior and management strategies. *Neurosurgery* 1995;**37**:591–605.

4. Muras, I., Conforti, R., Scuotto, A., Rinaldi, F. & Bernini, F. P. Cerebral cavernous angioma. Diagnostic considerations. *J Neuroradiol* 1993;**20**:34–41.

5. Zimmerman, R. S., Spetzler, R. F., Lee, K. S., Zabramski, J. M. & Hargraves, R. W. Cavernous malformations of the brain stem. *J Neurosurg* 1991;**75**:32–39.

6. Del Curling, O., Jr., Kelly, D. L., Jr., Elster, A. D. & Craven, T. E. An analysis of the natural history of cavernous angiomas. *J Neurosurg* 1991;**75**:702–708.

7. Kida, Y., Kobayashi, T. & Mori, Y. Radiosurgery of angiographically occult vascular malformations. *Neurosurg Clin N Am* 1999;**10**:291–303.

8. Nyary, I., Major, O., Hanzely, Z. & Szeifert, G. T. Pathological considerations to irradiation of cavernous malformations. *Prog Neurol Surg* 2007;**20**:231–234.

9. Labauge, P., Brunereau, L., Levy, C., Laberge, S. & Houtteville, J. P. The natural history of familial cerebral cavernomas: a retrospective MRI study of 40 patients. *Neuroradiology* 2000;**42**:327–332.

10. Liscak, R., Vladyka, V., Simonova, G., Vymazal, J. & Novotny, J., Jr. Gamma knife surgery of brain cavernous hemangiomas. *J Neurosurg* 2005;**102** Suppl:207–213.

11. Mitchell, P., Hodgson, T. J., Seaman, S., Kemeny, A. A. & Forster, D. M. Stereotactic radiosurgery and the risk of haemorrhage from cavernous malformations. *Br J Neurosurg* 2000;**14**:96–100.

12. Pollock, B. E., Garces, Y. I., Stafford, S. L., *et al.* Stereotactic radiosurgery for cavernous malformations. *J Neurosurg* 2000;**93**:987–991.

13. Amin-Hanjani, S., Ogilvy, C. S., Candia, G. J., Lyons, S. & Chapman, P. H. Stereotactic radiosurgery for cavernous malformations: Kjellberg's experience with proton beam therapy in 98 cases at the Harvard Cyclotron. *Neurosurgery* 1998;**42**:1229–1236; discussion 1236–1228.

14. McLaughlin, M. R., Kondziolka, D., Flickinger, J. C., Lunsford, S. & Lunsford, L. D. The prospective natural history of cerebral venous malformations. *Neurosurgery* 1998;**43**:195–200; discussion 200–191.

15. Otten, P., Pizzolato, G. P., Rilliet, B. & Berney, J. [131 cases of cavernous angioma (cavernomas) of the CNS, discovered by retrospective analysis of 24,535 autopsies]. *Neurochirurgie* 1989;**35**:82–83, 128–131.

16. Porter, P. J., Willinsky, R. A., Harper, W. & Wallace, M. C. Cerebral cavernous malformations: natural history and prognosis after clinical deterioration with or without hemorrhage. *J Neurosurg* 1997;**87**:190–197.

17. Kondziolka, D., Lunsford, L. D. & Kestle, J. R. The natural history of cerebral cavernous malformations. *J Neurosurg* 1995;**83**:820–824.

18. Moriarity, J. L., Wetzel, M., Clatterbuck, R. E., *et al.* The natural history of cavernous malformations: a prospective study of 68 patients. *Neurosurgery* 1999;**44**:1166–1171; discussion 1172–1163.

19. Aiba, T., Tanaka, R., Koike, T., *et al.* Natural history of intracranial cavernous malformations. *J Neurosurg* 1995;**83**:56–59.

20. Gewirtz, R. J., Steinberg, G. K., Crowley, R. & Levy, R. P. Pathological changes in surgically resected angiographically occult vascular malformations after radiation. *Neurosurgery* 1998;**42**:738–742; discussion 742–733.

21. Liu, K. D., Chung, W. Y., Wu, H. M., *et al.* Gamma knife surgery for cavernous hemangiomas: an analysis of 125 patients. *J Neurosurg* 2005;**102** (Suppl):81–86.

22. Mathiesen, T., Edner, G. & Kihlstrom, L. Deep and brainstem cavernomas: a consecutive 8-year series. *J Neurosurg* 2003;**99**:31–37.

23. Nyary, I., Major, O., Hanzely, Z. & Szeifert, G. T. Histopathological findings in a surgically resected thalamic cavernous hemangioma 1 year after 40-Gy irradiation. *J Neurosurg* 2005;**102** Suppl:56–58.

24. Porter, R. W., Detwiler, P. W., Spetzler, R. F., *et al.* Cavernous malformations of the brainstem: experience with 100 patients. *J Neurosurg* 1999;**90**:50–58.

25. Bertalanffy, H., Benes, L., Miyazawa, T., *et al.* Cerebral cavernomas in the adult. Review of the literature and analysis of 72 surgically treated patients. *Neurosurg Rev* 2002;**25**:1–53; discussion 54–55.

26. Kondziolka, D., Lunsford, L. D., Flickinger, J. C. & Kestle, J. R. Reduction of hemorrhage risk after

stereotactic radiosurgery for cavernous malformations. *J Neurosurg* 1995;**83**:825–831.

27. Chang, S. D., Steinberg, G. K., Levy, R. P., *et al.* Microsurgical resection of incompletely obliterated intracranial arteriovenous malformations following stereotactic radiosurgery. *Neurol Med Chir (Tokyo)* 1998;**38**(Suppl):200–207.

28. Karlsson, B., Kihlstrom, L., Lindquist, C., Ericson, K. & Steiner, L. Radiosurgery for cavernous malformations. *J Neurosurg* 1998;**88**:293–297.

29. Samii, M., Eghbal, R., Carvalho, G. A. & Matthies, C. Surgical management of brainstem cavernomas. *J Neurosurg* 2001;**95**:825–832.

30. Hasegawa, T., McInerney, J., Kondziolka, D., *et al.* Long-term results after stereotactic radiosurgery for patients with cavernous malformations. *Neurosurgery* 2002;**50**:1190–1197; discussion 1197–1198.

31. Kim, D. G., Choe, W. J., Paek, S. H., *et al.* Radiosurgery of intracranial cavernous malformations. *Acta Neurochir (Wien)* 2002;**144**:869–878; discussion 878.

32. García-Muñoz, L., Velasco-Campos, F., Lujan-Castilla, P., *et al.* [Radiosurgery in the treatment of brain cavernomas. Experience with 17 lesions treated in 15 patients]. *Neurochirurgie* 2007;**53**:243–250.

33. Lindquist, C., Guo, W. Y., Karlsson, B. & Steiner, L. Radiosurgery for venous angiomas. *J Neurosurg* 1993;**78**:531–536.

34. Barker, F. G., Amin-Hanjani, S., Butler, W. E., *et al.* Temporal clustering of hemorrhages from untreated cavernous malformations of the central nervous system. *Neurosurgery* 2001;**49**:15–24; discussion 24–25.

Genetic counseling

Leslie Morrison

Diagnosis of CCM encompasses patient neurological history and family history, neurological and cutaneous examinations, and brain imaging with MRI (brain and spinal cord depending on history and examination) or cranial CT. The finding of multiple lesions on MRI, a single lesion combined with strong family history (especially in Hispanic families with origins in the south-west USA or northern Mexico) and cutaneous or spinal cord lesions is strongly suggestive of diagnosis. Confirmatory testing with DNA is encouraged to obtain a specific diagnosis for prognosis since the various types of CCM have differing severity [1]. Genetic testing has opened many diagnostic possibilities for patients with CCM. The use of this powerful tool has also resulted in ethical dilemmas in the care of patients. Physicians and genetic counselors have been guided by the recommendation of several groups, including the American Association of Pediatrics and the American Society for Human Genetics. A recent standard of care document has been developed by the European Society of Human Genetics that provides detailed advice in the management of patients with autosomal dominant disorders, as seen in all familial forms of CCM.

CCM1, 2, 3, and a probable CCM4 are inherited in an autosomal dominant manner. Affected individuals have a 50% chance of passing on the disease gene to their offspring. Sexes are equally affected. The *de novo* mutation rate is unknown; however, there are some reports of this occurrence [2,3]. Approximately 25% of patients who carry the disease mutation may remain unaffected. Affected patients are likely to have inherited the disease from one of their parents who may be asymptomatic and unaware of the diagnosis. Family history provides additional information, but due to wide variability of the clinical phenotype it does not provide adequate diagnostic information about potentially affected family members [4–6]. This is in part due to the range of phenotypes from entirely asymptomatic members without MRI lesions, to those with MRI lesions without clinical symptoms, to a smaller percentage with permanent neurological impairments including pharmaco-resistant epilepsy and neurological disability. In addition, family history may include members with epilepsy, headaches, and neurological impairment from other causes as these sequelae are relatively prevalent in the general population. CCM lesions are often mistakenly referred to as arteriovenous malformations, aneurysms, brain tumors, or hemorrhagic strokes by both physicians and family members. Given these limitations, genetic testing can be a valuable tool for obtaining an accurate diagnosis when combined with clinical observation, family history, and brain imaging.

Index cases

Most index cases in a family will present with acute neurological symptoms or chronic headache. Brain MRI or cranial CT is performed in the acute setting and is available for review by the genetic counselor or clinician considering testing. In general, symptomatic patients should be offered a specific diagnosis through DNA testing. This is important for at least the index case in a family to provide confirmation of diagnosis and to assist other family members with the diagnosis. Once an index case has been confirmed as a disease-causing mutation (CHM), family members with negative testing can be reassured that they are not at risk for inheritance.

Examination of the index case for cutaneous lesions, retinal or other system involvement is paramount. Other affected family members may display cutaneous lesions even if neurologically asymptomatic, and the family history should include a query for skin or other involvement in other family members [7,8].

The current cost of the common Hispanic mutation (CHM) test is less than $200 and at least in the southwestern USA and with families of Mexican heritage is justifiable to most insurance companies. In non-Hispanic patients or in Hispanic patients with negative CHM testing, a progressive approach can be employed to screen for the most common mutations, and then searching for less common mutations. It is considerably more costly if the mutation is not identified in the first or second gene screening. As such, if brain imaging has not been performed in asymptomatic family members, this may be the next step.

When gene testing has identified a mutation in a patient, brain MRI with at least gradient-echo sequence (GRE) should be performed to identify the number, size, and location of lesions to serve as a baseline to detect future hemorrhage with MRI. The quality of MRI varies with regard to specific type of MRI performed, magnet size, and sequences performed, with susceptibility-weighted imaging (SWI) and GRE showing the greatest sensitivity to lesion burden. Where possible, the baseline and any subsequent MRIs should be of the same quality for best comparisons.

Founder mutations

The Hispanic cohort originating in New Mexico is the only large cohort in the world with familial CCM, the type CCM1 with the common Hispanic mutation (CHM). Interestingly, this is not found in Spain [9] or southern Mexico, but has been reported in Arizona patients with ancestry from Sonora [10], and more recently found in new immigrants from Chihuahua, Mexico, to New Mexico (Morrison, personal communication).

Children

Predictive testing or presymptomatic testing is discouraged by the majority of organizations involved in genetic testing of children, unless a direct benefit to the minor can be justified based on potential medical intervention or preventive measures [11,12]. This process should always involve informed consent, and assent by the minor even when performed for clinical purposes. In some situations, parents or guardians present justified reasons to perform testing on their asymptomatic children, such as the death of an affected sibling or parent. Young children usually need sedation or anesthesia for MRI scanning, which

poses additional risk for this alternative diagnostic test. In older cooperative children, MRI scanning in a family with known index mutation may be the most effective way to diagnose, since it also provides the necessary information regarding lesion number, size, and location in addition to any other information derived from the scan.

In asymptomatic children, it is reasonable to delay gene testing until they reach majority age so that they may make their own decision about knowing or not knowing their status. In families with known CCM, children with acute neurological events, seizures, and headaches will need evaluation with brain MRI (GRE or SWI) and if no other family members have had DNA testing, it will confirm the type of CCM and specific mutation if found. This then will serve as the index case for that family.

Prenatal testing

Prenatal testing and preimplantation genetics can be performed if the disease-causing mutation is known in a family.

Recommendations:

(1) While obtaining the family history, inquire about family members affected by brain tumors, arteriovenous malformations (AVMs), aneurysms, epilepsy or unexplained loss of consciousness, chronic or severe headaches, and unexplained deaths.
(2) If the obligate carrier parent is suspected on the basis of family members with the above concerns, it would be reasonable to perform a brain MRI with GRE and /or SWI on that parent or to offer DNA testing if an index case has been identified with a specific mutation.
(3) For patients with a single CCM, consider genetic testing and counseling, especially if patients have ancestry from the Hispanic southwest or family history of epilepsy, migraine or other headaches, early strokes or severe acute neurological events.

References

1. Denier, C., Labauge, P., *et al.* Genotype-phenotype correlations in cerebral cavernous malformations patients. *Ann Neurol* 2006;**60**:550–556.

2. Surucu, O., Sure, U., *et al.* Clinical impact of CCM mutation detection in familial cavernous angioma. *Childs Nerv Syst* 2006;**22**:1461–1464.

3. Surucu, O., Sure, U., *et al.* Cavernoma of the trochlear nerve. *Clin Neurol Neurosurg* 2007;**109**:791–793.

4. Lucas, M., Costa, A. F., *et al.* Variable expression of cerebral cavernous malformations in carriers of a premature termination codon in exon 17 of the Krit1 gene. *BMC Neurol* 2003;**3**:5.

5. Gianfrancesco, F., Cannella, M., *et al.* Highly variable penetrance in subjects affected with cavernous cerebral angiomas (CCM) carrying novel CCM1 and CCM2 mutations. *Am J Med Genet B Neuropsychiatr Genet* 2007;**144**:691–695.

6. Ortiz, L., Costa, A. F., *et al.* Study of cerebral cavernous malformation in Spain and Portugal: high prevalence of a 14 bp deletion in exon 5 of MGC4607 (CCM2 gene). *J Neurol* 2007;**254**:322–326.

7. Eerola, I., McIntyre, B., *et al.* Identification of eight novel 5'-exons in cerebral capillary malformation gene-1 (CCM1) encoding KRIT1. *Biochim Biophys Acta* 2001;**1517**:464–467.

8. Zlotoff, B. J., Bang, R. H., *et al.* Cutaneous angiokeratoma and venous malformations in a Hispanic-American patient with cerebral cavernous malformations. *Br J Dermatol* 2007;**157**:210–212.

9. Lucas, M., Solano, F., *et al.* Spanish families with cerebral cavernous angioma do not bear 742C–>T Hispanic American mutation of the KRIT1 gene. *Ann Neurol* 2000;**47**:836.

10. Polymeropoulos, M. H., Hurko, O., *et al.* Linkage of the locus for cerebral cavernous hemangiomas to human chromosome 7q in four families of Mexican-American descent. *Neurology* 1997;**48**:752–757.

11. Borry, P., Stultiens, L., *et al.* Presymptomatic and predictive genetic testing in minors: a systematic review of guidelines and position papers. *Clin Genet* 2006;**70**:374–381.

12. Borry, P. Coming of age of personalized medicine: challenges ahead. *Genome Med* 2009;**1**:109.

Special problems in cavernous malformations: migraine, pregnancy, hormonal replacement, anticoagulation, NSAIDs, stress, and altitude elevation changes

Richard Leigh and Robert J. Wityk

Introduction

Cerebral cavernous malformations (CCM) of the nervous system are relatively rare and can be symptomatic or incidentally discovered. Factors leading to their discovery are varied and not always causally associated. While a seizure may lead to discovery of a symptomatic CCM, a headache may lead to an incidental discovery of an asymptomatic CCM. Cerebrovascular neurologists and neurosurgeons are often asked about the safety and relationship of various medical issues with the CCM. The problem of epilepsy is covered in another chapter. In this chapter, we focus on some common questions that have arisen during consultation, such as the relationship to migraine, effects of pregnancy, and particularly the safety of use of antithrombotic agents in CCM patients.

With the widespread use of brain MRI and the more frequent use of hemosiderin-sensitive sequences, the discovery of asymptomatic CCMs will probably increase. This book contains current information concerning the pathology, diagnosis and natural history and treatment of CCMs, but a number of medical and neurological issues arise in patients with CCMs that have not been as well studied. These issues will eventually present to the practitioner, and we have reviewed the literature to give the best guidance on management.

Methods

The search strategy was formed by combining the appropriate database-specific controlled vocabulary terms with keyword phrases for each concept. These terms were then combined using Boolean operators and adapted for each database searched. The databases searched were PubMed, Embase and SCOPUS. The search terms used for each concept were: "cavernous malformation", "cavernous malformations", "cavernous angioma", "cavernous angiomas", "cavernoma", "cavernomas", "cavernous hemangioma", "cavernous hemangioma, diffuse", "cavernous angioma", "cavernous haemangioma", "diffuse cavernous hemangioma", "haemangioma cavernosum", "hemangioma cavernosum", "hemangioma, cavernous", "polypoid cavernous hemangioma", "angioma, brain", "brain angioma", "brain haemangioma", "brain microangioma", "central nervous system venous angioma", "cerebral angioma", "cerebral haemangioma", "cerebral hemangioma", "hemangioma, brain", "hemangioma, cavernous, central nervous system", "intracranial haemangioma", "intracranial hemangioma", "venous angioma, central nervous system", "brain hemangioma". Citations were then reviewed to select ones relevant to CCM. Only English-language references were reviewed. References within papers were also examined to find citations missed by the database search.

Where the literature is sparse or even non-existent, we supply suggestions based upon our own personal experience. Review of clinical records of patients seen by one of the co-authors (RJW) over the previous 13 years revealed 56 patients with a diagnosis of CCM confirmed by an experienced neuroradiologist who reviewed all the available imaging studies. All cases were reviewed with regard to the issues described below, and, where appropriate, are offered as anecdotal information.

Cavernous Malformations of the Nervous System, ed. Daniele Rigamonti. Published by Cambridge University Press.
© Cambridge University Press 2011.

Migraine disorder

Migraine is a common disorder affecting approximately 10% of the population. Because of its high prevalence, determining its role in patients with a rare disorder, such as intracranial CCMs, can be difficult. Multiple series have demonstrated that headache is one of the more common presenting symptoms leading to the discovery of CCMs after seizures, focal neurological deficits, and overt hemorrhage [1–8]. The percentage of patients presenting with headache ranges from 3 to 31.4% in these series. The mechanism of headache could certainly be secondary to superficial bleeding of a CCM causing local dural irritation.

Whether CCMs cause recurrent headaches and migraine disorder in particular is less clear. The proportion of CCM patients who have a history of a migraine disorder is not reported in any study; however, in one natural history study of 32 patients, 34% reported a history of chronic headache [9]. In another study the headaches were classified according to the International Classification of Headache Disorders [6]. Of the 11 patients with headache, 36% were classified as migraine, half of which had an associated aura. However, during the follow-up period, the number of patients with headache classified as migraine increased from four to eight. This finding suggests that migraine disorder may be caused by CCMs in some cases.

The hemorrhagic nature of CCMs, often evolving over time, makes them a possible source of chronic headaches even in the absence of a migraine disorder. However, one series reported that of the 11 patients who presented with headache and were treated non-surgically, five had resolution of symptoms at follow-up [1]. Another series identified 18 patients out of a cohort of 145 patents with CCMs whose lesions exhibited aggressive behavior defined as growth, bleeding or *de novo* appearance [2]. Of these 18 patients, only one complained of recurrent headaches. In a study of the natural history of patients with CCMs, a history of headache was associated with an increased risk of subsequent hemorrhage [3]. In a study of familial CCM patients, 41 patients had a hemorrhage, of whom three complained of headache, and none of these headaches was felt to be migrainous by the authors [4]. While little can be concluded from these studies about the role of migraine in CCMs they illustrate that while these lesions may cause headaches, unrelated headache syndromes will occur in this population as well. In a study of familial CCMs in 31 patients from six families, 52% complained of recurrent headaches [10]. Numerous case reports have described migraine-like headaches in patients with brainstem CCMs [11–16]. In all cases the authors felt that the migrainous symptoms were secondary to the lesion itself rather than any independent association.

In the authors' opinion, the apparent high frequency of headache and migraine disorder in patients with CCMs is likely biased by the fact that CCMs can only be diagnosed by brain imaging studies (e.g. CT and MRI), and these studies are being done because of the headache. A true study of the association of migraine and CCM would need to take into account individuals with CCM who are asymptomatic and do not have migraine, but are unknown because they have not had a brain imaging study.

In the authors' experience, patients with CCM and chronic or intermittent migraine headaches respond to standard treatments for migraine disorder. Although there has been no case-controlled study of headache characteristics in patients with and without CCM, clinical experience suggests that CCM patients with headache are similar to general migraineurs in terms of response to medications, triggering events, and the characteristics of the headache.

Gender, pregnancy, hormone replacement

There is a general perception that CCMs are more malignant in women than in men. Estrogen and pregnancy are thought to play a role in this asymmetry. However, these notions remain controversial, particularly in their etiology. A review of the literature reveals some common themes between studies, but also some contradictory findings.

The incidence of CCM has been shown to be equal between the genders in multiple natural history studies [1,3,4,6,7,9]. However, male [8] and female [17] weightings have also been reported. Multiple studies suggest a more malignant course for women, often associated with pregnancy. In a study of 66 patients in which less than half the patients were female, 86% of the hemorrhages were in females [1]. In a natural history study of 110 patients, half of whom were female, there were 18 instances of hemorrhage or neurological deterioration over the 427 patient-years of follow-up, but none of them occurred during pregnancy; however, the number of asymptomatic pregnancy years was not reported [7].

In a series of 62 women with brainstem CCMs, 11% suffered a hemorrhage during pregnancy [17]. The authors state that they have identified estrogen receptors in "a few" CCMs obtained in women. However, another pathological study of 12 cerebral CCMs examined by immunohistochemistry for estrogen or progesterone receptors found no evidence of either in any of their samples [18].

In a study of 145 patients with cavernous angiomas where 18 patients were identified as having an aggressive course, 72% were female, two of whom were pregnant. Although there were also two pregnant women in the non-malignant group, both of them presented with overt hemorrhage [2]. In a natural history study of 110 patients who were divided by presentation into a hemorrhage group, a seizure group, and an incidental group, investigators found that the hemorrhage group was 60% female while the incidental group was 82% male, suggesting a potentially more malignant nature of these lesions in the female population [19].

While CCMs are known to increase in size during pregnancy, it is unclear whether this confers an increased risk of hemorrhage. Some case reports of pregnant women with cavernous malformations have documented increased hemorrhages [20–23] and worsening or new onset of seizures [24–26]. Estrogen itself is thought to be epileptogenic and since patients with CCMs have a lower seizure threshold, new-onset seizures in a pregnant patient may not be a direct interaction of the hormonal changes with the CCM itself. Other studies have found no increased risk of hemorrhage in the female population as compared to the male population; however, the incidence of pregnancy in the population is usually not reported or is unknown [4,7]. In one series where hemorrhage was more prominent in the male population, the pregnancy rate was known to be zero [6]. We are not aware of any study examining the risk of hormone replacement therapy on the rate of bleeding or neurological symptoms.

In conclusion, the existing literature supports the generally perceived notion of there being a greater risk of neurological complications from CCM in female patients particularly in the setting of pregnancy.

Anticoagulation, antiplatelet agents, and NSAIDs

A common concern in clinical practice is the risk of using antiplatelet agents or anticoagulants in a person with a CCM. Clearly, situations will arise in which a patient with a CCM may need antithrombotic therapy because of concurrent medical illnesses, such as coronary artery disease, deep venous thrombosis, or a prothrombotic state. The hemorrhagic nature of CCMs makes them seem particularly susceptible to iatrogenic progression in the setting of these medications. However, given their lack of arterial supply and the hypothesized low blood flow state, the magnitude of effect of antithrombotic agents might be small. Thus the risk of hemorrhage in the setting of anticoagulation or antiplatelet therapy is unknown.

A review of the literature turns up only one report of anticoagulation-associated bleeding of a CCM [28]. In our review of the Hopkins experience, we identified 23 patients who were taking antiplatelet or anticoagulant medications at some point in their medical history. Most patients who were on antithrombotic agents at the time of their diagnosis were told to discontinue the medication if medically possible. However, in several cases the risk of withholding antithrombotic medication was felt to outweigh the risk of increased bleeding of a CCM.

Review of our database revealed 14 patients who had been on aspirin, seven patients on anticoagulation (warfarin or intravenous heparin), and nine patients who were taking non-steroidal anti-inflammatory drugs (NSAIDs) at some point in their medical history. Of the patients who had been on ASA three had serial imaging available for review, two of which showed no progression of disease. The third had been on aspirin for coronary artery disease, but was switched to warfarin due to paroxysmal atrial fibrillation. He developed a new but asymptomatic hemorrhagic lesion on repeat brain imaging. Another patient was admitted for chest pain and while receiving low molecular weight heparin, he developed a headache. Imaging revealed a CCM-associated hemorrhage. On the other hand, another patient with a known CCM treated with both aspirin and later warfarin has been asymptomatic for two years, and has had no bleeding detected on yearly brain imaging studies. Of the patients known to have taken NSAIDs, all have been asymptomatic. Three of these patients had serial brain imaging; two were stable and one developed new but asymptomatic lesions.

Our clinical impression is that the risk of bleeding from a CCM is not excessively high with use of antithrombotic agents, and the risk from use of aspirin in particular seems quite modest. Clearly, further studies are needed to compare rates of bleeding or progression of CCMs in patients treated with antithrombotic agents with the natural history of the disorder, and explore associated factors such as the size or location of the CCM, or other medical factors such as hypertension, on the risk of bleeding.

We did not find any report in the literature of a patient with a known CCM being treated with thrombolytic therapy (e.g. intravenous or intraarterial), nor are we aware anecdotally of such a case. During treatment of acute ischemic stroke with intravenous tissue plasminogen activator, intracranial bleeding occurs in about 6% of patients (NINDS study, NEJM 1995). Occasionally, the site of bleeding is found to be outside the region of acute ischemia. One may speculate that these cases could be due to bleeding of an occult CCM.

Psychological stress or altitude changes

We found no literature commenting on these issues in relation to CCMs. Patients with a recent neurological event often raise the question about whether psychological or personal stress plays a role. There is little study of the role of stress in neurological disorders, and none that we could find related to CCMs. In clinical practice, patients with cerebrovascular conditions frequently fly in commercial airlines without problems. The authors are not aware of any patient with a CCM having complications during a commercial airline flight, but the risk of flying in smaller airplanes or in planes without cabin pressurization is not known.

Conclusions

The topics reviewed in this chapter are common clinical problems that might affect management of a patient with CCM, but are poorly understood because of the rarity of CCMs. Further studies need larger numbers of patients and standardization of endpoints during follow-up, particularly in terms of imaging studies. A better estimate of the risk of pregnancy or antithrombotic medication use would be valuable to the physician and patient making decisions.

References

1. Robinson, J. R., Awad, I. A. & Little, J. R. Natural history of the cavernous angioma. *J Neurosurg* 1991;**75**:709–714.

2. Pozzati, E., Acciarri, N., Tognetti, F., Marliani, F. & Giangaspero, F. Growth, subsequent bleeding, and de novo appearance of cerebral cavernous angiomas. *Neurosurgery* 1996;**38**:662–669.

3. Kondziolka, D., Lunsford, L. D. & Kestle, J. R. The natural history of cerebral cavernous malformations. *J Neurosurg* 1995;**83**:820–824.

4. Labauge, P., Laberge, S., Brunereau, L., Levy, C. & Tournier-Lasserve, E. Hereditary cerebral cavernous angiomas: clinical and genetic features in 57 French families. Societe Francaise de Neurochirurgie. *Lancet* 1998;**352**:1892–1897.

5. Rigamonti, D., Hadley, M. N., Drayer, B. P., *et al.* Cerebral cavernous malformations. Incidence and familial occurrence. *New Engl J Med* 1988;**319**:343–347.

6. Ebrahimi, A., Etemadifar, M., Ardestani, P. M., *et al.* Cavernous angioma: a clinical study of 35 cases with review of the literature. *Neurol Res* 2009;**31**:785–793.

7. Porter, P. J., Willinsky, R. A., Harper, W. & Wallace, M. C. Cerebral cavernous malformations: natural history and prognosis after clinical deterioration with or without hemorrhage. *J Neurosurg* 1997;**87**:190–197.

8. Kim, D. S., Park, Y. G., Choi, J. U., Chung, S. S. & Lee, K. C. An analysis of the natural history of cavernous malformations. *Surg Neurol* 1997;**48**:9–17.

9. Del, C. O., Jr., Kelly, D. L., Jr., Elster, A. D. & Craven, T. E. An analysis of the natural history of cavernous angiomas. *J Neurosurg* 1991;**75**:702–708.

10. Zabramski, J. M., Wascher, T. M., Spetzler, R. F., *et al.* The natural history of familial cavernous malformations: results of an ongoing study. *J Neurosurg* 1994;**80**:422–432.

11. Malik, S. N. & Young, W. B. Midbrain cavernous malformation causing migraine-like headache. *Cephalalgia* 2006;**26**:1016–1019.

12. Obermann, M., Gizewski, E. R., Limmroth, V., Diener, H. C. & Katsarava, Z. Symptomatic migraine and pontine vascular malformation: evidence for a key role of the brainstem in the pathophysiology of chronic migraine. *Cephalalgia* 2006;**26**:763–766.

13. Afridi, S. & Goadsby, P. J. New onset migraine with a brain stem cavernous angioma. *J Neurol Neurosurg Psychiatry* 2003;**74**:680–682.

14. Goadsby, P. J. Neurovascular headache and a midbrain vascular malformation: evidence for a role of the brainstem in chronic migraine. *Cephalalgia* 2002;**22**:107–111.

15. Bruti, G., Mostardini, C., Pierallini, A., *et al.* Neurovascular headache and occipital neuralgia secondary to bleeding of bulbocervical cavernoma. *Cephalalgia* 2007;**27**:1074–1079.

16. Katsarava, Z., Egelhof, T., Kaube, H., Diener, H. C. & Limmroth, V. Symptomatic migraine and sensitization of trigeminal nociception associated with contralateral pontine cavernoma. *Pain* 2003;**105**:381–384.

17. Porter, R. W., Detwiler, P. W., Spetzler, R. F., *et al.* Cavernous malformations of the brainstem: experience with 100 patients. *J Neurosurg* 1999;**90**:50–58.

18. Kaya, A. H., Ulus, A., Bayri, Y., *et al.* There are no estrogen and progesterone receptors in cerebral cavernomas: a preliminary immunohistochemical study. *Surg Neurol* 2009;**72**:263–265.

19. Aiba, T., Tanaka, R., Koike, T., *et al.* Natural history of intracranial cavernous malformations. *J Neurosurg* 1995;**83**:56–59.

20. Flemming, K. D., Goodman, B. P. & Meyer, F. B. Successful brainstem cavernous malformation resection after repeated hemorrhages during pregnancy. *Surg Neurol* 2003;**60**:545–547.

21. Safavi-Abbasi, S., Feiz-Erfan, I., Spetzler, R. F., *et al.* Hemorrhage of cavernous malformations during pregnancy and in the peripartum period: causal or coincidence? Case report and review of the literature. *Neurosurg Focus* 2006;**21**:e12.

22. Warner, J. E., Rizzo, J. F., III, Brown, E. W. & Ogilvy, C. S. Recurrent chiasmal apoplexy due to cavernous malformation. *J Neuroophthalmol* 1996;**16**:99–106.

23. Maruoka, N., Yamakawa, Y. & Shimauchi, M. Cavernous hemangioma of the optic nerve. Case report. *J Neurosurg* 1988;**69**:292–294.

24. Awada, A., Watson, T. & Obeid, T. Cavernous angioma presenting as pregnancy-related seizures. *Epilepsia* 1997;**38**:844–846.

25. Hoeldtke, N. J., Floyd, D., Werschkul, J. D., Calhoun, B. C. & Hume, R. F. Intracranial cavernous angioma initially presenting in pregnancy with new-onset seizures. *Am J Obstet Gynecol* 1998;**178**:612–613.

26. Aladdin, Y. & Gross, D. W. Refractory status epilepticus during pregnancy secondary to cavernous angioma. *Epilepsia* 2008;**49**:1627–1629.

27. Gazzaz, M., Sichez, J., Capelle, L. & Fohanno, D. [Recurrent bleeding of thalamic cavernous angioma under hormonal treatment. A case report]. *Neurochirurgie* 1999;**45**:413–416.

28. Pozzati, E., Zucchelli, M., Marliani, A. F. & Riccioli, L. A. Bleeding of a familial cerebral cavernous malformation after prophylactic anticoagulation therapy. Case report. *Neurosurg Focus* 2006;**21**:e15.

Index